AF896616

Parathyroid Imaging

Petra Petranović Ovčariček
Luca Giovanella • Martin W. Huellner
Editors

Parathyroid Imaging

Springer

Editors
Petra Petranović Ovčariček
Department of Oncology and Nuclear Medicine
University Hospital Center Sestre Milosrdnice
Zagreb, Croatia

Luca Giovanella
Department of Nuclear Medicine
Clinica Luganese Moncucco
Lugano, Switzerland

Martin W. Huellner
Department of Nuclear Medicine
University Hospital Zurich / University of Zurich
Zurich, Switzerland

ISBN 978-3-032-14177-4 ISBN 978-3-032-14178-1 (eBook)
https://doi.org/10.1007/978-3-032-14178-1

© The Editor(s) (if applicable) and The Author(s), under exclusive license to Springer Nature Switzerland AG 2026

This work is subject to copyright. All rights are solely and exclusively licensed by the Publisher, whether the whole or part of the material is concerned, specifically the rights of translation, reprinting, reuse of illustrations, recitation, broadcasting, reproduction on microfilms or in any other physical way, and transmission or information storage and retrieval, electronic adaptation, computer software, or by similar or dissimilar methodology now known or hereafter developed.
The use of general descriptive names, registered names, trademarks, service marks, etc. in this publication does not imply, even in the absence of a specific statement, that such names are exempt from the relevant protective laws and regulations and therefore free for general use.
The publisher, the authors and the editors are safe to assume that the advice and information in this book are believed to be true and accurate at the date of publication. Neither the publisher nor the authors or the editors give a warranty, expressed or implied, with respect to the material contained herein or for any errors or omissions that may have been made. The publisher remains neutral with regard to jurisdictional claims in published maps and institutional affiliations.

This Springer imprint is published by the registered company Springer Nature Switzerland AG
The registered company address is: Gewerbestrasse 11, 6330 Cham, Switzerland

If disposing of this product, please recycle the paper.

To our families, whose unwavering love, patience, and enduring support make all our work possible.

Foreword

Even in contemporary medicine, the parathyroid glands remain somewhat enigmatic. First identified by Sir Richard Owen in 1852 during his dissection of an Indian rhinoceros, they were later described in humans and formally named "glandulae parathyroidae" by the Swedish medical student Ivar Viktor Sandström in 1882. Despite their minute size—often no larger than a grain of rice—these glands can exert profound systemic effects in a patient unlucky enough to have one (or more) of the four glands dysregulated and beginning excessive secretion of parathyroid hormone.

To date, surgical excision remains the only curative therapy for hyperfunctioning parathyroid glands. Although typically found adjacent to the thyroid, as their name implies, ectopic parathyroid glands may reside anywhere from the mandibular angle to the pericardium.

This is where medical imaging assumes a pivotal role. Advances in imaging have dramatically enhanced our ability to locate abnormal parathyroid tissue—from conventional ultrasonography to sophisticated [^{18}F]Fluorocholine PET/MR. While numerous reviews and guidelines have summarized individual aspects of these methods, a comprehensive, multidisciplinary reference devoted entirely to parathyroid imaging has been notably absent—until now.

It is therefore a privilege to introduce this volume, authored and edited by distinguished experts in the field of parathyroidology. The book provides an in-depth overview of available imaging modalities, with particular emphasis on nuclear medicine techniques, and places them in the broader clinical, anatomical, physiological, and pathological context of parathyroid disease. It will serve as an invaluable resource not only for nuclear medicine physicians but also for radiologists, endocrinologists, and endocrine surgeons. Even seasoned veterans in the field will find new insights and a reliable reference within these pages—as I did myself, despite having co-authored several guidelines and reviews on the subject!

I trust that you, dear reader, will find this work as enlightening and practical as I have, and that it will serve as a lasting reference for your clinical and academic endeavors in parathyroid imaging.

Frederik A. Verburg
Professor of Translational Nuclear Medicine
Department of Radiology and Nuclear Medicine
Erasmus Medical Centre Rotterdam
Rotterdam, The Netherlands
October of 2025

Preface

The field of parathyroid imaging has undergone a profound transformation over the past several decades, progressing from rudimentary anatomical localization methods to sophisticated functional and molecular imaging approaches that now represent essential pillars of modern endocrine surgery. This trajectory reflects not only the rapid evolution of imaging technologies but also an expanding understanding of parathyroid pathophysiology and the pivotal role that precise preoperative localization plays in optimizing patient outcomes.

Parathyroid disorders, particularly primary hyperparathyroidism, remain among the most common endocrine diseases encountered in clinical practice. However, the small size, variable anatomical location, and complex embryological origins of the parathyroid glands have historically posed significant challenges for both diagnostic imaging and surgical management.

This volume synthesizes the expertise of nuclear medicine physicians, radiologists, endocrine surgeons, biochemists, and pathologists to provide a comprehensive overview of contemporary parathyroid imaging. It covers the established roles of [^{99m}Tc]Tc-MIBI scintigraphy and ultrasonography, as well as more advanced techniques, including four-dimensional computed tomography, magnetic resonance imaging, and positron emission tomography. Both the technical principles and clinical applications of each modality are thoroughly discussed.

The multidisciplinary perspective of this work underscores the necessity of integrating imaging findings with clinical presentation, biochemical profiles, histopathological correlation, and surgical strategy. Looking ahead, the incorporation of artificial intelligence, novel radiopharmaceuticals, and hybrid imaging technologies promises to further advance diagnostic precision and clinical utility.

This book is intended as both a practical guide for current practice and a reference point for understanding future innovations in this dynamic and rapidly evolving field. We hope that it will serve clinicians across disciplines involved in care of patients with parathyroid disease, ultimately fostering greater diagnostic accuracy, improved surgical outcomes, and enhanced quality of life for the patients entrusted to us.

Zagreb, Croatia — Petra Petranović Ovčariček
Lugano, Switzerland — Luca Giovanella
Zurich, Switzerland — Martin W. Huellner

Acknowledgments

The successful completion of this comprehensive volume on parathyroid imaging would not have been possible without the contributions of our distinguished co-authors—radiologists, nuclear medicine physicians, endocrine surgeons, biochemists, and pathologists—who generously shared their expertise and devoted their valuable time to make this multidisciplinary collaboration a reality.

We are deeply indebted to our colleagues in the imaging departments, clinical laboratories, pathology services, and operating theaters, whose provision of exemplary case material, high-quality images, and meticulous clinical correlations form the foundation of this work.

Our sincere gratitude extends to the medical students, residents, and fellows whose thoughtful questions and fresh perspectives have challenged us to clarify complex concepts and to continually refine our explanations.

We are equally grateful to our publisher and editorial team for their professionalism, patience, and unwavering commitment to ensuring the highest standards of quality.

Most importantly, we acknowledge our patients, whose trust in our care and willingness to contribute to academic and educational endeavors make continued progress in this field possible.

Finally, we extend our heartfelt thanks to our families and loved ones, whose understanding, encouragement, and sacrifice throughout the many hours devoted to this project enabled its successful realization.

Contents

1 Anatomy and Embryology of Parathyroid Glands

Gürsan Kaya and Murat Tuncel

Definitions The parathyroid glands are small endocrine organs derived from the third and fourth pharyngeal pouches, responsible for maintaining calcium homeostasis through secretion of parathyroid hormone (PTH). Variations in their embryologic development lead to differences in number, size, and location. These anatomic variations have direct clinical relevance, as they influence both diagnostic evaluation and surgical management of hyperparathyroidism.

Learning Objectives

After reviewing this chapter, the reader should be able to:

1. Describe the embryologic origin and migratory pathways of the parathyroid glands.
2. Identify the typical and variant anatomic locations of the glands, including their vascular supply.
3. Recognize key histological features of parathyroid tissue and their clinical significance.
4. Understand how developmental anomalies and ectopic localizations affect imaging interpretation and surgical strategy.

G. Kaya
Department of Nuclear Medicine, Yozgat City Hospital, Yozgat, Turkey
e-mail: gursan.kaya@hacettepe.edu.tr; kayagursan@gmail.com

M. Tuncel (✉)
Department of Nuclear Medicine, Faculty of Medicine, Hacettepe University, Ankara, Turkey
e-mail: muratmtx@yahoo.com; murat.tuncel@hacettepe.edu.tr

1.1 Embryologic Development

1.1.1 Pharyngeal Pouch Origins and Migration

The parathyroid glands develop from the endoderm of the pharyngeal (branchial) pouches during early embryogenesis. By the fifth to sixth week of gestation, the third and fourth pharyngeal pouches form the parathyroid primordia, which initiates their differentiation and subsequent migration [1]. The inferior parathyroid glands arise from the dorsal wing of the third pharyngeal pouch, whereas the ventral wing of the same pouch gives rise to the thymus [1, 2].

As embryonic development progresses, the thymus migrates caudally into the anterior mediastinum, carrying the paired inferior parathyroid

© The Author(s), under exclusive license to Springer Nature Switzerland AG 2026
P. Petranović Ovčariček et al. (eds.), *Parathyroid Imaging*,
https://doi.org/10.1007/978-3-032-14178 1_1

primordia along its path. By the seventh to eighth week of gestation, this descent positions the inferior parathyroid glands just caudal to the developing thyroid, typically near its lower poles or occasionally within the thymic tongue in the lower neck. In contrast, the superior parathyroid glands originate from the dorsal wing of the fourth pharyngeal pouch. During development, they detach from the pharyngeal wall and associate with the descending thyroid gland, which migrates caudally from the foramen cecum. This relatively shorter migratory path results in a more consistent final position near the upper poles of the thyroid. By the end of the second month of gestation, all parathyroid glands generally reach their definitive cervical positions. Notably, the parathyroids become functionally active during fetal life [1, 3–5].

1.1.2 Molecular Regulation of Organogenesis

Parathyroid development is regulated by a coordinated network of transcription factors and signaling pathways that shape the patterning of the pharyngeal endoderm. A key regulator in this process is the transcription factor GCM2 (Glial Cells Missing-2), which begins to express in the dorsal endoderm of the third and fourth pharyngeal pouches as the parathyroid domain becomes specified. GCM2 is essential for parathyroid organogenesis; experimental models show that mice lacking GCM2 do not form parathyroid glands, leading to congenital hypoparathyroidism. In humans, loss-of-function mutations in GCM2 similarly cause familial isolated hypoparathyroidism, highlighting its critical role in parathyroid development and function [6]. Another key transcriptional regulator is TBX1, a member of the T-box family that is implicated in the pathogenesis of 22q11 deletion syndrome (DiGeorge syndrome). TBX1 is essential for the proper development of the third and fourth pharyngeal pouches; its absence or mutation leads to agenesis or hypoplasia of the thymus and parathyroid glands [7]. This mechanistic disruption explains why individuals with DiGeorge syndrome are typically born without parathyroid glands, resulting in neonatal hypocalcemia. Additional genes implicated in parathyroid embryogenesis include HOXA3, PAX1, and EYA1/SIX1, among others. HOXA3 and PAX1 play pivotal roles in pharyngeal pouch patterning and contribute to the upregulation of GCM2; mutations in these genes can impair GCM2 expression and induce apoptosis of parathyroid progenitor cells, thereby arresting gland development [8, 9]. In addition to transcription factors, local signaling molecules play a critical role in parathyroid morphogenesis. Fibroblast Growth Factors (FGFs) and Bone Morphogenetic Protein 4 (BMP4) facilitate the separation of the thymus-parathyroid complex from the pharyngeal endoderm and help define the distinct cellular identities of parathyroid and thymic lineages. These coordinated molecular cues collectively instruct the endoderm of the third and fourth pharyngeal pouches to differentiate into mature, hormone-producing parathyroid glands located in the cervical region [10–12].

1.2 Macroscopic Anatomy of the Parathyroid Glands

1.2.1 Number and Location

The overwhelming majority of individuals have four PTGs, two superior and two inferior, whereas between 2.5% and 13.0% have supernumerary glands, and 3% have fewer than four glands. These glands typically appear as small, soft, yellow-tan ovoid structures embedded in the fat overlying the thyroid capsule. The superior and inferior parathyroid glands are located on the dorsal surface of the thyroid, generally adjacent to the upper and lower poles, respectively [13]. The superior glands are most commonly identified at the level of the upper thyroid pole, within a 2 cm zone centered approximately 1 cm above the junction of the recurrent laryngeal nerve (RLN) and the inferior thyroid artery, as demonstrated in surgical series [5, 14]. In contrast, the inferior glands—owing to their longer embryologic migration with the thymus—are more vari-

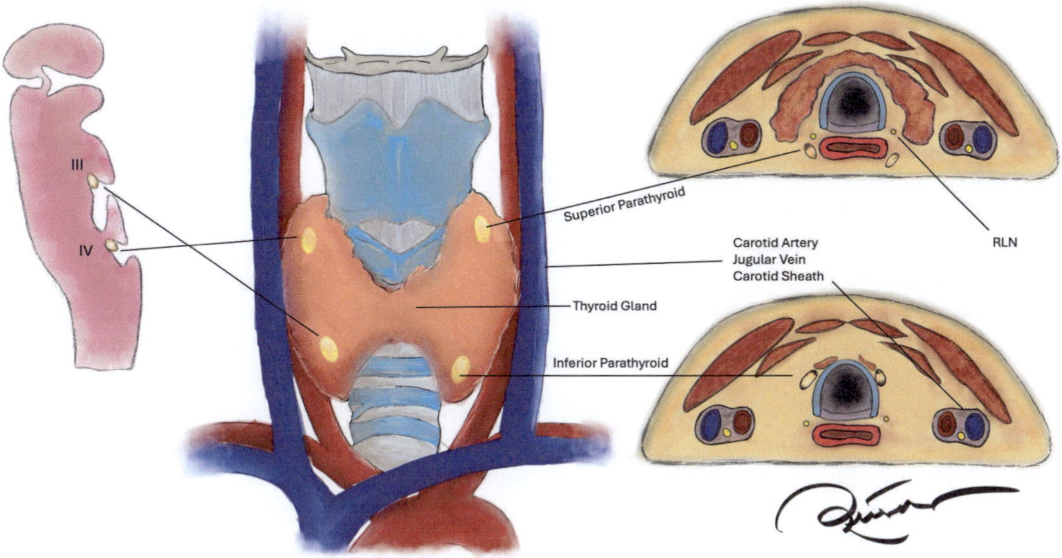

Fig. 1.1 Brief summary of parathyroid gland embryology and typical location of parathyroid glands

able in position, typically found near the lower thyroid pole or along the thyrothymic ligament, but may be located anywhere from just below the thyroid gland to the superior mediastinum [1, 3, 15]. The upper PTGs are located behind the tracheoesophageal groove, the upper parts of the thyroid lobes (80–95%), and the retropharyngeal and retroesophageal area (3%) and, less frequently, in the carotid sheath (<1%), in the thyroid parenchyma (<1%), or in the fatty tissue adjacent to the scalene muscles (<1%). The inferior glands are located near the lower thyroid lobe (50–60%), along the thyrothymic ligament (25%) and in the mediastinum (3%) and, less commonly, carotid sheath (<1%) or intrathyroidal (<1%) [16] (Fig. 1.1).

1.2.2 Size and Vascular Supply

Each normal parathyroid gland typically measures 4–6 mm in length, 3–4 mm in width, and 1–2 mm in thickness, with an average weight of approximately 30–40 mg; those located at the inferior poles tend to be slightly larger on average [17]. The arterial supply of the parathyroid glands arises predominantly from the inferior thyroid arteries, which provide branches to both the superior and inferior glands in approximately 76–86% of individuals. In the remaining cases, vascular supply may arise from anastomoses or direct branches of the superior thyroid artery. Venous drainage is directed into the thyroid venous plexus. The parathyroid stroma is richly vascularized, reflecting the high metabolic demand required for continuous parathyroid hormone (PTH) secretion. Lymphatic drainage of the parathyroid glands generally follows thyroid lymphatics, primarily draining into the deep cervical and paratracheal lymph node chains [18–20].

1.3 Histology and Cellular Composition

1.3.1 Parenchymal Cells

Histologically, the parathyroid gland consists of tightly packed cords and nests of epithelial cells embedded within a richly vascularized stroma, interspersed with abundant adipocytes. Notably, the adipocyte content is generally higher in women, a variation that may reflect hormonal or age-related influences on stromal composition. The predominant cell type is the chief cell (or principal cell), which serves as the primary functional unit responsible for parathyroid hormone (PTH) secretion. Chief cells are small and polygonal in shape (8–12 μm in diameter), with centrally located nuclei and pale, finely granular cytoplasm. They synthesize and release PTH in response to declining serum calcium levels, thereby playing a critical role in calcium homeostasis.

In contrast, oxyphil cells are larger (12–20 μm), and acidophilic epithelial cells typically emerge after puberty and progressively increase in number with age. Their densely granular, eosinophilic cytoplasm reflects a high mitochondrial content; however, they lack significant secretory function and do not contribute meaningfully to PTH production. Transitional forms between chief and oxyphil cells are frequently observed, suggesting a gradual oncocytic transformation. Additionally, fetal parathyroid tissue and pathological forms such as adenomas may contain water-clear cells—chief cells laden with glycogen—but these are not present in normal adult glands [1, 4, 17, 21].

1.3.2 Stromal Features

A distinctive feature of parathyroid histology is the presence of adipose tissue within the stromal compartment. In normal adults, adipocytes can comprise approximately 30–50% of the gland's volume. Fat content is minimal during infancy, begins to accumulate after puberty, and progressively increases with age. This stromal fat contributes to the characteristic yellow coloration of the gland observed during gross inspection and serves as a key histologic hallmark. The supporting stroma also contains delicate fibrous septa and a dense capillary network that ensures efficient perfusion of the parenchymal cells. As age advances, there is a corresponding increase in both stromal fat and the proportion of oxyphil cells, although the glandular architecture remains optimized for calcium sensing and parathyroid hormone secretion [1, 4, 17, 21, 22].

1.4 Anatomical Variations and Anomalies

1.4.1 Variations in Number: Supernumerary or Absent Glands

While four is the typical number of parathyroid glands, a significant proportion of individuals exhibit variations due to developmental anomalies. Supernumerary glands—most commonly a fifth and rarely a sixth—arise from the division of a single primordial gland or the persistence of accessory parathyroid tissue. Conversely, some individuals have only three glands, reflecting agenesis or regression during development. Most supernumerary glands are small (<5 mg) and are often located adjacent to a normally positioned gland, occasionally appearing as a "double" gland within the same anatomical region [18, 19]. In otherwise healthy individuals, the presence of an additional or absent parathyroid gland typically has no physiological consequence, as overall PTH output adjusts accordingly. However, in cases of hyperparathyroidism, undetected supernumerary glands may contribute to persistent or recurrent disease if they are not identified and excised during surgery. True congenital absence of parathyroid tissue is rare, except in the previously mentioned syndromic contexts [23, 24]. In summary, approximately 10–15% of individuals have a variant number of PTGs. This usually presents as either one supernumerary gland or, less frequently, a missing gland compared to the typical count of four [13].

1.4.2 Ectopic Locations of Parathyroid Tissue

Beyond numerical variation, the location of the parathyroid glands can vary significantly due to deviations in embryonic migration. Ectopic parathyroid glands occur when normal descent is disrupted, causing a gland to settle in an abnormal position outside its typical location adjacent to the thyroid. As previously mentioned, approximately 10–15% of PTGs are found in ectopic sites within the general population [13]. The inferior parathyroids have a longer migratory path with the thymus and are especially prone to ectopia along that course [1, 3]. Common ectopic sites for inferior PTGs include the thymus, the shallow recess of the thyrothymic ligament, and the anterior superior mediastinum. These sites essentially span the entire path of thymic descent from the lower cervical region to the upper anterior mediastinum [15, 25].

Using the recurrent laryngeal nerve as a reference (coronal RLN plane), the surgical neck can be divided into anterior and posterior planes. Superior ectopic PTGs typically lie posterior (dorsal) to the RLN, often located along the carotid sheath, retroesophageal space, or posterior mediastinum. These glands migrate only a short distance during embryonic development, which explains their relatively consistent deep positioning. In contrast, inferior ectopic glands are generally located anterior (ventral) to the RLN, following the path of thymic descent. Common locations for these glands include the thyrothymic ligament, cervical thymus, anterior superior mediastinum, carotid sheath, and, less frequently, the aortopulmonary window and intrathyroidal localization. Awareness of these spatial patterns—superior glands being dorsal and cephalad and inferior glands ventral and caudal—is crucial for guiding both preoperative imaging and targeted surgical exploration, especially in cases of nonlocalized disease [16, 26, 27].

The superior parathyroids are more often near their expected location, but can occasionally be ectopic in locations such as the retroesophageal (paraesophageal) space, the posterior superior mediastinum, the carotid sheath, or high in the neck near the pharynx [28]. A particularly important variant is the intrathyroidal parathyroid, in which a gland is embedded within the thyroid parenchyma itself. Intrathyroidal parathyroid glands are uncommon (occurring in roughly 0.7–3.6% of cases). But they represent a critical pitfall as they may be overlooked during surgery or imaging. Both superior glands that fail to detach from the thyroid anlage or inferior glands dragged into the thyroid capsule can lead to intrathyroidal placement [29].

A non-recurrent laryngeal nerve (NRLN) is a rare anatomical variant, most commonly observed on the right side and nearly always associated with an aberrant right subclavian artery (ARSA) that arises directly from the aortic arch. This vascular anomaly alters the embryologic course of the fourth branchial arch derivatives and may impact adjacent structures, including the trajectory of the inferior parathyroid glands. The absence of a normal subclavian loop eliminates the caudal migration path of the right recurrent laryngeal nerve (RLN), resulting in a horizontally oriented NRLN that enters the larynx directly. Surgically, this variation can obscure typical neurovascular landmarks, increasing the risk of injury or misidentification during parathyroidectomy, especially when ectopic inferior glands are located in unusual areas such as the carotid sheath or high tracheoesophageal groove. Preoperative identification of an ARSA via CT angiography or US can alert the surgeon to the likely presence of an NRLN and potential alterations in parathyroid migration patterns [16, 30].

Recognizing the spectrum of potential ectopic sites is critical, as any parathyroid gland located outside its typical anatomical position may lead to diagnostic uncertainty and significant surgical difficulty if not anticipated during preoperative planning or exploration.

1.4.3 Developmental Anomalies and Syndromes

In rare instances, as previously discussed, parathyroid glands may be congenitally absent or exhibit marked atypia due to developmental arrest or genetic perturbations. DiGeorge syndrome (22q11.2 deletion) serves as the prototypical example, where maldevelopment of the third and fourth pharyngeal pouches results in complete agenesis of the parathyroids and thymus, leading to neonatal hypocalcemia and congenital hypoparathyroidism. Other syndromic entities, such as HDR syndrome (hypoparathyroidism, deafness, renal dysplasia), caused by GATA3 mutations, similarly involve parathyroid hypoplasia or aplasia due to disrupted embryologic differentiation [6]. At the opposite end of the developmental spectrum, chronic stimulation of the parathyroid glands—most notably in the context of longstanding secondary hyperparathyroidism due to end-stage renal disease—leads to diffuse multiglandular hyperplasia. In this setting, previously unrecognized supernumerary parathyroid glands, often arising from embryologic rests, may become hyper-functional and macroscopically apparent. Surgical series have documented up to seven or even eight glands in some patients with refractory disease. These cases illustrate a challenging spectrum of anatomical variation that, although congenital in origin, becomes clinically relevant through acquired hyperplasia—posing significant obstacles to complete resection and durable disease control [13, 31].

Although such extreme presentations are uncommon, any deviation in parathyroid number or location becomes clinically significant in the setting of hyperparathyroidism, as unrecognized or ectopic glands can result in persistent or recurrent disease following surgery.

1.5 Surgical Anatomy Insights from Clinical Series

Contemporary surgical and imaging series have provided detailed quantitative data on parathyroid anatomical variation, offering valuable context for operative planning and localization strategy. The most comprehensive analysis to date—a 2019 meta-analysis aggregating findings from 26 studies encompassing 7005 patients—characterizes both typical and ectopic gland distributions with high granularity, informing preoperative expectations and guiding intraoperative decision-making. In this meta-analysis, approximately 81% of patients exhibited the typical complement of four parathyroid glands. The remaining ~19% demonstrated numerical variation, either supernumerary or fewer glands. Most deviations involved a single additional or missing gland. True extremes—such as the presence of six or more glands—were exceedingly uncommon, underscoring their rarity in routine surgical practice but emphasizing the need for vigilance during reoperative exploration. The same meta-analysis reported that approximately 15.9% of all parathyroid glands examined were in ectopic positions. When broken down by region, 11.6% of glands were found in ectopic cervical locations—outside the typical posterior surface of the thyroid—while 4.3% were identified within the mediastinum. These findings underscore the clinical relevance of ectopy, particularly in cases of non-localizing imaging or failed initial surgery. In other words, nearly one in six parathyroid glands may reside outside the expected posterior thyroid location. Notably, within the ectopic cervical group, more than half were located either in a retroesophageal or paraesophageal position or within the thyroid parenchyma itself. These findings highlight the importance of considering both deep cervical and intrathyroidal sites during preoperative localization and intraoperative exploration [13].

Large autopsy series by Gilmour and later by Wang in the twentieth century were among the first to systematically quantify the prevalence of supernumerary and ectopic parathyroid glands. More recent analyses, including the aforementioned meta-analysis, have refined these estimates with larger pooled data. Similarly, the incidence and distribution of ectopic glands have been well characterized in surgical literature. For example, Akerström's 1984 operative series highlighted that the thymus and mediastinum commonly harbor inferior parathyroids, while a small but consistent proportion of superior glands were identified in paraesophageal locations or high cervical positions, reflecting their shorter migratory pathway during embryologic development. An anatomical analysis of 645 parathyroid glands from 160 cadavers reported that while the vast majority of superior glands (approximately 80%) were localized within a 2 cm zone posterior to the upper thyroid pole, inferior glands displayed much greater positional variability. Only about 42% of inferior glands were found at the lower thyroid pole, with the remainder distributed along the thyrothymic tract—including ~39% in the lower neck near thymic remnants and approximately 2% within the upper mediastinum. These findings underscore the more extensive migratory pathway and broader ectopic potential of inferior parathyroid glands [5, 32, 33].

Importantly, certain ectopic locations have been consistently identified as frequent culprits in surgical failures. Intrathyroidal parathyroid glands, although accounting for only 1–3% of all parathyroid glands, are a well-documented cause of persistent or recurrent hyperparathyroidism. Surgical series report that intrathyroidal parathyroid adenomas are encountered in approximately 0.7–3.6% of parathyroidectomies, underscoring the need for a high index of suspicion when conventional imaging and exploration fail to localize the offending gland [25, 29].

These findings from high-volume surgical centers underscore that while focused, minimally invasive parathyroidectomy achieves high success rates in the majority of patients, the physicians must remain vigilant for supernumerary and ectopic glands. Failure to identify and remove all hyperfunctioning parathyroid tissue—such as an unrecognized fifth gland or an ectopic gland concealed within the mediastinum—can result in persistent or recurrent hyperparathyroidism, often necessitating re-operation with increased surgical complexity and morbidity.

1.6 Clinical Significance of Parathyroid Anatomy Variations

A detailed understanding of parathyroid anatomy—including its variations and embryologic basis—is essential for clinicians in nuclear medicine, radiology, and surgery to accurately localize and manage parathyroid lesions, particularly in the context of minimally invasive or targeted therapeutic approaches.

1.6.1 Intraoperative Considerations

A thorough understanding of embryologic migration patterns is essential for guiding intraoperative decision-making when a parathyroid gland is not found in its expected location. For example, if a superior gland is missing during exploration, the surgeon should systematically inspect known ectopic sites such as the paraesophageal space, posterior pharyngeal wall, or high cervical positions, given the tendency of superior glands to remain undescended or migrate posteriorly along the carotid sheath or retropharyngeal tract. Conversely, when an inferior gland is absent from its typical position near the lower thyroid pole, attention should shift toward the thymus and anterior mediastinum, often warranting partial excision of cervical thymic tissue or exploration along the thyrothymic ligament to identify a gland that followed the thymic descent path. In cases of suspected intrathyroidal parathyroid adenoma, a high index of suspicion is necessary; when three glands are accounted for but one remains elusive, inspection of the thyroid parenchyma and, in select cases, thyroid lobectomy may be required. Although minimally invasive parathyroidectomy typically focuses on a single adenoma identified on preoperative imaging, conversion to bilateral neck exploration becomes necessary if intraoperative PTH levels fail to fall as expected or if preoperative imaging was non-localizing. In such scenarios, familiarity with the full spectrum of ectopic locations—including the carotid sheath, retroesophageal space, and substernal thymus—is often the decisive factor between surgical success and failure [34].

1.7 Conclusions

With the advent of minimally invasive surgical techniques, accurately detecting diseased parathyroid glands has become increasingly crucial. Although the anatomy of these glands may seem straightforward, significant variability exists due to their complex embryology. Disturbances in the molecular regulation of organogenesis can lead to a wide range of numbers and ectopic locations of parathyroid glands. Understanding the different anatomical locations resulting from this embryologic variation will aid physicians in making accurate interpretations.

References

1. Sadler TW. Langman's medical embryology, 14e. Lippincott Williams & Wilkins, a Wolters Kluwer business; 2019.
2. Lofrese JJBH, Lappin SL. Physiology, Parathyroid. [Updated 2023 Jul 17]. In: StatPearls [internet]. Treasure Island: StatPearls Publishing.
3. Mansberger AR Jr, Wei JP. Surgical embryology and anatomy of the thyroid and parathyroid glands. Surg Clin North Am. 1993;73(4):727–46.
4. Schoenwolf GC, Bleyl SB, Brauer PR, Francis-West PH, Larsen WJ. Larsen's human embryology. 6th ed. Philadelphia: Elsevier; 2021.
5. Wang C-A. The anatomic basis of parathyroid surgery. Ann Surg. 1976;183(3):271–5.
6. Peissig K, Condie BG, Manley NR. Embryology of the parathyroid glands. Endocrinol Metab Clin N Am. 2018;47(4):733–42.
7. Jerome LA, Papaioannou VE. DiGeorge syndrome phenotype in mice mutant for the T-box gene, Tbx1. Nat Genet. 2001;27(3):286–91.
8. Günther T, Chen Z-F, Kim J, Priemel M, Rueger JM, Amling M, et al. Genetic ablation of parathyroid glands reveals another source of parathyroid hormone. Nature. 2000;406(6792):199–203.
9. Liu Z, Yu S, Manley NR. Gcm2 is required for the differentiation and survival of parathyroid precursor cells in the parathyroid/thymus primordia. Dev Biol. 2007;305(1):333–46.
10. Gordon J, Wilson VA, Blair NF, Sheridan J, Farley A, Wilson L, et al. Functional evidence for a single endodermal origin for the thymic epithelium. Nat Immunol. 2004;5(5):546–53.
11. Gardiner JR, Jackson AL, Gordon J, Lickert H, Manley NR, Basson MA. Localised inhibition of FGF signalling in the third pharyngeal pouch is required for normal thymus and parathyroid organogenesis. Development. 2012;139(18):3456–66.
12. Gordon J, Patel SR, Mishina Y, Manley NR. Evidence for an early role for BMP4 signaling in thymus and parathyroid morphogenesis. Dev Biol. 2010;339(1):141–54.
13. Taterra D, Wong LM, Vikse J, Sanna B, Pękala P, Walocha J, et al. The prevalence and anatomy of parathyroid glands: a meta-analysis with implications for parathyroid surgery. Langenbeck's Arch Surg. 2019;404(1):63–70.
14. Akerstrom G, Malmaeus J, Bergstrom R. Surgical anatomy of human parathyroid glands. Surgery. 1984;95(1):14–21.
15. Kurtay M, Crile G Jr. Aberrant parathyroid glands in relationship to the thymus. Am J Surg. 1969;117(5):705.
16. Bunch PM, Randolph GW, Brooks JA, George V, Cannon J, Kelly HR. Parathyroid 4D CT: what the surgeon wants to know. Radiographics. 2020;40(5):1383–94.
17. Lindberg. Diagnostic pathology – normal histology. 3rd ed. Elsevier Science Health Science.
18. Alveryd A. Parathyroid glands in thyroid surgery. I. Anatomy of parathyroid glands. II. Postoperative hypoparathyroidism–identification and autotransplantation of parathyroid glands. Acta Chir Scand. 1968;389:1–120.
19. Fancy T, Gallagher D 3rd, Hornig JD. Surgical anatomy of the thyroid and parathyroid glands. Otolaryngol Clin N Am. 2010;43(2):221–7. vii
20. Mohebati A, Shaha AR. Anatomy of thyroid and parathyroid glands and neurovascular relations. Clin Anat. 2012;25(1):19–31.
21. Mills SE. Histology for pathologists, 5e. Lippincott Williams & Wilkins, a Wolters Kluwer business; 2020.
22. Chen RA, Goodman WG. Role of the calcium-sensing receptor in parathyroid gland physiology. Am J Physiol Renal Physiol. 2004;286(6):F1005–F11.
23. Pattou FN, Pellissier LC, Noël C, Wambergue F, Huglo DG, Proye CA. Supernumerary parathyroid glands: frequency and surgical significance in treatment of renal hyperparathyroidism. World J Surg. 2000;24(11):1330–4.
24. Chen W, Chen L, Wei T, Li Z, Lei J, Zhu J. Idiopathic hypoparathyroidism with papillary thyroid carcinoma in a young male: a rare case report. Front Endocrinol (Lausanne). 2020;11:569308.
25. Goodman A, Politz D, Lopez J, Norman J. Intrathyroid parathyroid adenoma. Otolaryngol Head Neck Surg. 2011;144(6):867–71.
26. Noussios G, Anagnostis P, Natsis K. Ectopic parathyroid glands and their anatomical, clinical and surgical implications. Exp Clin Endocrinol Diabetes. 2012;120(10):604–10.
27. Phitayakorn R, McHenry CR. Incidence and location of ectopic abnormal parathyroid glands. Am J Surg. 2006;191(3):418–23.
28. Mohebati A, Shaha AR. Imaging techniques in parathyroid surgery for primary hyperparathyroidism. Am J Otolaryngol. 2012;33(4):457–68.
29. Bahar G, Feinmesser R, Joshua B-Z, Shpitzer T, Morgenstein S, Popovtzer A, et al. Hyperfunctioning intrathyroid parathyroid gland: a potential cause of failure in parathyroidectomy. Surgery. 2006;139(6):821–6.
30. Henry JF, Audiffret J, Denizot A, Plan M. The nonrecurrent inferior laryngeal nerve: review of 33 cases, including two on the left side. Surgery. 1988;104(6):977–84.
31. Tai TS, Hsu YH, Chang JM, Chen CC. Recurrent tertiary hyperparathyroidism due to supernumerary parathyroid glands in a patient receiving long-term hemodialysis: a case report. BMC Endocr Disord. 2019;19(1):16.
32. Akerström G, Malmaeus J, Bergström R. Surgical anatomy of human parathyroid glands. Surgery. 1984;95:14.
33. Gilmour JR, Martin WJ. The weight of the parathyroid glands. J Pathol Bacteriol. 1937;44(2):431–62.
34. Wilhelm SM, Wang TS, Ruan DT, Lee JA, Asa SL, Duh Q-Y, et al. The American Association of Endocrine Surgeons guidelines for definitive management of primary hyperparathyroidism. JAMA Surg. 2016;151(10):959–68.

2 Histopathology of Parathyroid Glands

Maria Gloor and Niels J. Rupp

Definitions

Parathyroid glands: Endocrine glands (typically four) which are usually located dorsally of the thyroid. They are responsible for parathyroid hormone (PTH) production, which is involved in calcium homeostasis.

Parathyroid hormone (PTH): A hormone produced by the parathyroid glands. It regulates calcium and phosphate metabolism by acting on the bone, kidneys, and indirectly intestine.

Chief cells (principal cells): The most abundant parenchymal cell type in the parathyroid glands. They are small cells with a centrally located, round nucleus and slightly eosinophilic cytoplasm. Their main function is parathyroid hormone (PTH) production.

Oxyphil cells (oncocytic cells): Large parathyroid cells with small nuclei and intensely eosinophilic cytoplasm due to their high mitochondrial content. They occur in clusters among the other parenchymal cells.

Parathyroid hyperplasia: A non-neoplastic proliferative disorder of the parathyroid glands, characterized by an increase in mass of parenchymal cells with more than one gland involved. Histologically, it shows enlargement with reduced stromal fat and may consist of one or several parenchymal cell types.

Parathyroid adenoma: A benign neoplasm of the parathyroid glands and the most common cause of primary hyperparathyroidism. Typically, it affects a single gland, shows reduction of stromal fat, and is composed of one or more parenchymal cell types.

Parathyroid carcinoma: A rare and malignant neoplasm of the parathyroid glands, which can cause hyperparathyroidism. Required for diagnosis are invasive growth or metastasis.

Learning Objectives

- Recognizing the normal histological architecture and main cell types of the parathyroid glands.
- Describing the most common pathologies of the parathyroid glands, including hyperplasia, adenoma, and carcinoma.

(continued)

M. Gloor
Department of Pathology and Molecular Pathology, University Hospital Zurich, Zurich, Switzerland
e-mail: maria.gloor@usz.ch

N. J. Rupp (✉)
Department of Pathology and Molecular Pathology, University Hospital Zurich, Zurich, Switzerland

Faculty of Medicine, University of Zurich, Zurich, Switzerland
e-mail: niels.rupp@usz.ch

© The Author(s), under exclusive license to Springer Nature Switzerland AG 2026
P. Petranović Ovčariček et al. (eds.), *Parathyroid Imaging*,
https://doi.org/10.1007/978-3-032-14178-1_2

- Understanding the role of immunohistochemistry in the evaluation of parathyroid lesions.
- Relating histopathological findings to clinical presentation and endocrine function.

2.1 Gross Anatomy

The parathyroid glands are typically four in number and located posterior to the thyroid gland, yellowish to reddish-brown in color, lentil-sized, and weigh from 35 to 40 mg [25, 31].

2.2 Histology

The parathyroid glands are constituted of parenchymal cells with endocrine function as well as stromal adipocytes (Fig. 2.1). The endocrine cells are organized in nests and cords, enclosed by a fine fibrous capsule and separated into subtle lobules. Their main function is the production of parathyroid hormone (PTH).

Histologically, there are several cell phenotypes in the parathyroid parenchyma that are thought to be differentiated states of the same cell type, all of which appear to be involved in PTH production. The most abundant cell type is the *chief cell (principal cell)*. It is the smallest cell type, showing a centrally located, round nucleus and slightly eosinophilic cytoplasm, containing PTH secretory granules (Fig. 2.2) [8]. Organized in nests and cords, they make up most of the parathyroid tissue. The *oxyphil cells (oncocytic cells)* are larger, with small nuclei [6] and a more eosinophilic (oxyphilic) cytoplasm due to their increased mitochondria content (Fig. 2.2) [47]. They are organized in clusters throughout the plentiful chief cells. Oxyphil cells are rare in children; however, they increase in number with age and functional stress [15]. Although their physiological significance is still somewhat elusive, they seem to be involved in the PTH production based on immunohistochemical staining for PTH as well as gene expression analysis [47, 56]. The oxyphil cells are believed to develop out of chief cells since a transitional cell type, the *transient cells (transitional cells)*, has been described [47]. These cells are more similar to chief cells regarding size, but show a more eosinophilic cytoplasm, closer to oxyphil cells (Fig. 2.2). They can be found in small numbers, distributed between the chief cells [16]. In pathological parathyroid glands, a further cell type has been discovered, the *water clear cells (clear cells)*. This cell type presents slightly larger than common chief cells and has a distinct glycogen-rich cytoplasm appearing empty in histological sections. So far, they have only infrequently been observed in physiological parathyroid tissue of adults, found among the chief cells, and are more commonly associated with parathyroid hyperplasia and adenoma. It is assumed that they also develop from chief cells [8, 16, 22, 48].

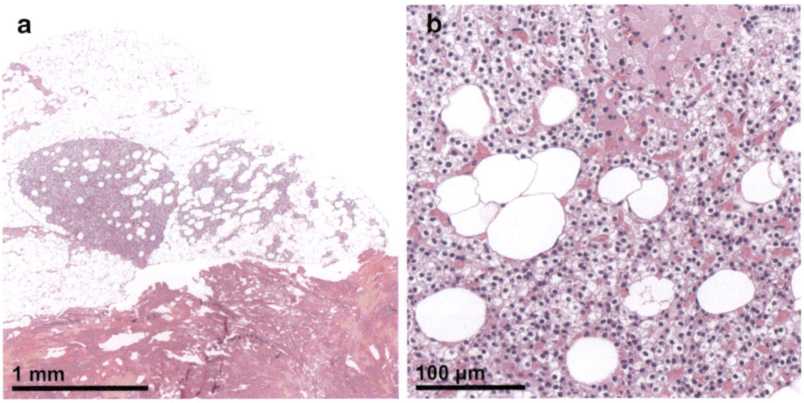

Fig. 2.1 Normal parathyroid gland cross section consisting of endocrine tissue scattered with adipocytes, H&E stainings. (**a**) Overview of the gland. (**b**) Closer view, which shows chief cells and a cluster of oxyphil cells with adipocytes scattered between the endocrine tissue

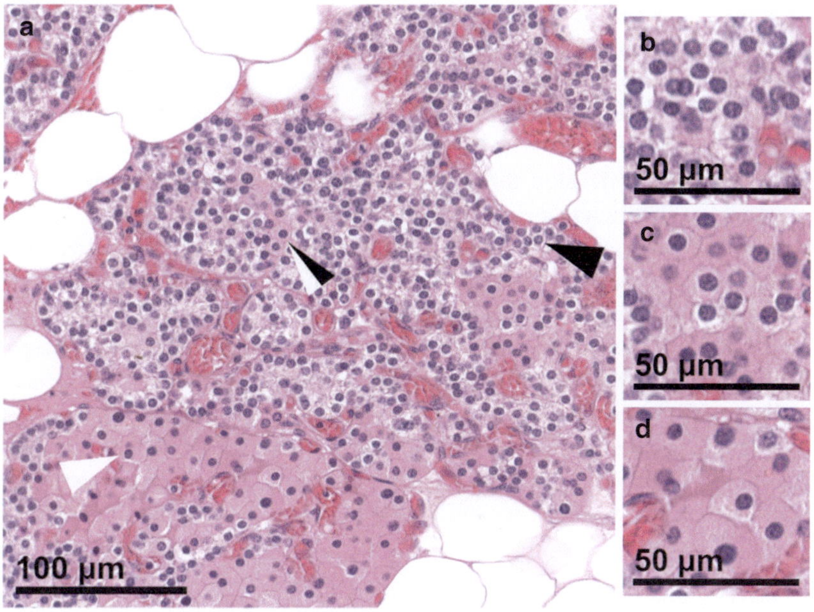

Fig. 2.2 Normal parathyroid tissue with physiological cell types, H&E stainings. (**a**) Overview consisting of chief cells (black arrowhead) with a few transient cells (striped arrowhead) and a cluster of oxyphil cells (white arrowhead). Adipocytes are visibly scattered between the endocrine tissue. (**b**) Chief cells (principal cell) organized in nests. (**c**) A grouping of transient cells (transitional cells). (**d**) Oxyphil cells (oncocytic cells)

Adipocytes are found in varying frequencies between the endocrine cells (Fig. 2.1). This stromal fat usually makes up around 20–25% of the parathyroid gland but can also be more pronounced or even completely absent in physiological glands [18].

2.3 Pathologies

2.3.1 Non-neoplastic

2.3.1.1 Innate Abnormalities

The location of *ectopic parathyroid glands* is determined by embryonic migration routes. The inferior parathyroid glands are more commonly affected than the superior ones. Possible locations differ between superior and inferior glands, but generally include mediastinum, along the tracheoesophageal groove, intrathyroidal or adjacent to the thymus, skull base or mandible angle, etc. [31].

A *variation in number* occurs in 16% of cases, whereas an increase in gland number is more common than a decrease (13% vs. 3%) [3].

Agenesis and *aplasia* are rare conditions of the parathyroid gland. In agenesis, the glands have not formed at all, whereas in aplasia they have formed, though not developed. Neither is compatible with life. *Hypoplasia* of the parathyroid glands on the other hand is indeed compatible with life but causes hypoparathyroidism. It can either occur sporadically or in the context of a genetic disorder, such as DiGeorge syndrome. DiGeorge syndrome, just like the chromosome 22q11.2 deletion syndrome, shows an impairment of the development of structures arising from the pharyngeal pouch. Not only the parathyroid glands are affected, but also craniofacial structures, the cardiac outflow tract, and the thymus, which leads to hypoparathyroidism, palatal anomalies, cardiac malformations, and immunodeficiency [39].

2.3.1.2 Developed Abnormalities

Parathyroid hyperplasia is a proliferative disorder which is defined as an increase in mass of non-neoplastic, parenchymal cells. Grossly, hyperplastic parathyroid glands are enlarged, reddish brown in color, and the cut surface is homogeneous with occasionally a slightly nodular configuration. The involvement of more than one gland is essential. This is also one of the most important features for distinguishing between hyperplasia and adenoma. Rarely, however, adenomas can also occur as multiglandular disease.

Typically, hyperplastic parathyroid tissue is made up of parenchymal cells with a reduction in stromal fat, consisting of either one cell type or a mix of cell types including chief, transient, oncocytic, and water clear cells [21, 43]. Parathyroid hyperplasia appears to develop through a polyclonal mechanism, although in specific cases like hyperparathyroidism due to renal failure, transformation into monoclonal growth has been suggested [49, 58]. To a lesser extent, hyperplasia may occasionally show features seen in atypical parathyroid tumors or parathyroid carcinoma, especially in the context of tertiary hyperparathyroidism. Such changes include fibrotic bands, nuclear pleomorphism or atypia, and degenerative changes (calcification, hemorrhage, fibrosis) [31].

Parathyromatosis is a rare cause of hyperparathyroidism in which parathyroid tissue is scattered across the tissue of the neck or even the mediastinum. It usually occurs through spillage of parathyroid tissue during surgery and can cause hyperparathyroidism through hyperfunctioning of these gland fragments [27]. Histologically, it is a hyperplastic parathyroid parenchyma that is not precisely circumscribed and involves the surrounding tissue [31]. Presenting in such a manner, it may be difficult to differentiate from parathyroid carcinoma [26].

Parathyroid cysts most commonly occur as a mass on the neck, with hyperparathyroidism or with symptoms of compression. They can either be functioning or non-functioning regarding hormone production. They are an important differential diagnosis in patients presenting with neck mass (accounting for 1–5%) or with a presumed thyroid cyst [46]. Evidence of PTH in the cyst fluid helps to confirm the diagnosis.

2.3.2 Neoplastic

2.3.2.1 Benign

Parathyroid adenoma is a benign neoplastic disease of the parathyroid glands and the leading cause of primary hyperparathyroidism, constituting up to 90% of cases [45]. Commonly one gland is affected, more frequently the inferior ones, but also adenomas can occur in ectopic locations. In up to 15% of cases, double adenomas affecting two glands are found [41]. In almost half of these cases, both are localized in the upper glands [41]. Compared to regular parathyroid glands, adenomas present with an increase in size and weight, with a more ovoid configuration and a thin pseudo capsule. An important feature, though not always found, is a slim rim of non-neoplastic tissue, aiding in differentiating an adenoma from a hyperplastic gland (Fig. 2.3). However, this is not a reliable diagnostic criterion, as hyperplasia can also occasionally have a rim-like area [19]. Adenomatous tissue can consist of one single or a mix of cell types. These include the chief, transient, oncocytic, and water clear cells. Accordingly, parathyroid adenomas can either be monoclonal or polyclonal [49, 52]. Usually they have a bland appearance, are well circumscribed, and show a reduction in stromal fat (Fig. 2.3) [3]. In some cases, they can depict subtle changes like follicular growth, cyst formation, hemorrhage, focal fibrosis, or occasionally a mitotic figure [29, 54, 62]. A clear distinction between adenoma and hyperplasia based on morphology alone is not possible, as many features overlap. Radiological and clinical correlation is therefore crucial. While parathyroid adenomas often occur sporadically, 10% of cases have a hereditary cause [57]. Syndromes involving parathyroid neoplasms include multiple endocrine neoplasia (types 1, 2, 4, and 5), familial-isolated hyperparathyroidism syndromes, and CDC73-related syndromes, such as hyperparathyroidism-jaw syndrome [17, 28, 37, 51].

Parathyroid lipoadenoma is an entity characterized by a neoplastic increase in parathyroid tissue and a high percentage of adipose tissue (>50%) [34]. Compared to common parathyroid adenomas, gross appearance mainly differs regarding color, since due to the increased fat content, the cut surface presents yellow [2]. Only a few cases have been reported so far, and this diagnosis should be differentiated from non-neoplastic parathyroid tissue with an increase in adipose tissue as well as from parathyroid adenomas containing adipose tissue [34, 36].

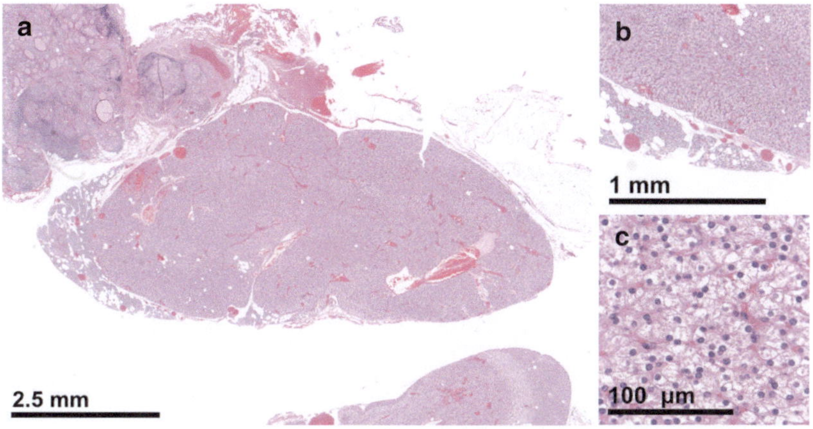

Fig. 2.3 Parathyroid adenoma cross section. Clinically, only one gland was suspicious. In the gross examination weighing 0.4 g and histologically measuring 8.9 mm. H&E stainings. (**a**) Overview showing an obvious reduction in stromal fat. Additionally, there is a rim of normal parathyroid tissue visible at the left corner. (**b**) Higher magnification depicting the adjacent rim of normal parathyroid tissue. (**c**) Further magnification shows almost exclusively chief cells with a solid growth pattern

2.3.2.2 Uncertain Malignant Potential

Atypical parathyroid tumors show significant atypical cytologic and architectural changes, but crucially no convincing invasion or metastases. They often reach a considerable size and, like parathyroid carcinomas, may show adhesions, fibrotic bands, mitotic activity, cytologic atypia, and even extension into the capsule. Their malignant potential is uncertain, but usually there is no recurrence after complete excision [13]. Only a few cases have been described in which a metastasis was diagnosed years after the initial diagnosis of an atypical parathyroid tumor, suggesting that the original neoplasm was more likely a carcinoma [42].

2.3.2.3 Malignant

Parathyroid carcinomas are rare malignancies and account for less than 1% of primary hyperparathyroidism [4]. Very rarely can they arise from tertiary hyperparathyroidism [40]. Essential for the diagnosis is either invasion or metastasis [20]. Like adenomas, carcinomas can develop sporadically or due to hereditary alterations. The most notable syndrome regarding parathyroid carcinomas is the hyperparathyroidism-jaw tumor syndrome, in which up to 15% of patients develop parathyroid carcinomas [53]. Clinically, parathyroid carcinomas often present with highly increased parathyroid hormone and calcium levels [14]. Another indication of a malignant disease is a palpable mass on the neck [44]. In general, parathyroid carcinomas present as large, poorly circumscribed tumors and often show adhesion to neighboring structures as well as varying or missing encapsulation [9]. The cut section is typically firm and appears lobulated [50]. Possible locations include not only anatomical parathyroid gland locations, but also ectopic locations [5, 11, 63]. Histologically, parathyroid carcinomas often show broad fibrous bands; however, they can lack a fibrous capsule surrounding the lesion [50]. Growth patterns mainly include trabecular or sheet-like growth [60]. Typically, cellular atypia can be appreciated but is not essential. Elevated mitotic activity (>5 mitoses/10 mm^2) often occurs, but singular mitoses can sporadically also be seen in non-malignant parathyroid changes [10]. Atypical mitotic figures as well as tumor necrosis are highly suspicious of carcinoma (Fig. 2.4) [10]. Histological evidence of either invasion of vessels, the perineurium, or adjacent structures or metastasis is essential [20]. To increase the chances of detecting invasive growth, the submission of the complete specimen is advised [24].

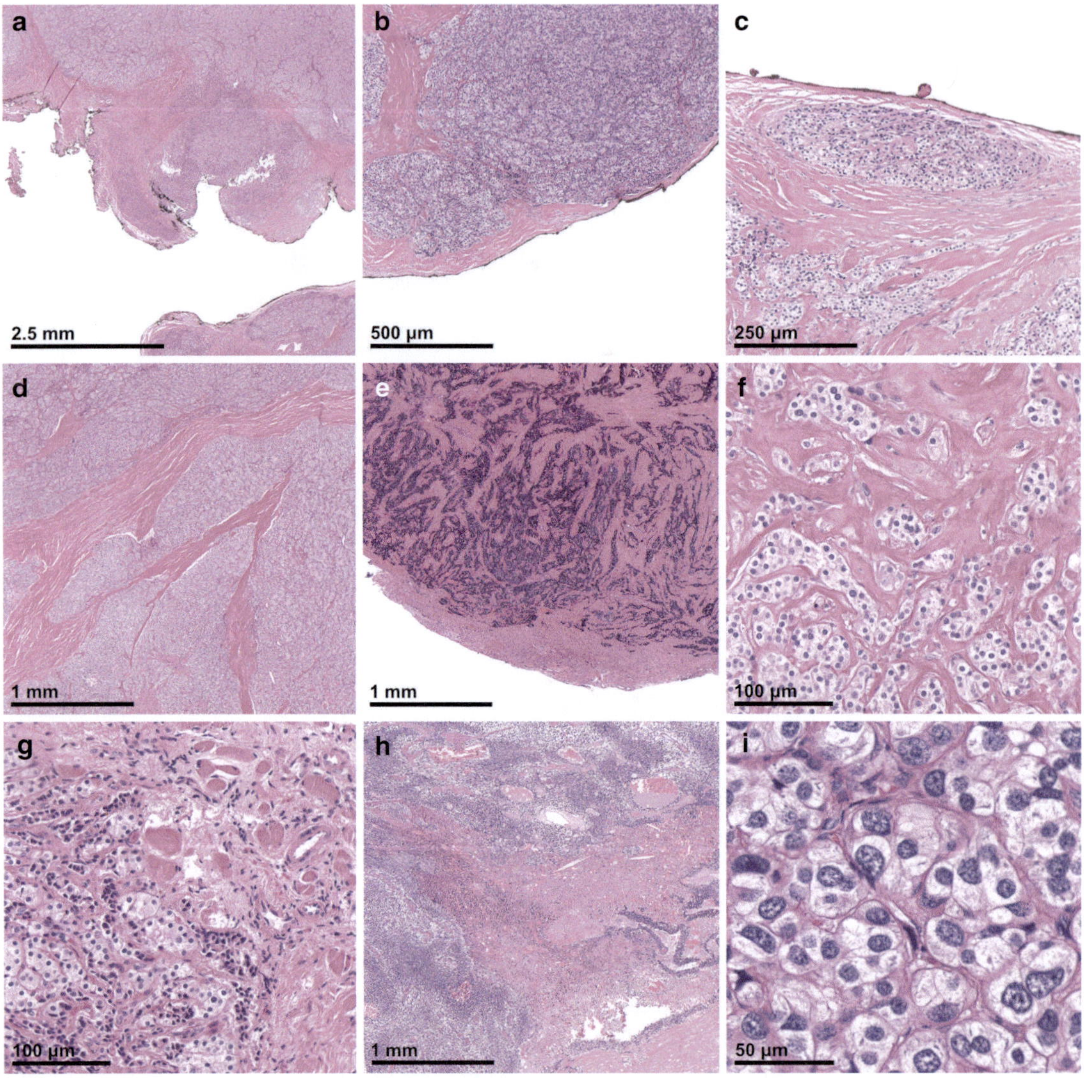

Fig. 2.4 Morphology and changes typically seen in atypical parathyroid tumors and parathyroid carcinomas, H&E stainings. (**a**) Poor circumscription. (**b**) Varying encapsulation. (**c**) Extension into capsule. (**d–f**) Broad fibrous bands. (**g**) Invasive growth into skeletal muscle. This is a diagnostic criterion for parathyroid carcinoma. (**h**) Necrosis. (**i**) Cellular atypia

Metastases to the parathyroid glands are exceedingly rare and most often emerge in the context of widely spread metastatic disease. Most prevalent primary tumors are breast carcinoma (67%), melanoma (12%), and lung carcinoma (6%). Metastases in the parathyroid glands severely disrupt calcium homeostasis and place an additional burden on patients who are often already severely exhausted by the disease [7].

2.4 Complementary Diagnostic Methods

2.4.1 Immunohistochemistry

Immunohistochemistry can be a useful tool to aid pathologists in their diagnostic workup. Regarding the parathyroid glands, there are several relevant markers.

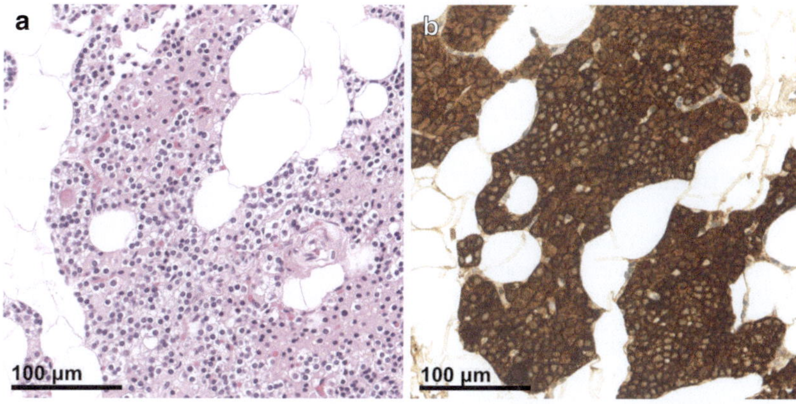

Fig. 2.5 Comparison of H&E versus PTH immunohistochemical staining of normal parathyroid tissue. (**a**) Normal parathyroid tissue with chief and oxyphil cells. (**b**) PTH immunohistochemical staining of the same section of normal parathyroid tissue. Strong positivity in all endocrine cells can be observed

In normal parathyroid glands as well as all parathyroid diseases, the tissue stains strongly positive for *parathyroid hormone* (Fig. 2.5). This can be helpful in the differential diagnosis of parathyroid and adenomatoid thyroid tissue, which can sometimes show remarkable similarities.

To aid in distinguishing between the different parathyroid pathologies, several markers have been studied, though many of which are limited in their use on their own. Even though they often show high specificity, they lack sensitivity [59]. To counteract this, it was proposed to use a panel of markers in combination [13, 23].

2.4.2 Molecular Pathology

Molecular pathology focuses on the submicroscopic component of diseases including genetic and molecular aspects. Some genetic changes are hinted at by specific morphological features or immunohistochemical characteristics, which should thus prompt further molecular investigation.

A common gene involved in parathyroid disease development is *MEN1*. It can show sporadic mutations or germline mutations, which cause multiple endocrine neoplasia type 1 (MEN1) [32]. It encodes the protein menin, which acts as tumor suppressor [1]. Mutations causing MEN1, MEN4, or MEN5 entail distinct morphological features, such as multinodular growth. In cases presenting with such morphology, it is reasonable to perform immunohistochemistry for menin, p27, or MAX, which are typically lost in these syndromes. However, morphology and immunohistochemistry alone are not sufficient to verify the diagnosis but are highly indicative [24].

Parafibromin deficiency in parathyroid tumors typically coincides with morphological features and strongly correlates with *CDC73* gene mutations as the underlying cause [30]. Such *CDC73* mutations can be observed in parathyroid carcinomas or atypical parathyroid tumors, but also in a subgroup of parathyroid adenomas, typically with a cystic configuration [33]. Germline mutation of *CDC73* causes hyperparathyroidism-jaw tumor syndrome [12]. Loss of parafibromin can be visualized using immunohistochemistry.

Cyclin D1 is encoded by the *CCND1* gene. This protein is overexpressed in many parathyroid carcinomas, a fraction of parathyroid adenomas, and even some parathyroid hyperplasia [61]. When mutated it acts as an oncogene by, among other things, inhibition of the retinoblastoma protein (RB) [35].

Interestingly, parathyroid adenomas and parathyroid carcinomas tend toward different genetic changes. Parathyroid adenomas are more commonly associated with *MEN1* alterations, while *CDC73* aberrancies are typically seen in parathyroid carcinomas and atypical parathyroid tumors [24, 38]. Moreover, epigenetic changes also vary between these entities. It has been observed that parathyroid adenomas and carcinomas show methylation patterns distinct from each other [55]. This all suggests there might generally be a different genetic background of formation, though their genetic relationship is not yet fully understood [24].

References

1. Agarwal SK, Guru SC, Heppner C, et al. Menin interacts with the AP1 transcription factor JunD and represses JunD-activated transcription. Cell. 1999;96(1):143–52. https://doi.org/10.1016/s0092-8674(00)80967-8.
2. Aggarwal A, Wadhwa R, Aggarwal V. Parathyroid lipoadenoma: a rare entity. Indian J Endocrinol Metab. 2018;22(1):174–6. https://doi.org/10.4103/ijem.IJEM_273_17.
3. Akerström G, Malmaeus J, Bergström R. Surgical anatomy of human parathyroid glands. Surgery. 1984;95(1):14–21.
4. Al-Kurd A, Mekel M, Mazeh H. Parathyroid carcinoma. Surg Oncol. 2014;23(2):107–14. https://doi.org/10.1016/j.suronc.2014.03.005.
5. Alharbi N, Asa SL, Szybowska M, Kim RH, Ezzat S. Intrathyroidal parathyroid carcinoma: an atypical thyroid lesion. Front Endocrinol (Lausanne). 2018;9:641. https://doi.org/10.3389/fendo.2018.00641.
6. Baloch ZW, LiVolsi VA. Pathology of the parathyroid glands in hyperparathyroidism. Semin Diagn Pathol. 2013;30(3):165–77. https://doi.org/10.1053/j.semdp.2013.06.003.
7. Bauer JL, Toluie S, Thompson LDR. Metastases to the parathyroid glands: a comprehensive literature review of 127 reported cases. Head Neck Pathol. 2018;12(4):534–41. https://doi.org/10.1007/s12105-017-0850-x.
8. Bilezikian JP, Marcus R, Levine MA. The parathyroids: basic and clinical concepts. 2nd ed. San Diego: Academic; 2001.
9. Black BK. Carcinoma of the parathyroid. Ann Surg. 1954;139(3):355–63. https://doi.org/10.1097/00000658-195403000-00014.
10. Bondeson L, Sandelin K, Grimelius L. Histopathological variables and DNA cytometry in parathyroid carcinoma. Am J Surg Pathol. 1993;17(8):820–9. https://doi.org/10.1097/00000478-199308000-00007.
11. Cao C, Dou C, Chen F, Wang Y, Zhang X, Lai H. An unusual mediastinal parathyroid carcinoma coproducing PTH and PTHrP: a case report. Oncol Lett. 2016;11(6):4113–6. https://doi.org/10.3892/ol.2016.4548.
12. Carpten JD, Robbins CM, Villablanca A, et al. HRPT2, encoding parafibromin, is mutated in hyperparathyroidism-jaw tumor syndrome. Nat Genet. 2002;32(4):676–80. https://doi.org/10.1038/ng1048.
13. Cetani F, Marcocci C, Torregrossa L, Pardi E. Atypical parathyroid adenomas: challenging lesions in the differential diagnosis of endocrine tumors. Endocr Relat Cancer. 2019;26(7):R441–r464. https://doi.org/10.1530/erc-19-0135.
14. Chen Q, Kaji H, Nomura R, et al. Trial to predict malignancy of affected parathyroid glands in primary hyperparathyroidism. Endocr J. 2003;50(5):527–34. https://doi.org/10.1507/endocrj.50.527.
15. Christie AC. The parathyroid oxyphil cells. J Clin Pathol. 1967;20(4):591–602. https://doi.org/10.1136/jcp.20.4.591.
16. Cinti S, Sbarbati A. Ultrastructure of human parathyroid cells in health and disease. Microsc Res Tech. 1995;32(2):164–79. https://doi.org/10.1002/jemt.1070320210.
17. Cristina EV, Alberto F. Management of familial hyperparathyroidism syndromes: MEN1, MEN2, MEN4, HPT-Jaw tumour, familial isolated hyperparathyroidism, FHH, and neonatal severe hyperparathyroidism. Best Pract Res Clin Endocrinol Metab. 2018;32(6):861–75. https://doi.org/10.1016/j.beem.2018.09.010.
18. Dekker A, Dunsford HA, Geyer SJ. The normal parathyroid gland at autopsy: the significance of stromal fat in adult patients. J Pathol. 1979;128(3):127–32. https://doi.org/10.1002/path.1711280303.
19. DeLellis RA. Parathyroid tumors and related disorders. Mod Pathol. 2011;24(Suppl 2):S78–93. https://doi.org/10.1038/modpathol.2010.132.
20. Duan K, Mete Ö. Parathyroid carcinoma: diagnosis and clinical implications. Turk Patoloji Derg. 2015;31(Suppl 1):80–97. https://doi.org/10.5146/tjpath.2015.01316.
21. Dufour DR, Wilkerson SY. The normal parathyroid revisited: percentage of stromal fat. Hum Pathol. 1982;13(8):717–21. https://doi.org/10.1016/s0046-8177(82)80293-1.
22. Emura S, Shoumura S, Isono H. Ultrastructure of the water-clear cell in the rabbit parathyroid gland. Arch Histol Cytol. 1992;55(2):159–66. https://doi.org/10.1679/aohc.55.159.
23. Erickson LA, Mete O. Immunohistochemistry in diagnostic parathyroid pathology. Endocr Pathol. 2018;29(2):113–29. https://doi.org/10.1007/s12022-018-9527-6.
24. Erickson LA, Mete O, Juhlin CC, Perren A, Gill AJ. Overview of the 2022 WHO classification of parathyroid tumors. Endocr Pathol. 2022;33(1):64–89. https://doi.org/10.1007/s12022-022-09709-1.
25. Fancy T, Gallagher D 3rd, Hornig JD. Surgical anatomy of the thyroid and parathyroid glands. Otolaryngol Clin North Am. 2010;43(2):221–7, vii. https://doi.org/10.1016/j.otc.2010.01.001.
26. Fernandez-Ranvier GG, Khanafshar E, Jensen K, et al. Parathyroid carcinoma, atypical parathyroid adenoma, or parathyromatosis? Cancer. 2007;110(2):255–64. https://doi.org/10.1002/cncr.22790.

27. Fitko R, Roth SI, Hines JR, Roxe DM, Cahill E. Parathyromatosis in hyperparathyroidism. Hum Pathol. 1990;21(2):234–7. https://doi.org/10.1016/0046-8177(90)90136-s.
28. Frank-Raue K, Leidig-Bruckner G, Lorenz A, et al. Hereditary variants of primary hyperparathyroidism–MEN1, MEN2, HPT-JT, FHH, FIHPT. Dtsch Med Wochenschr. 2011;136(38):1889–94. https://doi.org/10.1055/s-0031-1286358.
29. Ghandur-Mnaymneh L, Kimura N. The parathyroid adenoma. A histopathologic definition with a study of 172 cases of primary hyperparathyroidism. Am J Pathol. 1984;115(1):70–83.
30. Gill AJ, Lim G, Cheung VKY, et al. Parafibromin-deficient (HPT-JT type, CDC73 mutated) parathyroid tumors demonstrate distinctive morphologic features. Am J Surg Pathol. 2019;43(1):35–46. https://doi.org/10.1097/pas.0000000000001017.
31. Guilmette J, Sadow PM. Parathyroid pathology. Surg Pathol Clin. 2019;12(4):1007–19. https://doi.org/10.1016/j.path.2019.08.006.
32. Heppner C, Kester MB, Agarwal SK, et al. Somatic mutation of the MEN1 gene in parathyroid tumours. Nat Genet. 1997;16(4):375–8. https://doi.org/10.1038/ng0897-375.
33. Juhlin C, Larsson C, Yakoleva T, et al. Loss of parafibromin expression in a subset of parathyroid adenomas. Endocr Relat Cancer. 2006;13(2):509–23. https://doi.org/10.1677/erc.1.01058.
34. Juhlin CC, Falhammar H, Zedenius J, Nilsson IL, Höög A. Lipoadenoma of the parathyroid gland: characterization of an institutional series spanning 28 years. Endocr Pathol. 2020;31(2):156–65. https://doi.org/10.1007/s12022-020-09616-3.
35. Kato J, Matsushime H, Hiebert SW, Ewen ME, Sherr CJ. Direct binding of cyclin D to the retinoblastoma gene product (pRb) and pRb phosphorylation by the cyclin D-dependent kinase CDK4. Genes Dev. 1993;7(3):331–42. https://doi.org/10.1101/gad.7.3.331.
36. Krawitz R, Glover A, Koneru S, et al. The significance of histologically "large normal" parathyroid glands in primary hyperparathyroidism. World J Surg. 2020;44(4):1149–55. https://doi.org/10.1007/s00268-019-05302-6.
37. Lee M, Pellegata NS. Multiple endocrine neoplasia type 4. Front Horm Res. 2013;41:63–78. https://doi.org/10.1159/000345670.
38. Mao X, Wu Y, Yu S, Chen J. Genetic alteration profiles and clinicopathological associations in atypical parathyroid adenoma. Int J Genomics. 2021;2021:6666257. https://doi.org/10.1155/2021/6666257.
39. McDonald-McGinn DM, Sullivan KE. Chromosome 22q11.2 deletion syndrome (DiGeorge syndrome/velocardiofacial syndrome). Medicine (Baltimore). 2011;90(1):1–18. https://doi.org/10.1097/MD.0b013e3182060469.
40. Miki H, Sumitomo M, Inoue H, Kita S, Monden Y. Parathyroid carcinoma in patients with chronic renal failure on maintenance hemodialysis. Surgery. 1996;120(5):897–901. https://doi.org/10.1016/s0039-6060(96)80101-2.
41. Milas M, Wagner K, Easley KA, Siperstein A, Weber CJ. Double adenomas revisited: nonuniform distribution favors enlarged superior parathyroids (fourth pouch disease). Surgery. 2003;134(6):995–1003; discussion 1003-4. https://doi.org/10.1016/j.surg.2003.07.009.
42. Morand GB, Rupp NJ, Huellner MW, et al. Transnasal-transpterygoid endoscopic removal of an 18F-choline-avid parathyroid carcinoma metastasis in the skull base. JAMA Otolaryngol Head Neck Surg. 2019;145(10):978–80. https://doi.org/10.1001/jamaoto.2019.2352.
43. Obara T, Fujimoto Y, Aiba M. Stromal fat content of the parathyroid gland. Endocrinol Jpn. 1990;37(6):901–5. https://doi.org/10.1507/endocrj1954.37.901.
44. Okamoto T, Iihara M, Obara T, Tsukada T. Parathyroid carcinoma: etiology, diagnosis, and treatment. World J Surg. 2009;33(11):2343–54. https://doi.org/10.1007/s00268-009-9999-0.
45. Palmer JA, Brown WA, Kerr WH, Rosen IB, Watters NA. The surgical aspects of hyperparathyroidism. Arch Surg. 1975;110(8):1004–7. https://doi.org/10.1001/archsurg.1975.01360140148028.
46. Papavramidis TS, Chorti A, Pliakos I, Panidis S, Michalopoulos A. Parathyroid cysts: a review of 359 patients reported in the international literature. Medicine (Baltimore). 2018;97(28):e11399. https://doi.org/10.1097/md.0000000000011399.
47. Ritter CS, Haughey BH, Miller B, Brown AJ. Differential gene expression by oxyphil and chief cells of human parathyroid glands. J Clin Endocrinol Metab. 2012;97(8):E1499–505. https://doi.org/10.1210/jc.2011-3366.
48. Arrangoiz R, Cordera F, Caba D, Juárez MM, Moreno E, Luque E. Parathyroid embryology, anatomy, and pathophysiology of primary hyperparathyroidism. Int J Otolaryngol Head Neck Surg. 2017;6:39–58.
49. Sanjuan X, Bryant BR, Sobel ME, Merino MI. Clonality analysis of benign parathyroid lesions by human androgen receptor (HUMARA) gene assay. Endocr Pathol. 1998;9(1):293–300. https://doi.org/10.1007/bf02739689.
50. Schantz A, Castleman B. Parathyroid carcinoma. A study of 70 cases. Cancer. 1973;31(3):600–5. https://doi.org/10.1002/1097-0142(197303)31:3<600::aid-cncr2820310316>3.0.co;2-0.
51. Seabrook AJ, Harris JE, Velosa SB, et al. Multiple endocrine tumors associated with germline MAX

mutations: multiple endocrine neoplasia type 5? J Clin Endocrinol Metab. 2021;106(4):1163–82. https://doi.org/10.1210/clinem/dgaa957.
52. Shi Y, Hogue J, Dixit D, Koh J, Olson JA Jr. Functional and genetic studies of isolated cells from parathyroid tumors reveal the complex pathogenesis of parathyroid neoplasia. Proc Natl Acad Sci USA. 2014;111(8):3092–7. https://doi.org/10.1073/pnas.1319742111.
53. Simonds WF, James-Newton LA, Agarwal SK, et al. Familial isolated hyperparathyroidism: clinical and genetic characteristics of 36 kindreds. Medicine (Baltimore). 2002;81(1):1–26. https://doi.org/10.1097/00005792-200201000-00001.
54. Snover DC, Foucar K. Mitotic activity in benign parathyroid disease. Am J Clin Pathol. 1981;75(3):345–7. https://doi.org/10.1093/ajcp/75.3.345.
55. Starker LF, Svedlund J, Udelsman R, et al. The DNA methylome of benign and malignant parathyroid tumors. Genes Chromosomes Cancer. 2011;50(9):735–45. https://doi.org/10.1002/gcc.20895.
56. Tanaka Y, Funahashi H, Imai T, Seo H, Tominaga Y, Takagi H. Oxyphil cell function in secondary parathyroid hyperplasia. Nephron. 1996;73(4):580–6. https://doi.org/10.1159/000189144.
57. Thakker RV. Genetics of parathyroid tumours. J Intern Med. 2016;280(6):574–83. https://doi.org/10.1111/joim.12523.
58. Tominaga Y, Kohara S, Namii Y, et al. Clonal analysis of nodular parathyroid hyperplasia in renal hyperparathyroidism. World J Surg. 1996;20(7):744–50; discussion 750-2. https://doi.org/10.1007/s002689900113.
59. Truran PP, Johnson SJ, Bliss RD, Lennard TW, Aspinall SR. Parafibromin, galectin-3, PGP9.5, Ki67, and cyclin D1: using an immunohistochemical panel to aid in the diagnosis of parathyroid cancer. World J Surg. 2014;38(11):2845–54. https://doi.org/10.1007/s00268-014-2700-2.
60. Uljanovs R, Sinkarevs S, Strumfs B, Vidusa L, Merkurjeva K, Strumfa I. Immunohistochemical profile of parathyroid tumours: a comprehensive review. Int J Mol Sci. 2022;23(13) https://doi.org/10.3390/ijms23136981.
61. Vasef MA, Brynes RK, Sturm M, Bromley C, Robinson RA. Expression of cyclin D1 in parathyroid carcinomas, adenomas, and hyperplasias: a paraffin immunohistochemical study. Mod Pathol. 1999;12(4):412–6.
62. Walt J. Pathology of the parathyroid glands. Diagn Histopathol. 2012;18(6):221–33.
63. Xin Y, Zhao T, Wei B, et al. Intrapericardial parathyroid carcinoma: a case report. Endocrine. 2020;69(2):456–60. https://doi.org/10.1007/s12020-020-02283-8.

Biochemical Diagnosis of Hyperparathyroidism

3

Federica D'Aurizio, Marta Codrich, Marila De Luca, and Luca Giovanella

Abbreviations

AMR	Analytical measurement range
BMI	Body mass index
CaSR	Calcium-sensing receptor
CKD	Chronic kidney disease
CLIA	Chemiluminescent immunoassay
CMIA	Chemiluminescent microparticle immunoassay
CT	Calcitonin
ECLIA	Electrochemiluminescence assay
$H_2PO_4^-$	Dihydrogen phosphate
HPO_4^{2-}	Monohydrogen phosphate
IMAs	Immunoassays
FGF23	Fibroblast Growth Factor 23
FHH	Family hypocalciuric hypercalcemia
GFR	Glomerular filtrate rate
IFCC	International Federation of Clinical Chemistry and Laboratory Medicine
ISEs	Calcium specific ion-selective electrodes (ISEs)
LC-MS/MS	Liquid chromatography coupled to tandem mass spectrometry
LOD	Limit of detection
LOQ	Limit of quantification
ND	Not disclosed
P	Plasma
PEG	Polyethylene glycol
PHPT	Primary hyperparathyroidism
PTH	Parathyroid hormone
RI	Reference interval
RIA	Radioimmunoassay
S	Serum
SHPT	Secondary hyperparathyroidism
THPT	Tertiary hyperparathyroidism
VDBP	Vitamin D-binding protein
VDRs	Vitamin D receptors
$1,25(OH)_2D$	1,25-dihydroxyvitamin D
25(OH)D	25-hydroxyvitamin D

F. D'Aurizio (✉)
Institute of Clinical Pathology, Department of Laboratory Medicine, Academic Hospital "Santa Maria della Misericordia", Azienda Sanitaria Universitaria Friuli Centrale, Udine, Italy
e-mail: federica.daurizio@asufc.sanita.fvg.it

M. Codrich · M. De Luca
Department of Medicine (DMED), University of Udine, Udine, Italy
e-mail: marta.codrich@uniud.it; marila.deluca@asufc.sanita.fvg.it

L. Giovanella
Department of Nuclear Medicine and Thyroid Centre, Gruppo Ospedaliero Moncucco, Lugano, Switzerland

Department of Nuclear Medicine and Thyroid Centre, University Hospital of Zurich, Zurich, Switzerland
e-mail: luca.giovanella@moncucco.ch

© The Author(s), under exclusive license to Springer Nature Switzerland AG 2026

P. Petranović Ovčariček et al. (eds.), *Parathyroid Imaging*,
https://doi.org/10.1007/978-3-032-14178-1_3

Definitions

1. Primary Hyperparathyroidism (PHPT): PHPT is an endocrine disorder characterized by autonomous overproduction of parathyroid hormone (PTH) from one or more parathyroid glands, typically due to an adenoma, hyperplasia, or rarely carcinoma. This results in hypercalcemia and may lead to bone reabsorption, nephrolithiasis, and neuromuscular symptoms. Diagnosis is based on elevated serum calcium in conjunction with elevated or inappropriately normal PTH levels.
2. Serum Calcium: Serum calcium refers to the total concentration of calcium in the blood, which includes calcium bound to proteins (mainly albumin), calcium complexed with anions, and free (ionized) calcium. It is a routine biochemical marker assessed in evaluating parathyroid and bone metabolism.
3. Corrected Calcium: Corrected calcium accounts for variations in serum albumin levels that affect total calcium measurement. It provides a more accurate estimate of physiologically active calcium, especially important in assessing calcium status in patients with hypoalbuminemia.
4. Ionized Calcium: Ionized calcium represents the biologically active fraction of calcium in the serum, unbound to proteins. It is critical for cellular processes such as muscle contraction, nerve transmission, and blood coagulation. Ionized calcium is less affected by serum protein levels and provides a more accurate reflection of calcium status, especially in critically ill patients or when albumin is abnormal.
5. Parathormone (Parathyroid Hormone, PTH): PTH is an 84-amino acid peptide hormone secreted by the parathyroid glands. It plays a central role in calcium and phosphate homeostasis by stimulating bone resorption, increasing renal tubular calcium reabsorption, and promoting activation of vitamin D to enhance intestinal calcium absorption. PTH levels are measured to evaluate disorders of calcium metabolism, such as PHPT and secondary hyperparathyroidism.
6. Vitamin D: Vitamin D refers to a group of fat-soluble secosteroids essential for calcium and phosphate metabolism. The two main forms are vitamin D_2 (ergocalciferol) and vitamin D_3 (cholecalciferol). After hepatic and renal hydroxylation, the active form 1,25-dihydroxyvitamin D (calcitriol) enhances intestinal calcium absorption and modulates PTH secretion. Serum 25-hydroxyvitamin D [25(OH)D] is the preferred marker for assessing vitamin D status.
7. Immunoassay: An immunoassay is a biochemical test that uses the specific binding between an antigen and an antibody to detect and quantify substances, such as hormones, proteins, or drugs. Immunoassays are widely used in clinical laboratories for measuring PTH, vitamin D, and other analytes relevant to calcium and bone metabolism.

Learning Objectives

1. Explain the biochemical criteria for diagnosing primary hyperparathyroidism, including the interpretation of serum calcium and PTH levels.
2. Differentiate between primary, secondary, and tertiary hyperparathyroidism based on laboratory profiles of calcium, phosphate, PTH, and vitamin D.
3. Describe the role of serial testing and confirmatory laboratory evaluations in cases of hyperparathyroidism and borderline results.

3.1 Introduction

The parathyroid glands, typically four small endocrine glands located on the posterior surface of the thyroid gland, play a vital role in calcium and phosphate homeostasis. These glands secrete parathyroid hormone (PTH), which is the principal regulator of extracellular calcium levels. The maintenance of serum calcium within a narrow physiological range is critical for numerous cellular processes, including neuromuscular excitability, blood coagulation, and bone mineralization [1].

Dysfunction of the parathyroid glands, leading to hyperparathyroidism, results in significant clinical morbidity due to its multisystem effects. Hyperparathyroidism is a pathological condition characterized by excessive secretion of PTH, resulting in disturbances of calcium, phosphate, and bone metabolism. Understanding the physiology of the parathyroid glands is crucial to unravel the complex mechanisms behind the different forms of hyperparathyroidism, namely, primary, secondary, and tertiary, and is key to managing hyperparathyroid conditions [2].

Laboratory medicine plays a pivotal role in detecting and confirming hyperparathyroidism, discriminating different forms and characterizing target organ damage. This chapter aims to briefly summarize the normal physiology of the parathyroid gland and the pathophysiological alterations underlying hyperparathyroidism. Moreover, laboratory methods employed in the evaluation of parathyroid disease are illustrated, their limitations discussed, and a rational use of different methods is presented.

3.2 Physiology and Pathophysiology of the Parathyroid Glands

The parathyroid glands originate from the third and fourth pharyngeal pouches during embryogenesis. The inferior glands arise from the third pouch and descend further than the superior glands, which originate from the fourth pouch. This embryological origin accounts for the variable anatomical positions of the parathyroid glands ([3]).

Each parathyroid gland is composed predominantly of chief cells, which secrete PTH and a smaller population of oxyphil cells whose function is less well understood but may relate to mitochondrial metabolism and aging. PTH is synthesized as a preprohormone (preproPTH, 115 amino acids), processed in the endoplasmic reticulum to proPTH (90 amino acids) and then cleaved in the Golgi apparatus to the active 84-amino-acid hormone (PTH 1–84). PTH is stored in secretory granules and released in response to low extracellular ionized (free) calcium levels. PTH secretion is primarily regulated by the calcium-sensing receptor (CaSR), a G protein-coupled receptor located on the surface of chief cells. PTH acts to increase serum calcium levels and decrease serum phosphate through its effects on the bone, kidneys, and indirectly intestines [4].

Particularly, PTH stimulates osteoblasts to produce RANKL, which activates osteoclasts and promotes bone resorption; enhances renal calcium reabsorption while reducing phosphate reabsorption and stimulates 1α-hydroxylase in kidneys; and, finally, indirectly increases calcium and phosphate absorption via calcitriol in the intestine. PTH secretion is subject to complex feedback regulation by serum calcium via CaSR, calcitriol via vitamin D receptors (VDRs), and FGF23 which inhibits 1α-hydroxylase [5].

3.3 Hyperparathyroidism

Primary hyperparathyroidism (PHPT) is caused by autonomous overproduction of PTH, usually due to an adenoma and, less frequently, by multiple adenomas and parathyroid hyperplasia. It results in hypercalcemia and, frequently, hypophosphatemia [6].

Clinical features include nephrolithiasis, osteoporosis, and cardiac, neuromuscular, and neuropsychiatric symptoms. Depending on the clinical condition and laboratory parameters, PHPT can be managed by active surveillance or treated by surgery or calcimimetic drugs (i.e., cinacalcet) [7].

Secondary hyperparathyroidism (SHPT) is a response to chronic hypocalcemia, often from chronic kidney disease (CKD) or vitamin D deficiency. It leads to gland hyperplasia and elevated PTH levels despite low-normal calcium. SHPT is managed by phosphate binders, vitamin D analogs.

Tertiary hyperparathyroidism (THPT) occurs after long-standing SHPT, typically in post-

Table 3.1 Biochemical profiles of hyperparathyroidism

	PHPT				
Blood parameter	Classical	Inappropriate PTH secretion	Normocalcemic	SHPT	THPT
PTH	↑	↔	↑	↑	↑
Calcium	↑	↑	↔	↓ or ↔	↑

HPT hyperparathyroidism, *PHPT* primary hyperparathyroidism, *SHPT* secondary hyperparathyroidism, *THPT* tertiary hyperparathyroidism

transplant patients, leading to autonomous PTH secretion and hypercalcemia. THPT often requires parathyroidectomy [8].

3.4 Biochemical Markers in the Diagnosis of Hyperparathyroidism

Diagnosis of PHPT is suspected in patients with hypercalcemia with not adequately suppressed related PTH blood concentrations (inappropriately high or within the reference interval) [9].

PHPT must be distinguished from other causes which elevate PTH, such as SHPT or THPT (Table 3.1). Beyond the determination of blood concentration of calcium and PTH, biochemical tests useful for the diagnosis and the management of PHPT are as follows: 24-h urinary calcium (calciuria), phosphate, 25-hydroxyvitamin D [25(OH)D], and 1,25-dihydroxyvitamin D [1,25$(OH)_2$D].

3.5 Calcium

Calcium is the most common mineral in the human body amounting to approximately 1000–2000 g in adulthood. More than 99% of the total body calcium is present in the mineral form and stored in bone tissue as hydroxyapatite. Calcium in this form provides structural integrity as well as a reservoir exchangeable with the organism. The remaining 1% is called non-bone calcium, and it is allocated among the cellular organelles and the extracellular fluid through a turnover mechanism in a balance between production and degradation of bone matrix. This fraction plays an important role in muscle contraction, nerve transmission, hormone secretion, blood clotting, and enzyme reactions [10].

Calcium homeostasis is mainly maintained by the parathyroid glands and kidneys through the involvement of three hormones: 1,25$(OH)_2$D or calcitriol, PTH, and calcitonin (CT). PTH, synthetized and secreted by the parathyroid glands through the calcium-sensing receptor (CaSR), along with vitamin D, produced by a multi-step process involving the skin, liver, and kidneys, contributes to the increase in serum calcium, whereas CT, released by the parafollicular C cells in the thyroid, leads to serum calcium decreasing. In detail, PTH stimulates bone and renal reabsorption of calcium and secretion of vitamin D by the kidney. Vitamin D, for its part, stimulates gut calcium absorption. Conversely, CT promotes bone calcium deposition, inhibits kidney calcium reabsorption, increases urinary excretion of calcium, and prevents calcium absorption in the intestines. The normal plasma calcium concentration is typically between 8.8 and 10.4 mg/dL (2.2 and 2.6 mmol/L) in adults. Levels of calcium are tightly regulated since an elevation of calcium (hypercalcemia) is associated with osteoporosis, kidney stones, and kidney failure, whereas a reduction (hypocalcemia) can lead to life-threatening arrhythmias or seizures [11].

Calcium concentration represents the sum of the three circulating forms: ionized (free), complexed, and bound to protein (Fig. 3.1). A significant proportion of serum calcium (approximately 50%) is represented by the ionized (free) calcium and consists of the physiologically active form. Complexed calcium, which makes up 10% of the serum calcium, is chelated with anions to form ionic complexes (e.g., calcium oxalate, calcium phosphate, and calcium carbonate). This form, along with ionized calcium, is absorbed by tissues. Protein-bound calcium accounts for about

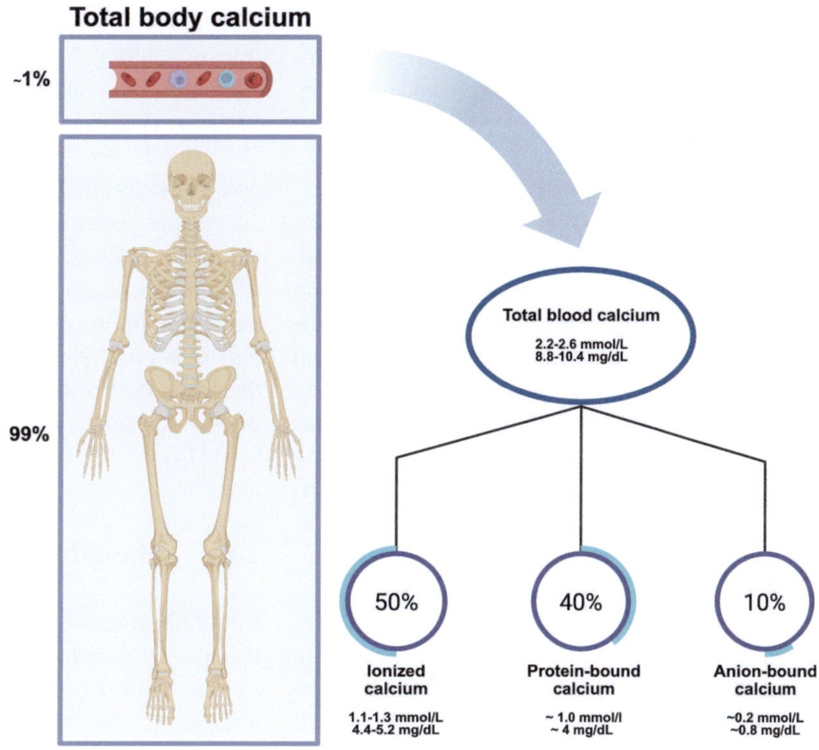

Fig. 3.1 Distribution of calcium. About 99% of the body's total calcium is stored in the bone, while the remaining 1% is allocated among the cellular organelles and the extracellular fluid. In the plasma, calcium exists in three forms: ionized, bound to proteins, and complexed to anions. (Created in BioRender. Codrich, M. (2025) https://BioRender.com/5g2sqzg)

40% of total calcium and is held physically to albumin (about 80%) and globulins (the remaining 20%). Protein-bound calcium is not metabolically active and cannot be used by tissues. In the blood, ionized and protein-bound calcium exist in a dynamic equilibrium. Many factors are capable of altering this balance such as blood pH and serum protein concentration. Indeed, acidosis enhances ionized calcium and decreases protein-bound calcium; vice versa, the opposite situation occurs in the case of alkalosis. In detail, there is an inverse shift of 0.2 mg/dL (0.05 mmol/L) in ionized calcium for each 0.1 unit change in pH. On the other hand, changes in albumin concentration affect the total calcium measurement provoking pseudohypocalcemia. There are different formulas to correct serum calcium in the case of low albumin. The corrected total calcium can be calculated if the albumin level is known as follows: total calcium = measured calcium mg/dL + 0.80 (4 − albumin g/dL). Other factors that alter calcium balance are drugs, free fatty acids, heparin, bilirubin, temperature, and presence of abnormal proteins, which can demonstrate a greater or lesser binding affinity. Total serum calcium (serum or plasma) is measured with colorimetric assays through spectrophotometric determination, which offers accurate and reproducible performance [10].

Calcium reference intervals can be slightly different between laboratories due to variations in measurement methods. Calcium specific ion-selective electrodes (ISEs) are used to directly determine the concentration of ionized calcium in a whole blood sample. The electrodes can detect slight variations in calcium ion concentration. When the protein concentration is highly altered (e.g., decreased plasma proteins as in the case of CKD or increased plasma globulins as with multiple myeloma) or in the case of disturbed acid-base equilibrium, it is recommended to rely on the direct measurement of ionized calcium, which demonstrates a higher sensitivity and specificity [12].

Venous blood samples are commonly used to measure total serum calcium levels. The use of tubes with anticoagulants such as K_2-EDTA/K_3-EDTA, potassium oxalate, or sodium citrate should be avoided because of their interference by complexing with calcium. Hemolyzed samples are unacceptable for testing because they produce unreliable laboratory results. Icteric and lipemic samples also interfere with the accurate measurement of calcium.

For the determination of ionized calcium, blood samples should be handled with great care by measuring within 30 min after collection and ensuring transport, refrigeration, and anaerobiosis to minimize pH changes, CO_2 loss, and changes in cellular metabolism [10].

Calciuria reflects blood calcium concentration, and its normal values range from 100 mg (2.5 mmol) to 300 mg (7.5 mmol) per day (24 h) [13]. The amount of calcium excretion is influenced by the diet and the intestinal ability of calcium absorption [14].

Determination of calcium in urine involves collection over 24 h, providing advantages in terms of result interpretation. However, literature data indicate that 24-h urine collection is a significant source of pre-analytical error mainly due to patient failure to adhere to the instructions [15].

When a 24-h sample is not available, the interpretation of urine calcium concentration should be done in relation to glomerular filtrate rate (GFR) and should be less than 0.16 mg/100 mL (0.04 mmol/L). Calciuria is calculated by the following equation: urinary calcium (mg/100 mL of GFR) = (urinary calcium mg/dL × serum creatinine mg/dL)/urinary creatinine mg/dL. Importantly, the urine container may be added with acids (HCl 6 mmol/L is commonly used) to prevent calcium salt precipitation or at least acidify the specimen after the collection without acid [10].

Hypercalciuria, more correctly defined as urinary excretion of calcium >4 mg/kg/24 h or alternatively as >250 mg/24 h in adult females and >300 mg/24 h in adult males is often found in PHPT [13].

Hypercalciuria, secondary to PTH stimulation, is caused by an increased filtered calcium load that exceeds the retention capacity of kidney. Among the PTH-dependent hypercalcemia that comes into differential diagnosis with PHPT, family hypocalciuric hypercalcemia (FHH) is genetically determined (dependent on an alteration of CaSR). The urinary calcium/creatinine clearance ratio less than 0.01 is suggestive of FHH, while a ratio value higher than 0.02 generally excludes this genetic condition; in cases with a ratio between 0.01 and 0.02, the mutational analysis of genes associated with FHH helps for a definitive diagnosis. Notably, in the evaluation of calciuria, it is important to carry out analysis under conditions of normal serum levels of vitamin D, regular dietary intake of calcium, and in the absence of confounding factors (e.g., thiazide diuretics, lithium, anti-resorptive bone therapies, etc.) [14].

3.6 Phosphate

Blood phosphate concentration is typically at the lower reference limit in PHPT patients, caused by the action of PTH which reduces phosphate absorption by the renal tubules. Phosphate metabolism is closely related to calcium since it is regulated by PTH, vitamin D (as for calcium), and Fibroblast Growth Factor 23 (FGF-23) in a process that involves kidneys, intestine, and skeleton [14].

In detail, PTH stimulates bone reabsorption and renal tubular secretion of phosphate. $1,25(OH)_2D$ induces phosphate intestinal absorption, and FGF-23 decreases phosphate renal tubular reabsorption [16].

An adult organism contains about 600 g (20 mmol) of phosphorus, expressed as phosphate, with about 85% present in bones (mainly complexed with calcium in the form of hydroxyapatite) and the remaining in other tissues [17].

In the human body, phosphate is responsible for several functions such as mineralization, muscle contractility, electrolyte transport, urinary buffer, and cellular functions (e.g., lipids/proteins/carbohydrates metabolism, gene transcription, and cell growth). The concentration of blood phosphate is closely regulated since alteration can be life-threatening. In detail, hyperphosphatemia results in vascular calcification and arteriopathy, while hypophosphatemia can lead to muscle weakness and respiratory or heart failure [18].

As calcium, blood phosphate levels depend upon circadian rhythm [19].

Moreover, phosphate concentration changes in relation to dietary intake and acid-base status and varies with age (higher in children than adults). The normal serum phosphate level ranges between 2.5 and 4.5 mg/dL (0.81–1.45 mmol/L) in adults. In blood, approximately 55% of phosphate exists as free (inorganic) phosphate, 10% is bound to proteins, and about 35% is complexed with cations such as sodium, calcium, and magnesium. Although both organic and inorganic phosphate compounds are present in plasma, only the inorganic phosphate compounds are measured: the dihydrogen phosphate ($H_2PO_4^-$) and its salt, monohydrogen phosphate (HPO_4^{2-}). The ratio between these two forms depends on the acid-base status of the blood. Phosphate is measured with colorimetric assays through spectrophotometric determination. Specimens of serum or heparinized plasma are commonly used to measure phosphate concentration. The use of other anticoagulants such as K_2-EDTA/K_3-EDTA, potassium oxalate, or sodium citrate is not recommended due to their interference by complexing with phosphate. Hemolyzed, icteric, and lipemic samples are unacceptable for testing phosphate laboratory results. Furthermore, it has been demonstrated that the presence of fluoride and monoclonal immunoglobulins may interfere with the measurement [17].

3.7 Parathormone

PTH is synthesized and released by parathyroid glands as a precursor of 115 amino acids, which undergoes two successive cleavages, leading to the formation of the biologically active peptide 1–84 [20].

PTH circulates not only as a whole peptide but also as multiple fragments, consisting mainly of the C-terminal part (Fig. 3.2) and deriving from both hepatic metabolism and direct secretion of parathyroid glands [21].

In addition, PTH undergoes post-translational modifications such as phosphorylation and oxidation, which render the molecule biologically inactive (Fig. 3.2). The plasma half-life of 1–84 PTH is very short (2–4 min) compared to the half-life of the fragments which is five to ten times longer under physiological conditions, further increasing in CKD [20].

As previously described, PTH is a hypercalcemic hormone that acts on target organs (kidney and bone) via the PTHR1 receptor. In contrast, hypercalcemia is the main inhibitor of PTH secretion: when levels of ionized calcium are high, CaSR inhibits the synthesis and secretion of PTH in the parathyroid gland in a negative feedback mechanism [22].

PTH measurement is particularly important in different clinical settings (i.e., classification of both hypocalcemia and hypercalcemia, assessment of SHPT and THPT, sequential PTH determination in parathyroid surgery) [20].

From a laboratory point of view, it is important to consider all the steps leading to the generation of the analytical data (pre-analytical, analytical, and post-analytical phases). Few studies have been published on the pre-analytical aspects of PTH determination (matrix type, sample stability, sample preservation, biological variability, etc.). In detail, both plasma and serum matrices can be used for PTH assay, although the stability of the hormone is higher in K_2-EDTA/K_3-EDTA plasma [23].

For example, a comparative study on 1–84 PTH molecule showed that Liaison® 1–84 PTH assay (DiaSorin, Saluggia, VC, Italy) reliably measured the biologically active hormone in plasma or serum, stored at room temperature for a maximum of 72 and 24 h, respectively. However, PTH concentration values determined in serum and plasma of the same subject were different, so the two matrices were not interchangeable [24].

PTH concentration is also influenced by the site of sampling: PTH concentrations are 30% higher in central blood than in peripheral blood. This is particularly relevant in hemodialysis patients, in whom blood samples are often drawn from a central line. Thus, to ensure reliable intra-

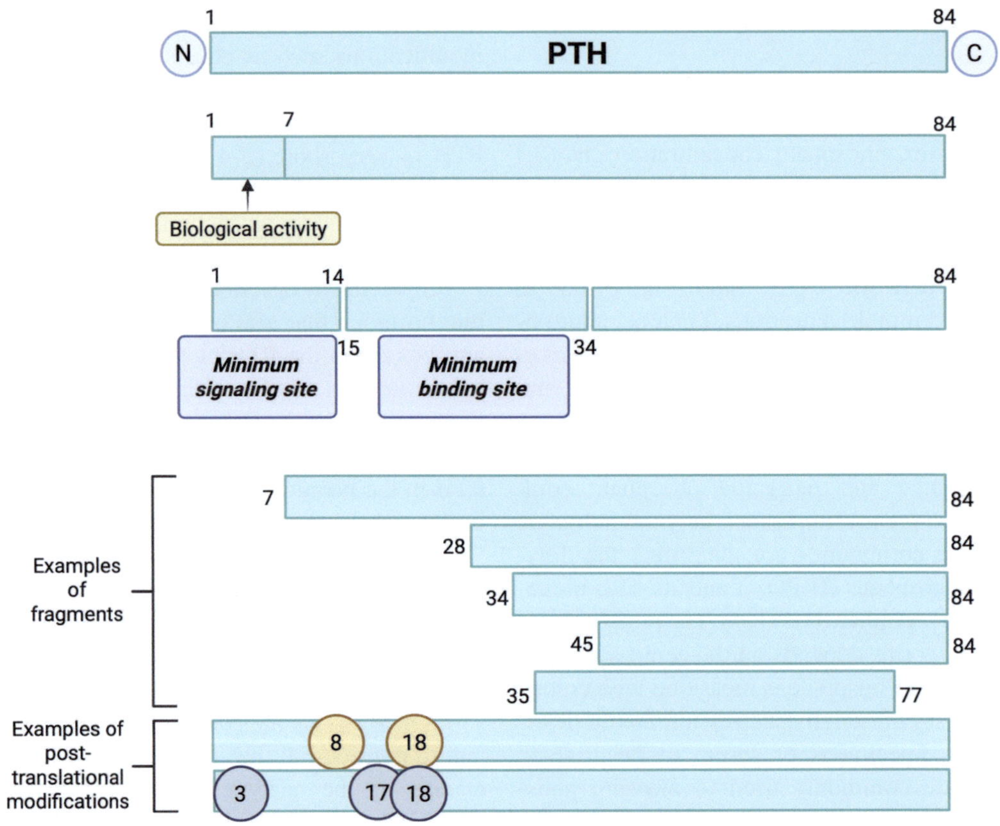

Fig. 3.2 PTH and its different forms. The whole form of PTH is composed of 84 amino acids. The first seven amino acids, at the N-terminal, have biological activity. Fragments 1–14 and 15–34 represent the minimum signalling portion and the minimum binding portion of the hormone, respectively. PTH circulates also as multiple fragments. In addition the whole molecule undergoes post-translational modifications (e.g., oxidation of amino acids 8 and 18 and phosphorylation of amino acids 3, 17, and 18). PTH, parathyroid hormone. (Created in BioRender. De Luca, M. (2025) https://BioRender.com/h46w876)

and inter-individual comparisons, it is advisable to consistently collect blood samples for PTH measurement from the same site [20].

Although not yet listed as a recommendation, apart from dialysis patients in whom PTH is measured before dialysis session, experts suggest that blood samples for PTH measurement should be collected early in the morning on fasting, using a reference interval obtained under the same sampling conditions for interpretation of the result. In fact, it is known that the blood concentrations of calcium, phosphate, and PTH present circadian variations and are influenced by food intake (especially foods reach in calcium) [23].

In addition to pre-analytical aspects, post-analytical issues, in particular the determination of reference intervals, are challenging because many factors influence PTH concentrations [25].

The most important factors to consider include vitamin D status, whose deficiency causes an increase in circulating PTH (see next paragraph), ethnicity (PTH concentration is higher in African than Caucasian subjects) [26], sex (PTH values are higher in males) [25], age (PTH values increase with age) [13, 27, 28], and body mass index (BMI) (higher PTH values are found in obese patients) [29].

The selection of subjects for the determination of the reference intervals should therefore meet well-defined inclusion and exclusion criteria. At present, most manufacturers do not take the above parameters into account when recruiting control group subjects, thus obtaining reference intervals that are not always adequately applicable to the population under consideration [28].

In addition, an important aspect to consider is that third-generation assays, due to their higher specificity, give on average lower results than those obtained with second-generation methods, by about 50–60% and 15% in subjects with and without CDK, respectively [24, 30].

As a result, the second and third generations have different reference intervals. In this respect, a recent work published by Gannagé-Yared et al. determined the reference intervals of PTH for the second- and third-generation assay, considering a selected sample from 339 healthy adult (18–63 years) subjects (230 males and 109 females), with normal blood calcium levels and an GFR higher than 60 mL/min. The reference intervals obtained were obviously different between the two assay generations, with PTH values 1–84 lower than those obtained by the second generation [31].

Concerning the analytical phase, immunoassays (IMAs) based on antigen-antibody reactions are used for PTH determination (Fig. 3.3).

The first method dates back to the 1960s (first generation): Berson et al. developed a competitive radioimmunoassay (RIA) using a polyclonal antibody, able to interact with the central and C-terminal region of the PTH molecule. Unfortunately, this type of assay measured many biologically inactive C-terminal fragments. Thus, first-generation competitive assays were dropped in favor of second-generation non-competitive methods which were more specific for the bioactive form (Table 3.2).

Initially, it was thought that the second generation of IMAs using an antibody for the C-terminal end and an antibody for the N-terminal end would be able to identify exclusively the whole molecule (intact PTH, iPTH). However, very soon, cross-reactivity was demonstrated even with non-1–84 fragments and with modified forms at the post-translational

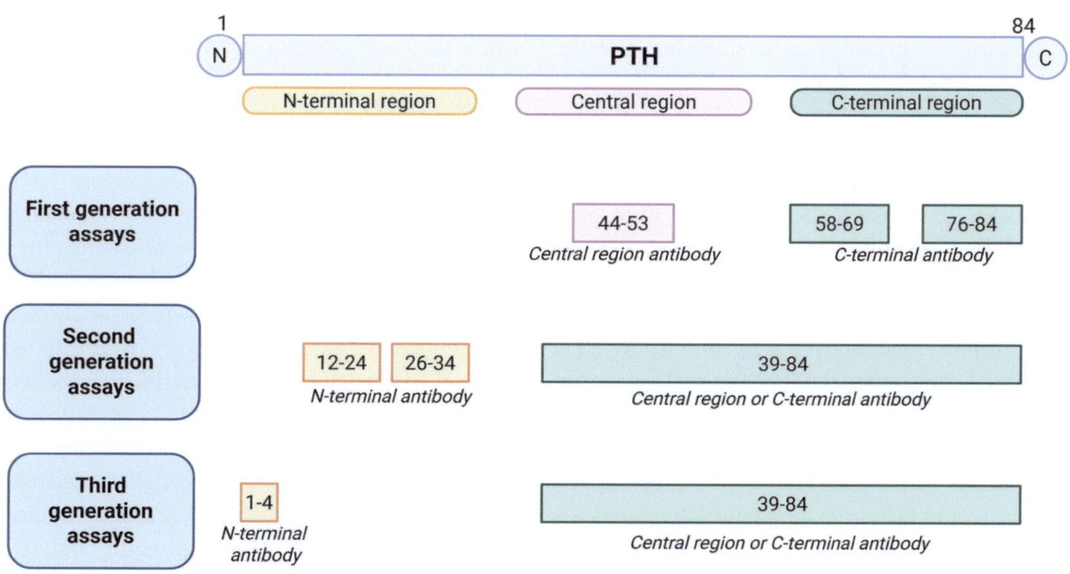

Fig. 3.3 Technical evolution of PTH assays. First-generation assays used a single polyclonal antibody against the central or the C-terminal region of the molecule in a competitive single site radioimmunoassay. Second-generation assays are based on the use of two monoclonal antibodies, one binding the C-terminal (AA 39–84) and the other ("signal") binding the N-terminal (AA 12–24, AA 26–34) in a non-competitive immunoassay. Third-generation assays involved the use of a C-terminal antibody and another antibody directed against first four amino acids (AA 1–4) of PTH at the N-terminal, allowing the determination of the biologically active 1–84 PTH. AA, amino acids; CLIA, chemiluminescent immunoassays; PTH, parathyroid hormone; RIA, radioimmunoassays. Figure adapted from ref 30. Created in BioRender. D'Aurizio, F. (2025) https://BioRender.com/8yp9mwk)

Table 3.2 Main analytical characteristics of the most used second generation of PTH automated immunoassays as quoted by manufacturers

Manufacturer/analyzer	Assay principle	LOD (pg/mL)	LOQ (pg/mL)	AMR (pg/mL)	RI (pg/mL)
Abbott/Alinity I	CMIA/ non-competitive	0.5	0.9	3.0–3000.0	15.0–68.3
Beckman Coulter/UniCel DxI	CLIA/ non-competitive	1.0	4.0	1.0–3500.0	12.0–88.0
DiaSorin/Liaison XL	CLIA/ non-competitive	1.5	3.0	3.0–1900.0	14.5–87.1
Immunodiagnostic Systems/iSYS	CLIA/ non-competitive	2.5	4.5	5.0–5000.0	11.5–78.4
Mindray/CL-series	CLIA/ non-competitive	3.0	6.0	1.2–5000.0	12.0–88.0
Roche Diagnostics/Cobas e	ECLIA/ non-competitive	2.4	6.0	2.4–5000.0	17.3–74.1
Siemens Healthineers/Atellica® CI Analyzer	CLIA/ non-competitive	1.6	1.6	4.6–2000.0	S: 18.5–88.0 P: 18.4–80.1
SNIBE Diagnostic/MAGLUMI	CLIA/ non-competitive	1.5	ND	1.0–1500.0	15.0–65.0

AMR analytical measurement range, *CLIA* chemiluminescent assay, *CMIA* chemiluminescent microparticle immunoassay, *ECLIA* electrochemiluminescence assay, *LOD* limit of detection, *LOQ* limit of quantification, *ND* not disclosed, *P* plasma, *RI* reference interval, *S* serum. To convert results to SI units: pmol/L = pg/mL × 0.106. Information updated to May 2025

level, particularly in patients with CKD. The third-generation IMAs are more specific and differ from the previous generation because the N-terminal binding antibody is directed exclusively to the first four amino acids of PTH, thus allowing determination of PTH 1–84 (PTH bioactive) (Table 3.3) [20].

Despite this greater specificity, the third generation also interacts with post-translated modified forms of PTH, in particular the nontruncated amino-terminal PTH [32].

To improve the analytical specificity of PTH assay by better understanding the real impact of the C-terminal fragment on total PTH concentrations, liquid chromatography coupled to tandem mass spectrometry (LC-MS/MS) has been developed in recent years for the quantitative analysis of PTH. This technology is able to detect various molecular forms of PTH including non-1–84 PTH, carboxy-terminal PTH fragments, amino-PTH, and oxidized PTH. However, these are complex methods both in the preparation and analysis of the sample (e.g., analysis and quantification of fragments obtained from enzymatic digestion of protein) and thus not routinely used in clinical laboratories [33].

Despite technological progress, PTH measurement still has a lot of inter-method variability, even within the same generation [24, 30]. In this respect, a study comparing serum PTH levels measured by 13 different IMAs in patients with CKD reported a median bias ranging from 44.9% to 123% between the various methods and the Allegro assay, which was used as the reference [34]. Understandably, these differences should be considered when interpreting PTH concentrations. In a subsequent study, Almond et al. observed up to 4.2-fold variations in PTH concentrations measured by five different methods in plasma samples from dialysis patients, although the proposed reference intervals were similar [35]. The causes of inter-method variability are due to various factors including different antibody specificities, different tracers, different sensitivities of the method, and possible analytical interferences (described below) [30].

In addition, a relevant aspect to consider is the presence of inadequate calibration with respect to an internationally recognized reference material and the failure to identify a reference measurement procedure [34]. For this reason, given the clinical importance of PTH determination, the International Federation of Clinical Chemistry

Table 3.3 Main analytical characteristics of the third generation of PTH (1–84 PTH) automated immunoassays as quoted by manufacturers

Manufacturer/analyzer	Assay principle	LOD (pg/mL)	LOQ (pg/mL)	AMR (pg/mL)	RI (pg/mL)
DiaSorin/Liaison XL	CLIA/non-competitive	1.7	4.0	4.0–1800.0	S: 6.5–36.8 P: 6.7–38.8
Roche Diagnostics/Cobas e	ECLIA/ non-competitive	5.5	10.0	5.5–2300.0	14.9–56.9

AMR analytical measurement range, *CLIA* chemiluminescent assay, *ECLIA* electrochemiluminescence assay, *LOD* limit of detection, *LOQ* limit of quantification, *ND* not disclosed, *P* plasma, *RI* reference interval, *S* serum. To convert results to SI units: pmol/L = pg/mL × 0.106. Information updated to May 2025

and Laboratory Medicine (IFCC) has set up a working group to improve the comparability of methods (IFCC Working Group for PTH, now referred to as the IFCC Committee for Bone Metabolism) [30].

As mentioned before, PTH measurements can be subject to analytical interferences like most IMAs. In a study of 743 patients with PTH blood levels higher than the upper reference limit, 3.4% of cases were due to heterophilic antibodies and 1.2% to rheumatoid factor [36]. In sandwich assays, heterophilic antibodies and rheumatoid factor form a bridge between the capture antibody and the marked antibody, resulting in signal amplification (positive interference). This type of interference is more likely to develop in patients suffering from autoimmune diseases or in subjects who recently received immunization, transfusion, or monoclonal therapy [37]. The presence of possible interference by heterophilic antibodies/rheumatoid factor can be assessed with the following approaches, although a shared and universal strategy for detecting assay interference is not available:

- Treatment of the sample with commercially available test tubes containing heterophilic blocking agents.
- Serial dilutions of the sample as the lack of linearity is suspected due to interference.
- Polyethylene glycol (PEG) precipitation to remove any interfering antibody.
- Use of A/G protein-coated magnetic beads to adsorb the crystallizable fragment of interfering antibody.
- Alternative analytical assay platform.

In literature, some cases of PTH analytical interference caused by biotin have also been described [38–40].

Due to the strong non-covalent binding interaction with avidin and its derivatives, biotin is widely used in current IMAs for the capture of solid-phase antigen-antibody complexes. At physiological plasma concentrations (0.1–0.8 ng/mL), biotin is not able to influence immunometric determinations. In contrast, when biotin is present in the circulation at high concentrations, as a result of oral administration of high doses, it may cause negative analytical interference in sandwich assays using the biotin-streptavidin complex. Most of the manufacturers have improved the tolerance of their biotin assays, indicating the cutoff of blood biotin concentration beyond which there may be interference. However, awareness of the risks of potential interactions with exogenous biotin is important for clinicians. If such interference is suspected, it is recommended that a new sample be taken after the biotin withdrawal (8–72 h depending on the daily dose of biotin and the duration of treatment). If it is not possible to collect a second sample after discontinuing the biotin intake, the interference can be confirmed by:

- Performing serial dilution test.
- Treating the sample with streptavidin-coated microspheres which remove biotin.
- Using an alternative analytical assay platform not based on biotin-streptavidin bond [41].

Considering the architecture of the assay, it could be assumed that other types of interferences exist as well, including antibodies anti-streptavidin and anti-ruthenium antibodies.

The use of multiple strategies for interference assessment is the most effective approach. However, it should be noted that these techniques are used to identify interference and not to obtain true values. In this respect, according to the study by Cavalier et al., only 52.9% of patients returned to the normal range after treatment of the sample to remove interferences. This suggests that results exceeding the upper limit of the reference range do not necessarily indicate pathological PTH levels in the patient [36].

The presence of positive analytical interferences should be considered in differential diagnosis with normocalcemic PHPT and SHPT or in all cases where blood levels of PTH are unusually high compared to levels of calcemia, 25(OH)D, and kidney function data [37].

In these cases, communication between the clinician and the laboratory is crucial. In fact, the results of interference can lead to misdiagnosis, redundant blood tests, and unnecessary imaging, with delayed or inappropriate medical intervention.

3.8 Vitamin D

Concentrations of 25(OH)D are usually normal or tend to the lower reference limit in PHPT. This is the result of the action of PTH which increases the conversion of 25(OH)D into 1,25(OH)$_2$D whose concentration is high or toward the upper reference limit in PHPT. In addition, in the diagnosis of PHPT, the serum concentration of 25(OH)D should be considered since the concomitant presence of a vitamin D deficiency could lead to an increase in PTH values and a decrease in calcemia, although in the normal range, suggesting wrongly a normocalcemic PHPT instead of a classical one [42].

Determination of 25(OH)D shows several analytical issues due to (1) the strong binding with the specific transport protein (Vitamin D-Binding Protein, VDBP), (2) the need to determine the quantity of both 25(OH)D$_2$ and 25(OH)D$_3$ of vegetable and animal origin, respectively, (3) the co-existence of numerous substances with similar chemical compositions which may cause cross-reactions, and finally (4) the possible interferences (matrix effects for changes in protein composition, heterophile antibodies, etc.) which may lead to over- or under-estimation of the data [43–45].

Most clinical laboratories use IMAs for 25(OH)D measurement due to progressive automation (Table 3.4).

IMAs differ in primary antibody specificity, assay architecture, and type of tracer used in the reaction, generating a variability of results between tests of 10–15% on average, even in the same samples [46]. Moreover, IMAs suffer from a lack of specificity cross-reacting with vitamin D metabolites such as 24,25-dihydroxyvitamin D. LC-MS/MS technology represents the gold standard method for 25(OH)D measurement. It exhibits high specificity able to distinguish between 25(OH)D$_2$, 25(OH)D$_3$, and other metabolites [44]. However, LC-MS/MS is less widespread because of the complexity of this type of technology which requires more expertise and longer turnaround time than IMAs. LC-MS/MS also presents variability of results attributable to differences in instrumentation, chromatographic separation, and calibration. Thus, methodological standardization is crucial for the correct definition of 25(OH)D clinical decision levels. Intensive efforts over the last 15 years to achieve this have resulted in three LC-MS/MS-based reference measurement procedures which, by providing reference (target) values, can facilitate standardization or re-measurement of standardization of methods used in clinical practice, making the results more comparable [45].

The current guidelines consistently recommend measuring 25(OH)D to assess vitamin D status. Results are usually interpreted using universal cutoffs that rely primarily on bone health [44]. However, the recommended decision limits vary depending on the studies considered [43]. The most commonly suggested definition of vitamin D sufficiency, particularly in the general population, is 50 nmol/L (20 ng/mL), while a value below 30 nmol/L (12 ng/ml) is considered to be indicative of severe deficiency [45].

Table 3.4 Main analytical characteristics of the most used 25-hydroxyvitamin D automated immunoassays as quoted by manufacturers

Manufacturer/analyzer	Assay principle	LOD (nmol/L)	LOQ (nmol/L)	AMR (nmol/L)	RI (nmol/L)
Abbott/Alinity I	CMIA/competitive	8.8	8.8	8.8–385.5	16.5–124.6
Beckman Coulter/UniCel DxI	CLIA/competitive	5.6	11.0	11.0–525.0	35.0–124.4
DiaSorin/Liaison XL	CLIA/competitive	ND	10.0	10.0–374.4	23.3–119.8
Immunodiagnostic Systems/iSYS	CLIA/competitive	4.95	8.83	10.0–275.0	26.0–149.0
Roche Diagnostics/Cobas e	ECLIA/competitive	7.5	15.0	7.5–300.0	25.4–123.0
Siemens Healthineers/Atellica CI Analyzer	CLIA/competitive	8.0	10.5	10.5–375.0	18.5–110.0
SNIBE Diagnostic/MAGLUMI	CLIA/non-competitive	1.3	3.8	3.7–374.4	16.3–125.7

AMR analytical measurement range, *CLIA* chemiluminescent assay, *CMIA* chemiluminescent microparticle immunoassay, *ECLIA* electrochemiluminescence assay, *LOD* limit of detection, *LOQ* limit of quantification, *ND* not disclosed, *RI* reference interval. To convert results to conventional units: ng/mL = nmol/L × 0.4. Information updated to May 2025

Nevertheless, the established value of 25(OH)D below 50 nmol/L should not be considered "universal." From a purely analytical point of view, the main arguments against the use of fixed cut-offs are (1) the variable analytical performance of widely used IMAs as described above with great impact on patient classification, especially when the serum concentration of 25(OH)D ranges from 40 to 60 nmol/L, and (2) the non-uniformity of units (nmol/L vs ng/mL) in publications, documents, and guidelines with possible sources of error and confusion. From a clinical point of view, 25(OH)D serum concentration depends on several factors (i.e., ethnicity, sun exposure, polymorphisms of VDBP which affect bond affinity, etc.) [45].

The association between vitamin D and PTH concentrations is well documented. Literature data show that PTH reference intervals in non-vitamin D deficient subjects are about 20% lower than those of hypovitaminosis subjects; this is particularly important in the diagnostic phase of hyperparathyroidism, particularly in SHPT where PTH levels are elevated due to hypocalcemia and/or vitamin D deficiency [20].

Serum concentration of 1,25$(OH)_2$D is strongly regulated by PTH, and it has little correlation with vitamin D status. Thus, its measurement is considered useful in the evaluation of patients with PHPT, characterized by 1,25$(OH)_2$D normal or increased values, hypercalcemia of unknown origin, sarcoidosis, rickets, and tumor-induced osteomalacia, and in the differential diagnosis of FGF23-dependent phosphopenic rickets [47].

Analytical determination of 1,25$(OH)_2$D is more challenging than that of 25(OH)D because its blood concentration is in the picomolar range and its half-life is very short (4–6 h); in addition, there are no available reference materials or reference measurement procedures which hampers the evaluation of the quality of existing methods [48].

Currently, for 1,25$(OH)_2$D determination, manual or automated IMAs are mainly used in clinical laboratories, while LC-MS/MS technology is still not widespread (Table 3.5).

Automated IMAs offer better analytical performance than manual ones, but they cannot distinguish between 1,25$(OH)_2D_2$ and 1,25$(OH)_2D_3$. LC-MS/MS improves both analytical sensitivity and specificity; however, there are discrepancies between different methods due to challenges in separating 1β-25-dihydroxyvitamin D_3 from its 3α-epimer [44].

Reference intervals are method-dependent, and, unlike 25(OH)D, decision levels have not yet been defined [45].

Overall, as a general suggestion, it is preferable to always use the same analytical methods and therefore always apply to the same laboratory as the analytical variability may concern not only PTH and vitamin D metabolites but also other biochemical parameters, useful for the diagnosis and the follow-up of patients with PHPT.

Table 3.5 Main analytical characteristics of the most used 1,25-dihydroxyvitamin D automated immunoassays as quoted by manufacturers

Manufacturer/analyzer	Assay principle	LOD (pmol/L)	LOQ (pmol/L)	AMR (pmol/L)	RI (pmol/L)
DiaSorin/Liaison XL	CLIA/non-competitive	1.8	12.5	12.5–500.0	49.8–198.3
Immunodiagnostic Systems/iSYS	CLIA/competitive	13.2	18.0	18.0–504.0	62.6–228.0

AMR analytical measurement range, *CLIA* chemiluminescent assay, *ECLIA* electrochemiluminescence assay, *LOD* limit of detection, *LOQ* limit of quantification, *ND* not disclosed, *RI* reference interval. To convert results to conventional units: pg/mL = pmol/L × 0.4. Information updated to May 2025

3.9 Conclusions

In summary, a laboratory medicine panel combining serum calcium, PTH, and adjunctive markers (phosphate, vitamin D, urinary calcium) when needed not only confirms the presence of hyperparathyroidism but also distinguishes primary, secondary, and tertiary forms, thereby ensuring timely and precise patient management. Laboratory tests are indispensable for guiding parathyroid imaging, monitoring post-surgical outcomes, and ensuring normalization of calcium and PTH after parathyroidectomy. In cases where surgery is delayed or contraindicated, serial laboratory tests—possibly with calcimimetic therapy—aid in medical management.

Declaration of Competing Interest The authors have no conflicts of interest to declare that are relevant to the content of this chapter.

Ethical Approval Not applicable.

References

1. Goltzman D. Physiology of parathyroid hormone. Endocrinol Metab Clin N Am. 2018;47:743–58. https://doi.org/10.1016/j.ecl.2018.07.003.
2. Mallick R, Chen H. Diagnosis and management of hyperparathyroidism. Adv Surg. 2018;52:137–53. https://doi.org/10.1016/j.yasu.2018.03.006.
3. Rosen RD, Bordoni B. Embryology, parathyroid. In: StatPearls. Treasure Island: StatPearls Publishing; 2025.
4. Khan M, Jose A, Sharma S. Physiology, parathyroid hormone. In: StatPearls. Treasure Island: StatPearls Publishing; 2025.
5. Vervloet MG, Brandenburg VM, CKD-MBD working group of ERA-EDTA. Circulating markers of bone turnover. J Nephrol. 2017;30:663–70. https://doi.org/10.1007/s40620-017-0408-8.
6. Brown EM. Calcium receptor and regulation of parathyroid hormone secretion. Rev Endocr Metab Disord. 2000;1:307–15. https://doi.org/10.1023/a:1026570518919.
7. Demir AD. A review of parathyroid mass and patients with nonspecific complaints. J Int Med Res. 2020;48:300060519827169. https://doi.org/10.1177/0300060519827169.
8. Pitt SC, Sippel RS, Chen H. Secondary and tertiary hyperparathyroidism, state of the art surgical management. Surg Clin North Am. 2009;89:1227–39. https://doi.org/10.1016/j.suc.2009.06.011.
9. Palermo A, Tabacco G, Makras P, et al. Primary hyperparathyroidism: from guidelines to outpatient clinic. Rev Endocr Metab Disord. 2024;25:875–96. https://doi.org/10.1007/s11154-024-09899-5.
10. Fraser WD. Bone and mineral metabolism. In: Tietz fundamentals of clinical chemistry and molecular diagnostics. 8th ed. St. Louis: Elsevier; 2019a. p. 744–52.
11. Yu E, Sharma S. Physiology, calcium. In: StatPearls. Treasure Island: StatPearls Publishing; 2025.
12. Pekar J-D, Grzych G, Durand G, et al. Calcium state estimation by total calcium: the evidence to end the never-ending story. Clin Chem Lab Med. 2020;58:222–31. https://doi.org/10.1515/cclm-2019-0568.
13. Bilezikian JP, Khan AA, Silverberg SJ, et al. Evaluation and management of primary hyperparathyroidism: summary statement and guidelines from the fifth international workshop. J Bone Miner Res. 2022;37:2293–314. https://doi.org/10.1002/jbmr.4677.
14. Bilezikian JP, Bandeira L, Khan A, Cusano NE. Hyperparathyroidism. Lancet. 2018;391:168–78. https://doi.org/10.1016/S0140-6736(17)31430-7.
15. Miler M, Simundić A-M. Low level of adherence to instructions for 24-hour urine collection among hospital outpatients. Biochem Med (Zagreb). 2013;23:316–20. https://doi.org/10.11613/bm.2013.038.
16. Erben RG. Physiological actions of fibroblast growth Factor-23. Front Endocrinol (Lausanne). 2018;9:267. https://doi.org/10.3389/fendo.2018.00267.
17. Fraser WD. Bone and mineral metabolism. In: Tietz textbook of clinical chemistry and molecular diagnostics. 8th ed. St. Louis: Elsevier; 2019b. p. 752–4.
18. Tinawi M. Disorders of calcium metabolism: hypocalcemia and hypercalcemia. Cureus. 2021;13:e12420. https://doi.org/10.7759/cureus.12420.
19. Kikyo N. Circadian regulation of bone remodeling. Int J Mol Sci. 2024;25:4717. https://doi.org/10.3390/ijms25094717.
20. Smit MA, van Kinschot CMJ, van der Linden J, et al. Clinical guidelines and PTH measurement: does assay generation matter? Endocr Rev. 2019;40:1468–80. https://doi.org/10.1210/er.2018-00220.
21. Jha S, Simonds WF. Molecular and clinical spectrum of primary hyperparathyroidism. Endocr Rev. 2023;44:779–818. https://doi.org/10.1210/endrev/bnad009.
22. Lemoine S, Figueres L, Bacchetta J, et al. Calcium homeostasis and hyperparathyroidism: nephrologic and endocrinologic points of view. Ann Endocrinol (Paris). 2022;83:237–43. https://doi.org/10.1016/j.ando.2022.05.003.
23. Sturgeon CM, Sprague S, Almond A, et al. Perspective and priorities for improvement of parathyroid hormone (PTH) measurement – a view from the IFCC working group for PTH. Clin Chim Acta. 2017;467:42–7. https://doi.org/10.1016/j.cca.2016.10.016.
24. Valcour A, Zierold C, Blocki FA, et al. Trueness, precision and stability of the LIAISON 1–84 parathyroid hormone (PTH) third-generation assay: comparison to existing intact PTH assays. Clin Chem

Lab Med. 2018;56:1476–82. https://doi.org/10.1515/cclm-2018-0217.
25. Censi S, Iacobone M, Simmini S, et al. PTH: redefining reference ranges in a healthy population-the role of interfering factors and the type of laboratory assay. Int J Endocrinol. 2020;2020:1053719. https://doi.org/10.1155/2020/1053719.
26. Aloia JF, Feuerman M, Yeh JK. Reference range for serum parathyroid hormone. Endocr Pract. 2006;12:137–44. https://doi.org/10.4158/EP.12.2.137.
27. Cavalcante LBCP, Brandão CMÁ, Chiamolera MI, et al. Big data-based parathyroid hormone (PTH) values emphasize need for age correction. J Endocrinol Investig. 2023;46:2525–33. https://doi.org/10.1007/s40618-023-02107-2.
28. Souberbielle J-C, Massart C, Brailly-Tabard S, et al. Serum PTH reference values established by an automated third-generation assay in vitamin D-replete subjects with normal renal function: consequences of diagnosing primary hyperparathyroidism and the classification of dialysis patients. Eur J Endocrinol. 2016;174:315–23. https://doi.org/10.1530/EJE-15-0595.
29. Drechsler C, Grootendorst DC, Boeschoten EW, Krediet RT, Wanner C, Dekker FW, NECOSAD Study Group. Changes in parathyroid hormone, body mass index and the association with mortality in dialysis patients. Nephrol Dial Transplant. 2011;26:1340–6. https://doi.org/10.1093/ndt/gfq541.
30. Cavalier E, Vasikaran S, Bhattoa HP, et al. The path to the standardization of PTH: is this a realistic possibility? A position paper of the IFCC C-BM. Clin Chim Acta. 2021;515:44–51. https://doi.org/10.1016/j.cca.2020.12.022.
31. Gannagé-Yared M-H, Kallas-Chémaly M-N, Sleilaty G. Parathormone levels in a middle-eastern healthy population using 2nd and 3rd generation PTH assays. Int J Endocrinol. 2020;2020:6302861. https://doi.org/10.1155/2020/6302861.
32. Ureña-Torres PA, Vervloet M, Mazzaferro S, et al. Novel insights into parathyroid hormone: report of the parathyroid day in chronic kidney disease. Clin Kidney J. 2019;12:269–80. https://doi.org/10.1093/ckj/sfy061.
33. Cavalier E. Determination of parathyroid hormone: from radioimmunoassay to LCMS/MS. Clin Chem Lab Med. 2023;61:946–53. https://doi.org/10.1515/cclm-2022-0942.
34. Souberbielle J-C, Boutten A, Carlier M-C, et al. Inter-method variability in PTH measurement: implication for the care of CKD patients. Kidney Int. 2006;70:345–50. https://doi.org/10.1038/sj.ki.5001606.
35. Almond A, Ellis AR, Walker SW, Scottish Clinical Biochemistry Managed Diagnostic Network. Current parathyroid hormone immunoassays do not adequately meet the needs of patients with chronic kidney disease. Ann Clin Biochem. 2012;49:63–7. https://doi.org/10.1258/acb.2011.011094.
36. Cavalier E, Carlisi A, Chapelle J-P, Delanaye P. False positive PTH results: an easy strategy to test and detect analytical interferences in routine practice. Clin Chim Acta. 2008;387:150–2. https://doi.org/10.1016/j.cca.2007.08.019.
37. Ohe MN, Takimoto RM, Ferrer CMA d F, et al. PTH immunoassay interference: differential diagnosis with normocalcemic primary hyperparathyroidism? Arch Endocrinol Metab. 2024;68:e230315. https://doi.org/10.20945/2359-4292-2023-0315.
38. Piketty M-L, Prie D, Sedel F, et al. High-dose biotin therapy leading to false biochemical endocrine profiles: validation of a simple method to overcome biotin interference. Clin Chem Lab Med. 2017;55:817–25. https://doi.org/10.1515/cclm-2016-1183.
39. Plasse RA, Olson SW, Yuan CM, Nee R. Biotin supplement interference with immunoassays for parathyroid hormone and 25-hydroxyvitamin D in a patient with metabolic bone disease on maintenance hemodialysis. Clin Kidney J. 2020;13:710–2. https://doi.org/10.1093/ckj/sfz134.
40. Waghray A, Milas M, Nyalakonda K, Siperstein AE. Falsely low parathyroid hormone secondary to biotin interference: a case series. Endocr Pract. 2013;19:451–5. https://doi.org/10.4158/EP12158.OR.
41. Li D, Ferguson A, Cervinski MA, et al. AACC guidance document on biotin interference in laboratory tests. J Appl Lab Med. 2020;5:575–87. https://doi.org/10.1093/jalm/jfz010.
42. Zavatta G, Clarke BL. Normocalcemic hyperparathyroidism: a heterogeneous disorder often misdiagnosed? JBMR Plus. 2020;4:e10391. https://doi.org/10.1002/jbm4.10391.
43. Alonso N, Zelzer S, Eibinger G, Herrmann M. Vitamin D metabolites: analytical challenges and clinical relevance. Calcif Tissue Int. 2023;112:158–77. https://doi.org/10.1007/s00223-022-00961-5.
44. Cavalier E, Makris K, Heijboer AC, et al. Vitamin D: analytical advances, clinical impact, and ongoing debates on health perspectives. Clin Chem. 2024;70:1104–21. https://doi.org/10.1093/clinchem/hvae056.
45. Plebani M, Zaninotto M, Giannini S, et al. Vitamin D assay and supplementation: still debatable issues. Diagnosis (Berl). 2025;12:35–44. https://doi.org/10.1515/dx-2024-0147.
46. Le Goff C, Cavalier E, Souberbielle J-C, et al. Measurement of circulating 25-hydroxyvitamin D: a historical review. Pract Lab Med. 2015;2:1–14. https://doi.org/10.1016/j.plabm.2015.04.001.
47. Herrmann M. Assessing vitamin D metabolism – four decades of experience. Clin Chem Lab Med. 2023;61:880–94. https://doi.org/10.1515/cclm-2022-1267.
48. Giustina A, Bilezikian JP, Adler RA, et al. Consensus statement on vitamin D status assessment and supplementation: whys, whens, and hows. Endocr Rev. 2024;45:625–54. https://doi.org/10.1210/endrev/bnae009.

4 Ultrasonography and Fine-Needle Aspiration Cytology of Parathyroid Glands

Murat Tuncel

▶ **Definitions**

Fine-needle aspiration cytology of parathyroid lesion: Cytological examination of prepared slides with/without specific immunohistochemistry after puncturing a suspicious parathyroid lesion.

Parathyroid lesion: Includes all parathyroid lesions, such as normal parathyroid gland, adenoma, hyperplasia, atypical adenoma, and parathyroid carcinoma.

Learning Objectives

This chapter will:

- Define the ultrasonography technique necessary for parathyroid imaging.
- Outline the ultrasonographic features of parathyroid pathologies.
- Describe pitfalls in the interpretation of ultrasonography of the parathyroid glands.
- Discuss the strengths and limitations of fine-needle aspiration cytology.
- Examine the role of PTH assay and immunocytochemistry in aiding parathyroid cytology.

M. Tuncel (✉)
Department of Nuclear Medicine, Faculty of Medicine, Hacettepe University, Ankara, Turkey
e-mail: murat.tuncel@hacettepe.edu.tr

4.1 Parathyroid Ultrasonography

Ultrasound (US) is a first-line imaging modality for localizing abnormal parathyroid glands (PTG) in patients with primary hyperparathyroidism (PHPT). High-frequency neck US is a non-ionizing, cost-effective tool that can be performed in an office setting [1]. It is a readily available imaging modality with considerable accuracy when conducted by experienced professionals. US allows for real-time evaluation of both parathyroid and adjacent thyroid tissue, often detecting concurrent thyroid nodules, and facilitates minimally invasive focused parathyroidectomy [1, 2].

Lesions associated with primary hyperparathyroidism (HPT) include solitary adenoma (80–85%), multiglandular disease (15–20%), and carcinoma (<1%). Multiglandular parathyroid diseases are caused by hyperplasia of all parathyroid glands or, occasionally, double adenomas (5%). In patients with parathyroid hyperplasia, all four glands are enlarged but usually smaller than in patients with parathyroid adenomas. Hence, they are not as readily visible. Hyperplasia is commonly seen in patients with familial syndromes such as multiple endocrine neoplasia (MEN) 1 and MEN 2A [3].

© The Author(s), under exclusive license to Springer Nature Switzerland AG 2026

P. Petranović Ovčariček et al. (eds.), *Parathyroid Imaging*,
https://doi.org/10.1007/978-3-032-14178-1_4

4.2 Anatomy and Localization

PTGs are small, smooth, soft, flattened ovoid or bean-shaped structures measuring 4–6 mm in length, 3–4 mm in width, and 1–2 mm in thickness, with a yellow-tan color. Each gland typically weighs between 30 and 40 mg, but this weight can vary significantly. The inferior glands are slightly larger; any weight exceeding 40 mg may be considered abnormal [4].

The upper PTGs are located behind the tracheoesophageal groove, the upper thyroid lobes (80–95%), and the retropharyngeal and retroesophageal area (3%) and, less frequently, in the carotid sheath (<1%), in the thyroid parenchyma (<1%), or in the fatty tissue adjacent to the scalene muscles (<1%). The inferior glands are located near the lower thyroid lobe (50–60%), along the thyrothymic ligament (25%), and in the mediastinum (3%) and less commonly in the carotid sheath (<1%) or intrathyroidal (<1%) [5].

The overwhelming majority of individuals have four PTGs, two superior and two inferior, whereas between 2.5% and 13.0% have supernumerary glands, and 3% have fewer than four glands [6, 7].

Multiglandular diseases, particularly those resulting from secondary hyperparathyroidism (HPT) or genetic conditions like multiple endocrine neoplasia type 1 (MEN 1), are characterized by hyperplasia that typically affects all four parathyroid glands. In these cases, each hyperplastic gland is generally smaller than a solitary adenoma.

Ectopic parathyroid adenomas are found in approximately 20% of unexplored patients with primary hyperparathyroidism, but this rate can rise to as high as 66% in patients undergoing reoperation [8]. Ectopic locations for superior or inferior parathyroid glands include the tracheoesophageal groove, retroesophageal space, and, less commonly, within the thyroid. Additional sites for ectopic superior parathyroid glands include retropharyngeal locations and the posterior mediastinum. In contrast, ectopic inferior glands can also be found within the thymic capsule (38% of ectopic glands), carotid sheath, submandibular region, and extending into the mediastinum.

Preoperative localization of these lesions is crucial for minimally invasive surgery. Ultrasound is typically the initial localization test indicated, often used alongside Tc-99 m sestamibi scintigraphy, in patients with biochemically confirmed primary hyperparathyroidism (PHPT) [2, 9]. The goal is to find all hyperfunctioning glands and identify any concomitant thyroid disease to guide surgery.

4.3 Scanning Technique and Reporting

4.3.1 Transducer and Patient Positioning

A high-frequency (10–14 MHz) linear-array transducer is used for the best resolution, while the superior mediastinum can be evaluated with a curved-array transducer and beam steering [1]. The patient lies supine with the neck typically hyperextended, supported by a towel underneath the neck or a pillow beneath the shoulders. Both thyroid lobes should be scanned in transverse and longitudinal planes, including the paratracheal regions. The examination encompasses the neck area bordered by the carotid arteries bilaterally, the carotid artery bifurcations or the hyoid bone superiorly, and the thoracic inlet inferiorly. The focus of the sonographic assessment is on the conventional gland sites located posterior and inferior to the thyroid lobes. Additionally, the carotid sheath and superior mediastinum below the clavicles should be examined for ectopic sites. Observing the lower neck while the patient swallows and angling the probe behind the sternum can reveal mobile adenomas along the thyrothymic ligament or in the lower neck. Rotating the patient's head may assist in identifying ectopic glands within the tracheoesophageal groove and deep paraesophageal regions. Swallowing maneuvers can help differentiate the esophagus from the inferior glands. However, even with these maneuvers, the identification of these ectopic lesions is often hindered by poor beam penetration.

In cases of secondary or tertiary hyperparathyroidism, multiple glands are enlarged and may appear more irregular or nodular. Small or multigland disease is more frequently missed. Operator factors, such as experience and device-related image quality, strongly affect accuracy. False positives can occur: thyroid nodules (especially hypoechoic ones) and enlarged lymph nodes may mimic parathyroid adenomas. Lymph nodes have a fatty hilum and a hilar vessel, in contrast to the polar vessel found in parathyroid glands. An intrathyroidal parathyroid adenoma can resemble a thyroid nodule, so any indeterminate lesion near the thyroid capsule should raise suspicion. PTH-FNA can confirm the diagnosis if needed, but only in select cases due to the risk of seeding.

4.3.2 US Report

The US report includes the number of candidate lesions, as single gland disease may be treated less invasively than multiglandular disease. If multiple candidates are identified, prioritizing them based on diagnostic confidence can influence the surgical approach. The size of candidate lesions is also significant: a larger size (>13 mm) suggests a single adenoma, while a smaller size (<7 mm) indicates multiglandular disease. The US operator should report the lesion's location in relation to surgically visible landmarks, such as the cricoid cartilage, tracheoesophageal groove, thyroid gland, or suprasternal notch, but not the cervical vertebrae. Additionally, vascular anomalies that indicate the presence of a nonrecurrent laryngeal nerve, typically the aberrant right subclavian artery, along with thyroid nodules requiring further preoperative evaluation, should also be reported.

4.4 Sonographic Appearance

4.4.1 Normal Parathyroids

Normal parathyroid glands (approximately 4–5 mm) are difficult to visualize on ultrasound. Recent data suggest that when they are visualized, they appear as hyperechoic ovoid structures with homogeneous echogenicity in 91% of cases and isoechoic structures with homogeneous echogenicity in 9% [10] (Fig. 4.1). The stromal fat component of the PTG accounts for hyperechogenicity, whereas perithyroidal fat tissue can be distinguished by ill-defined margins and heterogeneous echotexture [11].

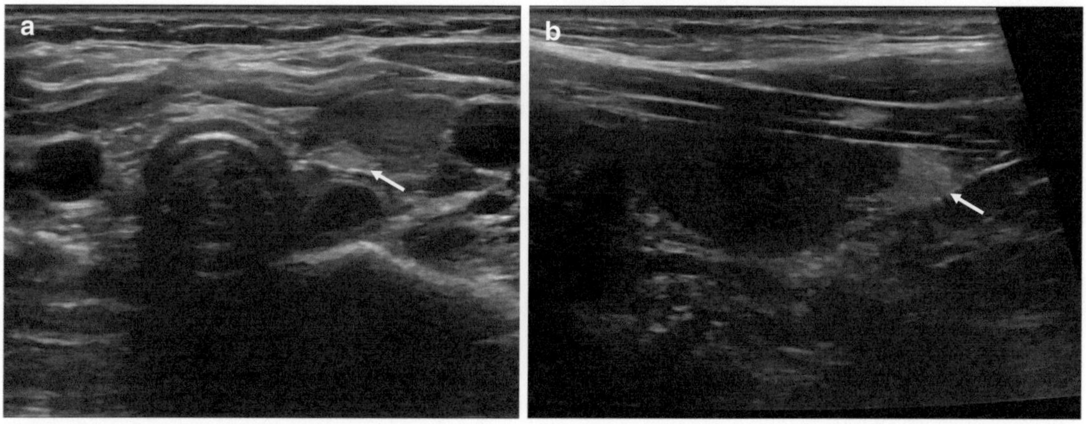

Fig. 4.1 US shows (**a** and **b**) small homogenous, hyperechoic lesions near the thyroid gland compatible with normal parathyroid glands (arrows) with fat content

4.4.2 Parathyroid Hyperplasia

Hyperplasia is characterized by the enlargement of multiple glands. US may reveal two or more hypoechoic ovoid glands instead of a single adenoma. Generally, hyperplastic glands are smaller and less uniform than solitary adenomas (Fig. 4.2). In cases of secondary or tertiary hyperparathyroidism, these glands may exhibit nodularity and irregular borders. It is virtually impossible to sonographically distinguish glandular hyperplasia from adenomatous formations. In instances of multiglandular disease, more than one enlarged lobulated gland, either symmetrically or asymmetrically, may be observed.

On the color Doppler US imaging, both adenoma and hyperplasia in most cases show prominent feeding polar vessels entering the pole and then extending around the periphery of the enlarged gland. Similarly to all the other imaging methods, US is less sensitive for the detection of multiglandular than of single-gland disease as hyperplastic PTGs are usually significantly smaller [12]. A systematic review by Ruda et al. including more than 20,000 patients with PHPT reported sensitivities of 78.5%, 16.2%, and 34.9% for single-gland, two-gland, and multiglandular parathyroid disease, respectively [13].

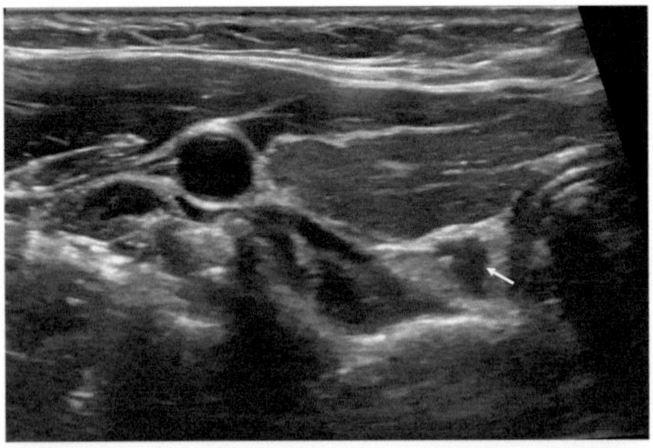

Fig. 4.2 US images showed a hypoechoic lesion with a diameter of 6 mm (arrow) which is found to be compatible with parathyroid hyperplasia

4.4.3 Parathyroid Adenomas

The characteristics of the PTG in the US reveal an abnormal presentation as an oval, bean-shaped, or occasionally multilobulated hypoechoic mass with well-defined margins, typically located posteriorly or inferiorly to the thyroid gland. Parathyroid lesions are generally very vascular, exhibiting a peripheral vascular arc and a prominent polar feeding vessel that arises from the branches of the inferior thyroid artery (Fig. 4.3). Identifying this polar feeding artery helps differentiate parathyroid glands from lymph nodes, which typically receive a hilar blood supply [14]. Although most adenomas are less than 2 cm in size, large adenomas greater than 5 cm can occur. Occasionally, parathyroid adenomas may be echogenic or heterogeneous in echotexture rather than displaying the typical homogenous hypoechoic appearance. This is commonly seen when the adenomas are larger than 2 cm. A typical parathyroid adenoma is solid with a less than 10% cystic component and appears uniformly hypoechoic relative to the thyroid at US [15]. Cystic adenomas occur in 2% of cases and may be difficult to differentiate from rare true parathyroid cysts. Cystic degeneration can range from minimal cystic change to mostly (>50%) cystic (~5%). Rarely calcification (~1.5%) can be observed [16, 17].

Recently published studies suggest that a relatively new technique contrast-enhanced ultrasound (CEUS) has high accuracy for the preoperative detection of parathyroid lesions, particularly due to its ability to dynamically visualize microvascularization and blood flow within the tissue. The CEUS evaluation is divided into the wash-in (0–30 s) and wash-out (30–120 s) periods; consequently, cine images are recorded immediately after the administration of the contrast agent, continuing through the complete wash-out phase. Based on previously published studies, parathyroid adenomas at CEUS exhibit early arterial hypervascularization (0–30 s) from the periphery to the center, followed by rapid

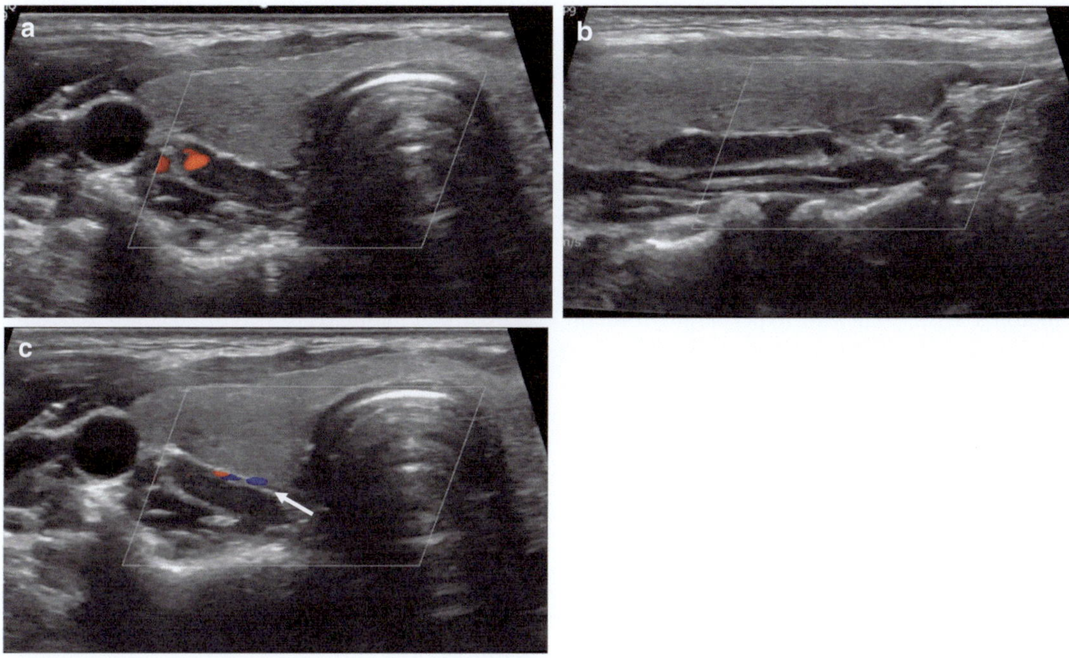

Fig. 4.3 Transverse (**a**) and longitudinal (**b**) images show a hypoechoic elongated lesion with a size of 20 × 7 mm compatible with parathyroid adenoma. Typical polar artery (**c**: arrow) and hypervascularity were noted

wash-out in the late phase (30–120 s). This pattern distinguishes them from physiologic lymph nodes and thyroid nodules. Findings are considered positive when the suspicious lesion demonstrates early arterial hypervascularization from the periphery to the center, along with wash-out in the late phase. In a study of 29 patients, CEUS revealed sensitivity of 66.7% (95% confidence interval [CI], 46–82.7%) for detection of single adenomas in comparison with 51.8% (95% CI, 32.3–70.8%) for high-resolution US. With CEUS, double adenomas could be detected in both cases (sensitivity, 100%); however, scintigraphy and high-resolution US did not detect any cases of double adenomas. In addition, CEUS allowed the differentiation of lymphatic nodes from parathyroid glands in two patients. No side effects were observed for CEUS [9, 18].

US elastography, particularly shear-wave elastography, allows assessment of tissue elasticity [19]. However the data on use of US elastography for detection of parathyroid adenomas are limited. One study concluded that shear-wave US elastography could allow differentiation of parathyroid adenomas from thyroid nodules, lymph nodes, and malignant parathyroid lesions with sensitivity of 46%, 78%, and 100% and specificity of 77%, 71%, and 95.4%, respectively [20].

At US elastography, parathyroid adenomas have lower tissue elasticity than thyroid nodules. The reported median shear wave velocity for parathyroid adenomas is 2.02 m/s with a range of 1.53–2.50 m/s; for thyroid nodules, it is 2.77 m/s with a range of 1.89–3.70 m/s [19]. At strain US elastography with a mean cut-off value of 2.58 kPa, malignant lesions were found to be stiffer than benign lesions, with reported stiffness of 1.77 kPa ± 0.54 for parathyroid adenomas and 3.47 kPa ± 0.77 for parathyroid carcinomas [12, 19]. Although these new US techniques show great promise, more validation and standardization of protocols are needed before they are adopted into guidelines and daily practice.

4.4.3.1 Parathyroid Cyst

A developmental or colloid retention cyst can present as an asymptomatic neck mass or with signs and symptoms of hyperparathyroidism. These cysts account for 1–5% of neck masses, with a slight female predominance, typically occurring in the fourth to fifth decades of life. Most of these cysts are nonfunctioning; however, a few may exhibit compressive symptoms or symptoms associated with hyperparathyroidism. On ultrasound, they appear as well-defined anechoic lesions with posterior acoustic enhancement (Fig. 4.4) [21]. Cystic appearance can complicate the accurate diagnosis and may be mistaken for a cystic thyroid nodule, making careful analysis of ultrasound images essential. The fluid aspirated from parathyroid cysts typically appears clear and watery during ultrasound-guided fine needle aspiration (FNA), although a small proportion of cysts may contain hemorrhagic, brown, or turbid fluid. An elevated level of parathyroid hormone (PTH) in the cyst fluid is pathognomonic. Management includes fluid aspiration, surgery, or sclerotherapy [22].

4.4.3.2 Parathyroid Carcinoma

Parathyroid carcinoma is a rare malignancy, accounting for less than 1% of hyperparathyroidism cases. It most commonly presents in individuals in their 40–50s, which is younger than the typical age for adenomas, and affects males and females equally [23]. Hyperparathyroidism due to parathyroid carcinoma typically presents with serum calcium levels greater than 14 mg/dL (3.5 mmol/L) and PTH levels three to ten times higher than normal. Clinically, the symptoms of parathyroid adenoma and carcinoma overlap; however, the symptoms of parathyroid carcinoma tend to be more severe, and no imaging features definitively distinguish carcinoma from adenoma.

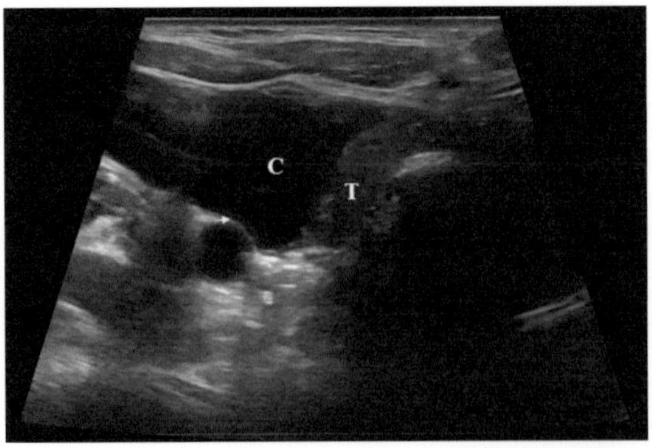

Fig. 4.4 US showed a cystic lesion (C) with an irregular thin mural component (arrow) near the right thyroid lobe (T)

On US, parathyroid carcinomas are generally larger (measuring over 2–3 cm) and exhibit a higher depth-to-width ratio, extensive heterogeneity, a thicker or irregular parathyroid capsule, calcifications, and increased vascularity. Additionally, they may show local tissue invasion and lymph node involvement. At CEUS, there is heterogeneous enhancement and early wash-out, whereas at US elastography the malignant lesions are stiffer than parathyroid hyperplasia and adenoma [24].

4.4.3.3 Diagnostic Performance

US is recognized as an excellent initial imaging modality for neck evaluation due to its speed, portability, cost-effectiveness, and lack of radiation risk. It is especially sensitive for detecting single-gland disease near the thyroid, with reported sensitivity varying widely (approximately 55–87%) based on operator experience, patient anatomy, and adenoma location.

When combined with ^{99m}Tc-sestamibi scintigraphy, US is a widely accepted first-line imaging approach for preoperative planning related to parathyroid pathologic conditions. This combination enhances sensitivity to 81%, compared to 70% with US alone and 64% with ^{99m}Tc-sestamibi scintigraphy alone.

US is less effective for detecting multigland disease; a systematic review of 20,225 cases showed sensitivity decreasing to 35%, as compared with a sensitivity of 78% for the detection of solitary adenomas [13]. Positive predictive value is high (93–97% in experienced hands), meaning that a lesion identified on US is very likely to be a true adenoma. In modern series, US often finds adenomas in 70–90% of first-time PHPT patients when performed skillfully [9]. In contrast, sensitivity drops in reoperative cases or multigland disease. In one study of patients with prior negative imaging, ultrasound identified only ~52% of adenomas. Thus, a negative US in a reoperative or complex case should prompt additional imaging (e.g., sestamibi, 4D-CT, or MRI). US can achieve sensitivity of 70–80% when performed by an experienced operator but shows lower sensitivity in detecting ectopic parathyroid lesions [25]. Multinodular goiter can distort the normal anatomy of the neck's soft tissues, causing parathyroid adenomas to shift to more lateral or deeper locations and reducing the sensitivity of US in their detection. In a study analyzing the factors that improve gland localization via US, multivariable analysis revealed that concomitant thyroid pathology was the only factor that decreased the success of US [26].

There are other limitations in US evaluation of parathyroid lesions, including operator experience, low sensitivity in localization of ectopic parathyroid lesions, intrathyroid lesions, and dependence on body habitus such as neck circumference and kyphosis, which can limit neck positioning [12]. The sensitivity of ultrasonography varies depending on the location of the parathyroid lesion; its overall sensitivity was reported to be 55–87%, and it is especially low in cases with ectopic parathyroid tissues or normocalcemic PHPT. The positive predictive value of ultrasonography ranges from 93% to 97%, and its specificity ranges from 40% to 98% [2].

4.5 Ultrasound Mimics of Parathyroid Glands

Overall, ultrasound (US) has limitations, especially in patients with inexperienced hands. Several benign or malignant structures may mimic the appearance of parathyroid adenomas, further complicating the diagnosis. Careful analysis of imaging features may aid in differential diagnosis (Table 4.1).

Adults with chronic lymphocytic thyroiditis typically have numerous reactive cervical lymph nodes that can mimic parathyroid adenomas. An abnormal small lymph node may lack a fatty hilum, appear enlarged or round, lose the hilar vascular pattern, and exhibit peripheral vascularity and chaotic vascularization. The esophagus, to inexperienced eyes, can be mistakenly identified as a parathyroid lesion due to its location. Its characteristic "gut signature," consisting of alternating layers of echogenicity, may assist in interpretation. Hypoechoic thyroid nodules near the capsule may also mimic parathyroid adenomas;

Table 4.1 Sonographic features of parathyroid lesions and mimics

Feature	Normal parathyroid	Parathyroid adenoma/hyperplasia	Parathyroid carcinoma	Lymph node
Size	≈4–6 mm (usually not seen)	~0.5–3 cm (variable)	Length > 3 cm	1–2 cm (variable)
Shape	Flat or oval, thin (<5 mm)	Ovoid/oblong, well-circumscribed	Depth/width ratio >1	Ovoid with fatty hilum
Echogenicity	Isoechoic or slightly hyperechoic (if visible)	Hypoechoic, homogeneous; may have cystic or calcific areas	Lobulated, heterogeneous, hypoechoic lesion	Hypoechoic; typically central echogenic hilum (fat)
Vascularity (color)	Minimal; glands are small	Prominent peripheral or central flow; a polar feeding vessel often seen at one pole	Intralesional disordered vascularity	Hilar flow only; vessel enters at hilum
Border/ capsule	Smooth, microscopic capsule	Well-circumscribed; echogenic capsule often visualized	Irregular borders Thick capsule	Sharp borders; distinct fatty hilum
Other features	–	May show cystic degeneration or calcifications in large adenomas	Intranodular calcifications Cystic inclusions may be seen	Fatty hilum with hyperechoic center

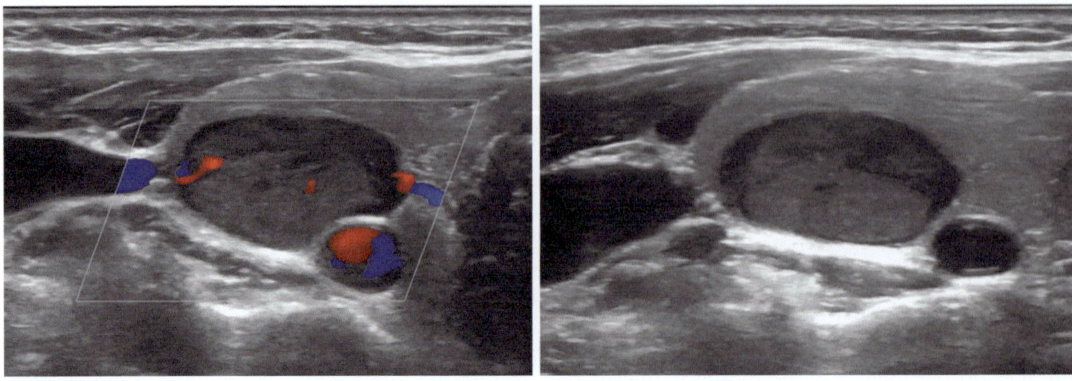

Fig. 4.5 An intrathyroidal parathyroid adenoma seen on US as a hypoechoic hypervascular lesion

the thyroid capsule and the absence of a polar feeding artery are differentiating features. Conversely intrathyroidal parathyroid adenomas may be falsely interpreted as thyroid nodules (Fig. 4.5). The longus colli muscle, located posterior to the thyroid, may mimic the appearance of parathyroid lesions. Striated muscle fibers and an elongated appearance on sagittal view may help in the differential diagnosis. Paragangliomas are a rare form of slowly growing but potentially locally invasive, highly vascularized neuroendocrine neoplasms arising from the chromaffin cells of sympathetic or parasympathetic paraganglia, accounting for 0.6% of all head and neck tumors [27]. At US, neck paragangliomas generally appear as well-defined oval to round, highly vascular, hypoechoic masses that displace the carotid bifurcation and mimic ectopic parathyroid adenomas [28].

4.6 Fine-Needle Aspiration Cytology of Parathyroid Glands

Despite using various imaging modalities, including US, to diagnose the etiology of hyperparathyroidism, the primary parathyroid lesion may not be identified, or only lesions lacking clear evidence of parathyroid origin may be detected. Parathyroid cytology through fine-needle aspiration (FNAC) is an important component of the diagnostic workup for these suspicious parathyroid lesions, especially in challenging or ambiguous cases. FNAC has been employed to localize suspected parathyroid adenomas and to differentiate between thyroid and parathyroid origins of neck nodules or incidental findings [29].

However, the sensitivity of the technique is variable. The smaller size and atypical localization of these suspicious lesions may hinder optimal sample collection. The results should always be interpreted alongside clinical and radiological data. In one study of 25 confirmed parathyroid aspirates, a cytologic diagnosis was correctly made in 18 out of 25 cases (~72%) when clinicoradiologic information was available; sensitivity decreased when that information was lacking. Major architectural findings of parathyroid lesions include scattered naked nuclei, loose clusters, a papillary pattern with a fibrovascular core, tight clusters, and a follicular pattern, which were often intermixed. Cytological features included anisokaryosis, stippled chromatin, well-defined cell borders, and oxyphilic cytoplasm. Seven patients were misdiagnosed with atypical cells ($n = 2$), benign follicular cells ($n = 2$), adenomatous goiter ($n = 2$), and metastatic carcinoma ($n = 1$) in FNAC. With clinicoradiologic data, the sensitivity of cytological diagnosis was 86.7%. Without this information, the sensitivity decreased to 50% [30].

In a larger series of 81 cases, the combination of cytology with PTH wash-out and/or immunostains significantly improved detection, enabling nearly all lesions to be accurately identified when these adjuncts were utilized. Key cytomorphologic features that favor parathyroid origin

Table 4.2 Commonly reported features in parathyroid cytology

Feature	Description	Relative frequency/diagnostic value
Architectural patterns	Scattered "naked" nuclei (cells stripped of cytoplasm in background) Loose clusters Papillary structures with fibrovascular cores Tight clusters Follicular-type (resembling thyroid follicles) arrangements Often a mix of these [30]	In 25 lesion series: Naked nuclei in 100% of cases; loose clusters in ~88%; papillary patterns in ~68%; follicular in ~44%
Nuclear features	Round to oval nuclei, generally regular Stippled or "salt-and-pepper" chromatin Mild to moderate anisokaryosis (variation in nuclear size) Eccentric nuclei rare Prominent nucleoli or intranuclear inclusions are uncommon but observed in a few cases [30]	Stippled chromatin in many cases; anisokaryosis present in majority; other features less frequent
Cytoplasmic features	Finely granular cytoplasm Oxyphilic cytoplasm in some lesions Well-defined cell borders (in some) Intracytoplasmic fat vacuoles (in some studies) [31]	Intracytoplasmic fat vacuolation: In one study ~53.3% sensitive, but very specific when present
Background features	Bare nuclei in the background Absence or scarcity of colloid (colloid-like material is more suggestive of thyroid) VASCULAR proliferation (capillaries, fibrovascular cores) Macrophages less common Sometimes "colloid-like" material may be misinterpreted when present [31]	The absence of background colloid and presence of vascular proliferation and bare nuclei, often help in discriminating parathyroid origin
Overlap/mimics	Papillary structures (with a fibrovascular core) can mimic thyroid papillary lesions Follicular patterns and colloid-like material may mislead toward thyroid follicular neoplasm or nodular goiter Tight clusters may simulate metastatic carcinoma Thyroid incidentalomas (intrathyroidal parathyroid tissue) complicate localization and interpretation [30]	

include high cellularity, scattered naked nuclei, cribriform and three-dimensional patterns, stippled chromatin, and oxyphilic cytoplasm (Table 4.2). The integration of these features with the FNA-PTH assay and/or GATA3, PTH, and chromogranin-A immunostains on cytologic specimens enhances the identification of parathyroid glands and helps differentiate parathyroid lesions from thyroid lesions [32].

Nonetheless, FNAC alone often has limitations: insufficient cellularity, contamination with thyroid tissue, presence of colloid or follicular structures that mimic thyroid lesions, etc. [33].

4.7 Method to Overcome the Limitations of Morphology Alone

1. *Parathyroid Hormone (PTH) Wash-out/FNA-PTH Assay:* The aspirate or needle-wash fluid is assayed for PTH. Elevated PTH levels in the wash-out compared to serum indicate a parathyroid origin, significantly improving sensitivity. This technique can be performed preoperatively under ultrasound guidance or intraoperatively. Index lesions are punctured 2–3 times with a 25-gauge syringe needle and

washed with 0.5 mL of normal saline to measure PTH levels. PTH concentrations were significantly higher in parathyroid tissues than in non-parathyroid tissues. Some authors reported that a PTH-FNA level of ≥100 pg/mL as a diagnostic test had a sensitivity of 93.7%, a specificity of 100%, a positive predictive value of 100%, and a negative predictive value of 71.4%. No complications were detected during or after the puncture, and no cases of parathyromatosis were identified [34]. The effectiveness of these methods decreased with the size of the thyroid gland, particularly when the thickness of the thyroid was ≥20 mm (50% vs. 87.5%, $p < 0.05$), and when the thickness of a lesion suspected of parathyroid pathology was ≤5 mm (66.7% vs. 93.3%, $p < 0.05$) [35].

2. *Immunocytochemistry/Cell Block-Based Staining*: Markers such as PTH, chromogranin A, GATA3, and/or negative thyroid markers such as thyroglobulin and TTF-1 are helpful. For instance, in some studies, all cytology-positive cases were chromogranin A positive, thyroglobulin negative [29].
3. *Radiologic and Clinical Correlation*: US findings (location posterior to thyroid, inferior location, intrathyroidal lesion, atypical localization), serum calcium and PTH levels, imaging (sestamibi, etc.) guide whether a given aspirate is likely parathyroid. Without these data, cytologic sensitivity drops significantly.

4.8 Diagnostic Pitfalls and Challenges

1. *Misdiagnoses*: Parathyroid lesions are often misinterpreted as thyroid follicular lesions, adenomatous goiter, benign thyroid nodules, or even metastatic carcinoma. In one series of 46 parathyroid lesions, about one-third were misdiagnosed initially [36].
2. *Insufficient cellularity*: Aspirates may be hypocellular, especially if the lesion is small or deep. Such samples are interpreted as nondiagnostic [33].
3. *Artifacts and Histologic Alterations from Prior FNA*: Prior FNAs may introduce fibrosis, hemorrhage, capsule distortion, pseudoinvasion, or implantation, which may confound later histologic assessment (especially when differentiating between benign adenoma, atypical adenoma, or carcinoma) [37].
4. *Overlap in Features*: Several cytologic features are shared between thyroid and parathyroid lesions (e.g., follicular architecture, presence of colloid-like material, papillary patterns). Thus, reliance on a single morphologic criterion is unsafe [31].
5. *Intrathyroidal Parathyroid Tissue*: When parathyroid tissue is located within thyroid parenchyma ("intrathyroidal parathyroid"), aspirates may sample intervening thyroid tissue, complicating interpretation [30].

4.9 Parathyroid Adenoma vs Hyperplasia vs Carcinoma in Cytology

Most studies find that cytology has a limited ability to distinguish between adenoma and hyperplasia reliably. Many morphologic features overlap. Features more suggestive of carcinoma include marked pleomorphism, irregular nuclear contours, prominent nucleoli, and increased mitotic activity, but these are rare and may only be evident on histology. Some series show that in cytology, carcinoma cases have more atypical features [33, 38].

4.10 Safety Considerations

FNA of suspected parathyroid lesions is generally safe, but histologic alterations resulting from FNA have been reported: fibrous bands, thickened capsule, pseudo-invasion, hemosiderin, etc. These may mimic malignant or atypical features on excision specimens. Recognizing the background of prior FNA is essential.

Risk of parathyromatosis (seeding of parathyroid tissue) is a theoretical concern, though literature suggests it's rare. However, to err from the side of safety, parathyroid FNA is discouraged in case of high pretest suspicious of parathyroid carcinoma as seeding of cancerous cells remains possible. Also, bleeding risk and patient discomfort should be considered [37].

4.11 Conclusion

Ultrasound is an excellent tool for evaluating PHPT. It offers numerous advantages, including low cost, high availability, no exposure to ionizing radiation, and effective visualization of neck morphology. In most cases, its sensitivity and specificity are comparable to those of other imaging techniques. However, interpretation requires expertise due to certain limitations, such as uncommon parathyroid gland features and locations, as well as the presence of various cervical structures and pathologies that can complicate the differential diagnosis of parathyroid diseases. Parathyroid cytology via fine-needle aspiration has a role in the diagnostic work-up of parathyroid lesions, particularly in challenging or ambiguous cases. While certain cytomorphologic features can indicate parathyroid origin, none are fully reliable on their own. The strength of this approach lies in integrating cytology with PTH wash-out assays, immunocytochemical markers, imaging, and clinical/laboratory data.

References

1. Morris MA, Saboury B, Ahlman M, Malayeri AA, Jones EC, Chen CC, et al. Parathyroid imaging: past, present, and future. Front Endocrinol (Lausanne). 2021;12:760419. https://doi.org/10.3389/fendo.2021.760419.
2. Park HS, Hong N, Jeong JJ, Yun M, Rhee Y. Update on preoperative parathyroid localization in primary hyperparathyroidism. Endocrinol Metab (Seoul). 2022;37(5):744–55. https://doi.org/10.3803/EnM.2022.1589.
3. Petranovic Ovcaricek P, Giovanella L, Carrio Gasset I, Hindie E, Huellner MW, Luster M, et al. The EANM practice guidelines for parathyroid imaging. Eur J Nucl Med Mol Imaging. 2021;48(9):2801–22. https://doi.org/10.1007/s00259-021-05334-y.
4. Elliott DD, Monroe DP, Perrier ND. Parathyroid histopathology: is it of any value today? J Am Coll Surg. 2006;203(5):758–65. https://doi.org/10.1016/j.jamcollsurg.2006.07.031.
5. Bunch PM, Randolph GW, Brooks JA, George V, Cannon J, Kelly HR. Parathyroid 4D CT: what the surgeon wants to know. Radiographics. 2020;40(5):1383–94. https://doi.org/10.1148/rg.2020190190.
6. Akerstrom G, Malmaeus J, Bergstrom R. Surgical anatomy of human parathyroid glands. Surgery. 1984;95(1):14–21.
7. Sawady J, Mendelsohn G, Sirota RL, Taxy JB. The intrathyroidal hyperfunctioning parathyroid gland. Mod Pathol. 1989;2(6):652–7.
8. Parikh AM, Suliburk JW, Moron FE. Imaging localization and surgical approach in the management of ectopic parathyroid adenomas. Endocr Pract. 2018;24(6):589–98. https://doi.org/10.4158/EP-2018-0003.
9. Amaral S, Rego T, Palha A, Carrilho N, Coutinho JM, Tavares P, et al. Preoperative location of parathyroid adenomas in primary hyperparathyroidism: the role of cervical Doppler ultrasound. Acta Medica Port. 2023;36(4):246–53. https://doi.org/10.20344/amp.18735.
10. Xia C, Zhu Q, Li Z, Hu M, Fang J, Zhong Q, et al. Study of the ultrasound appearance of the normal parathyroid using an intraoperative procedure. J Ultrasound Med. 2019;38(2):321–7. https://doi.org/10.1002/jum.14691.
11. Paik W, Lee JC, Noh BJ, Na DG. US features of the parathyroid glands: an intraoperative surgical specimen study. J Korean Soc Radiol. 2023;84(3):596–605. https://doi.org/10.3348/jksr.2022.0104.
12. Centello R, Sesti F, Feola T, Sada V, Pandozzi C, Di Serafino M, et al. The dark side of ultrasound imaging in parathyroid disease. J Clin Med. 2023;12(7) https://doi.org/10.3390/jcm12072487.
13. Ruda JM, Hollenbeak CS, Stack BC Jr. A systematic review of the diagnosis and treatment of primary hyperparathyroidism from 1995 to 2003. Otolaryngol Head Neck Surg. 2005;132(3):359–72. https://doi.org/10.1016/j.otohns.2004.10.005.
14. Sung JY. Parathyroid ultrasonography: the evolving role of the radiologist. Ultrasonography. 2015;34(4):268–74. https://doi.org/10.14366/usg.14071.
15. Kamaya A, Quon A, Jeffrey RB. Sonography of the abnormal parathyroid gland. Ultrasound Q. 2006;22(4):253–62. https://doi.org/10.1097/01.ruq.0000237260.33509.4f.
16. Mohammadi A, Moloudi F, Ghasemi-rad M. The role of colour Doppler ultrasonography in the preoperative localization of parathyroid adenomas. Endocr J.

2012;59(5):375–82. https://doi.org/10.1507/endocrj.ej11-0351.
17. Chandramohan A, Sathyakumar K, John RA, Manipadam MT, Abraham D, Paul TV, et al. Atypical ultrasound features of parathyroid tumours may bear a relationship to their clinical and biochemical presentation. Insights Imaging. 2014;5(1):103–11. https://doi.org/10.1007/s13244-013-0297-x.
18. Khot R, Santo ID d O, Shen L, Itani M, Sailer A, Kirsch JD, et al. US of the neck beyond the thyroid gland: parathyroid glands. Radiographics. 2025;45(6):e240182. https://doi.org/10.1148/rg.240182.
19. Azizi G, Piper K, Keller JM, Mayo ML, Puett D, Earp KM, et al. Shear wave elastography and parathyroid adenoma: a new tool for diagnosing parathyroid adenomas. Eur J Radiol. 2016;85(9):1586–93. https://doi.org/10.1016/j.ejrad.2016.06.009.
20. Isidori AM, Cantisani V, Giannetta E, Diacinti D, David E, Forte V, et al. Multiparametric ultrasonography and ultrasound elastography in the differentiation of parathyroid lesions from ectopic thyroid lesions or lymphadenopathies. Endocrine. 2017;57(2):335–43. https://doi.org/10.1007/s12020-016-1116-1.
21. Papavramidis TS, Chorti A, Pliakos I, Panidis S, Michalopoulos A. Parathyroid cysts: a review of 359 patients reported in the international literature. Medicine (Baltimore). 2018;97(28):e11399. https://doi.org/10.1097/md.0000000000011399.
22. Cappelli C, Rotondi M, Pirola I, De Martino E, Leporati P, Magri F, et al. Prevalence of parathyroid cysts by neck ultrasound scan in unselected patients. J Endocrinol Investig. 2009;32(4):357–9. https://doi.org/10.1007/BF03345727.
23. Shane E. Clinical review 122: parathyroid carcinoma. J Clin Endocrinol Metab. 2001;86(2):485–93. https://doi.org/10.1210/jcem.86.2.7207.
24. Liu J, Zhan WW, Zhou JQ, Zhou W. Role of ultrasound in the differentiation of parathyroid carcinoma and benign parathyroid lesions. Clin Radiol. 2020;75(3):179–84. https://doi.org/10.1016/j.crad.2019.10.004.
25. Nafisi Moghadam R, Amlelshahbaz AP, Namiranian N, Sobhan-Ardekani M, Emami-Meybodi M, Dehghan A, et al. Comparative diagnostic performance of ultrasonography and 99mTc-Sestamibi scintigraphy for parathyroid adenoma in primary hyperparathyroidism; systematic review and meta- analysis. Asian Pac J Cancer Prev. 2017;18(12):3195–200. https://doi.org/10.22034/APJCP.2017.18.12.3195.
26. Acin-Gandara D, Pereira-Perez F, Medina-Garcia M, Sebastian-Viana T. Factors influencing the sensitivity of ultrasound and gamma location of the parathyroid adenoma. Cir Esp (Engl Ed). 2020;98(1):18–25. https://doi.org/10.1016/j.ciresp.2019.09.002.
27. Pacini P, Polti G, Faggiano A, Giannetta E, Tarsitano MG, Cantisani V. Multiparametric ultrasound evaluation of a case of bilateral carotid body tumor. J Ultrasound. 2021;24(3):311–5. https://doi.org/10.1007/s40477-021-00581-z.
28. Jacobson JA, Middleton WD, Allison SJ, Dahiya N, Lee KS, Levine BD, et al. Ultrasonography of superficial soft-tissue masses: society of radiologists in ultrasound consensus conference statement. Radiology. 2022;304(1):18–30. https://doi.org/10.1148/radiol.211101.
29. Abati A, Skarulis MC, Shawker T, Solomon D. Ultrasound-guided fine-needle aspiration of parathyroid lesions: a morphological and immunocytochemical approach. Hum Pathol. 1995;26(3):338–43. https://doi.org/10.1016/0046-8177(95)90068-3.
30. Heo I, Park S, Jung CW, Koh JS, Lee SS, Seol H, et al. Fine needle aspiration cytology of parathyroid lesions. Korean J Pathol. 2013;47(5):466–71. https://doi.org/10.4132/KoreanJPathol.2013.47.5.466.
31. Kumari N, Mishra D, Pradhan R, Agarwal A, Krishnani N. Utility of fine-needle aspiration cytology in the identification of parathyroid lesions. J Cytol. 2016;33(1):17–21. https://doi.org/10.4103/0970-9371.175490.
32. Bakula-Zalewska E, Dlugosinska J, Stanek-Widera A, Goralski P, Galczynski J, Zylka A, et al. Fine needle aspiration biopsy of parathyroid; is it meaningful? A cytologic study of 81 cases with histological and clinical correlations. Cytopathology. 2024;35(3):362–70. https://doi.org/10.1111/cyt.13356.
33. Agarwal AM, Bentz JS, Hungerford R, Abraham D. Parathyroid fine-needle aspiration cytology in the evaluation of parathyroid adenoma: cytologic findings from 53 patients. Diagn Cytopathol. 2009;37(6):407–10. https://doi.org/10.1002/dc.21020.
34. Carral F, Jimenez AI, Tome M, Alvarez J, Diez A, Garcia C, et al. Safety and diagnostic performance of parathyroid hormone assay in fine-needle aspirate in suspicious parathyroid adenomas. Endocrinol Diabetes Nutr (Engl Ed). 2021;68(7):481–8. https://doi.org/10.1016/j.endien.2020.07.004.
35. Popowicz B, Klencki M, Sporny S, Jankiewicz-Wika J, Komorowski J, Pisarek H, et al. Usefulness of PTH measurements in FNAB washouts in the identification of pathological parathyroids–analysis of the factors that influence the effectiveness of this method. Endokrynol Pol. 2014;65(1):25–32. https://doi.org/10.5603/EP.2014.0004.
36. Ha HJ, Kim EJ, Kim JS, Shin MS, Noh I, Park S, et al. Major clues and pitfalls in the differential diagnosis of parathyroid and thyroid lesions using fine needle aspiration cytology. Medicina (Kaunas). 2020;56(11) https://doi.org/10.3390/medicina56110558.
37. Hirokawa M, Suzuki A, Higuchi M, Hayashi T, Kuma S, Miya A, et al. Histological alterations following fine-needle aspiration for parathyroid adenoma: incidence and diagnostic problems. Pathol Int. 2021;71(6):400–5. https://doi.org/10.1111/pin.13091.
38. Steen S, Hysek M, Zedenius J, Falhammar H, Juhlin CC. Cyto-morphological features of parathyroid lesions: fine-needle aspiration cytology series from an endocrine tumor referral center. Diagn Cytopathol. 2022;50(2):75–83. https://doi.org/10.1002/dc.24923.

Dual-Phase Parathyroid Scintigraphy

5

Alfredo Campennì, Rosaria Maddalena Ruggeri, Luca Giovanella, and Petra Petranović Ovčariček

Abbreviations

[11C]CH	[11C]2-hydroxy-N,N,N-trimethylethanamium
[11C]MET	L-[methyl-11C]methionine
[18F]FCH	N-[(18F)fluoromethyl]-2-hydroxy-N,N dimethylethanaminium
[18F]FCH	N-[(18F)fluoromethyl]-2-hydroxy-N,N dimethylethanaminium
[99mTc]Tc-MIBI	[99mTc]Tc-Methoxy-IsoButyl-Isonitrile
HPT	Hyperparathyroidism
LEHR	Low-energy high-resolution
MEN	Multiple endocrine neoplasia
MGD	Multiple-gland disease
NPV	Negative predictive value
nUS	Neck ultrasonography
PC	Parathyroid carcinoma
PET/CT	Positron emission tomography/computed tomography
PET/MRI	Positron emission tomography/magnetic resonance imaging
pHPT	Primary hyperparathyroidism
PPV	Positive predictive value
PTH	Parathyroid hormone
rHPT	Renal hyperparathyroidism
sHPT	Secondary hyperparathyroidism
SPECT	Single-photon emission computed tomography
SPECT/CT	Single-photon emission computed tomography/computed tomography

A. Campennì (✉)
Department of Biomedical and Dental Sciences and Morpho-Functional Imaging, University of Messina, Messina, Italy

Unit of Nuclear Medicine, University Hospital "Gaetano Martino", Messina, Italy
e-mail: acampenni@unime.it

R. M. Ruggeri
Endocrine Unit, Department of Human Pathology of Adulthood and Childhood DETEV, University of Messina, Messina, Italy
e-mail: rmruggeri@unime.it

L. Giovanella
Department of Nuclear Medicine, Gruppo Ospedaliero Moncucco SA, Clinica Moncucco, Lugano, Switzerland

Clinic for Nuclear Medicine, University Hospital of Zürich, Zürich, Switzerland
e-mail: luca.giovanella@moncucco.ch

P. Petranović Ovčariček
Department of Oncology and Nuclear Medicine, University Hospital Center Sestre Milosrdnice, Zagreb, Croatia

School of Medicine, University of Zagreb, Zagreb, Croatia
e-mail: p.petranovic@gmail.com

© The Author(s), under exclusive license to Springer Nature Switzerland AG 2026
P. Petranović Ovčariček et al. (eds.), *Parathyroid Imaging*,
https://doi.org/10.1007/978-3-032-14178-1_5

Definitions

1. Hyperparathyroidism (HPT): An endocrine disorder characterized by one or more hyperfunctioning parathyroid glands.
2. Primary Hyperparathyroidism (pHPT): The most frequent form of HPT, with hypercalcemia and elevated or inappropriately normal parathyroid hormone (PTH) levels; in rare cases, normocalcemic hyperparathyroidism is present.
3. Secondary Hyperparathyroidism (sHPT): A condition often associated with reduced vitamin D levels or chronic kidney disease, characterized by elevated PTH levels, hypocalcemia, and hyperphosphatemia.
4. Parathyroid Adenoma: A benign overgrowth of parathyroid tissue, accounting for 80–85% of primary hyperparathyroidism cases.
5. Parathyroid Hyperplasia: Multiple gland disorder affecting 15–20% of primary hyperparathyroidism cases and commonly seen in secondary hyperparathyroidism.
6. [^{99m}Tc]Tc-MIBI: Technetium-99 m hexakis-(2-methoxy-2-isobutyl isonitrile), a lipophilic cationic complex used as a radiotracer in parathyroid scintigraphy.
7. Dual-Phase Parathyroid Scintigraphy: An imaging technique using [^{99m}Tc]Tc-MIBI with image acquisition at early (10–15 min) and delayed (90–150 min) time points post-injection.
8. SPECT/CT: Single photon emission computed tomography/computed tomography, a hybrid imaging technique that combines functional ([^{99m}Tc]Tc-MIBI uptake) and anatomical information.
9. Differential Washout: The physiological principle exploited in dual-phase imaging, where [^{99m}Tc]Tc-MIBI washes out more slowly from hyperfunctioning parathyroid tissue than from normal thyroid tissue.

Learning Objectives

After studying this material, readers should be able to:

1. Explain the pathophysiology and classification of different types of hyperparathyroidism.
2. Describe the radiopharmaceutical characteristics of [^{99m}Tc]Tc-MIBI, including its uptake mechanism and biodistribution.
3. Outline the standard procedure for performing dual-phase parathyroid scintigraphy, including recommended activity, acquisition parameters, and imaging protocols.
4. Analyze and interpret dual-phase parathyroid scintigraphy images, recognizing patterns of normal distribution, hyperfunctioning parathyroid glands, and common causes of false-positive and false-negative results.
5. Compare the advantages and limitations of planar imaging versus SPECT and SPECT/CT in parathyroid imaging.
6. Identify patients for whom dual-phase parathyroid scintigraphy is appropriate as a first-line imaging technique and when alternative imaging methods should be considered.
7. Discuss the clinical significance of accurate preoperative localization of hyperfunctioning parathyroid glands in surgical planning.
8. Evaluate the comparative effectiveness of dual-phase parathyroid scintigraphy versus other imaging modalities in different clinical scenarios.

(continued)

9. Recognize potential pitfalls in image interpretation, including thyroid nodules, thyroiditis, and cervical lymphadenopathy.
10. Explain how patient-specific factors (multiglandular disease, prior neck surgery, thyroid abnormalities) affect the diagnostic performance of dual-phase parathyroid scintigraphy.

5.1 Introduction

Hyperparathyroidism (HPT) is a quite common endocrine disorder caused by one or more hyperfunctioning parathyroid glands. Primary hyperparathyroidism (pHPT) is the most frequent form of HPT, typically identified in postmenopausal women (female-to-male ratio 3–4:1) with hypercalcemia and parathyroid hormone (PTH) levels that can be either frankly increased (overt hyperparathyroidism) or inappropriately normal [8, 37, 46].

The prevalence of pHPT is estimated to be 1–7 cases per 1000 adults, while its incidence has significantly increased worldwide after a routine measurement of serum calcium levels has been introduced [17, 45].

pHPT is related to an overgrowth of parathyroid tissue [more frequently benign (i.e., parathyroid adenoma)] either as a single gland (80–85% of cases) or as a multiple gland disorder (i.e., parathyroid hyperplasia, 15–20% of cases). Noteworthy, parathyroid carcinoma (PC) should always be taken into account as a possible (even if rare) cause of pHPT, accounting up to 1% of all cases [1, 3].

Finally, pHPT is diagnosed as a sporadic disorder in most patients, but it can be observed as a part of genetic syndromes including multiple endocrine neoplasia (MEN) type 1, 2A, and 4, hyperparathyroidism-jaw tumor syndrome, familial isolated primary hyperparathyroidism, familial hypocalciuric hypercalcemia, and neonatal severe hyperparathyroidism [1, 7, 22, 36, 40].

In patients affected by chronic kidney disease, renal hyperparathyroidism (rHPT) is often one of the most common metabolic disorders [i.e., secondary hyperparathyroidism (sHPT)].

Multiple gland disorder (i.e., parathyroid hyperplasia) is the most common cause of sHPT that is usually diagnosed at first in 30–50% of patients with end-stage kidney disease, while, more rarely, a decreased serum vitamin D level can be the first cause of sHPT. The former (i.e., sHPT) is characterized by elevated parathyroid hormone (PTH) levels, hypocalcemia, reduced serum levels of vitamin D, and hyperphosphatemia [1, 11, 32, 50].

In patients with long-course renal failure, parathyroid hyperplasia, probably due to prolonged gland stimulation, can develop in autonomously secreting PTH, thus leading to hypercalcemia [5, 34, 43, 50].

The diagnosis of HPT, incidental in a not negligible number of patients (especially if affected by pHPT), is carried out through clinical evaluation for checking the presence (or not) of typical signs and/or symptoms (e.g., kidney stones, osteoporotic fractures) and laboratory tests [1].

Conversely, morphological [e.g., neck ultrasonography (nUS)] and/or functional [e.g., [^{99m}Tc]Tc-Methoxy-IsoButyl-Isonitrol ([^{99m}Tc]Tc-MIBI]) and/or choline PET/CT or PET/magnetic resonance imaging (MRI)] diagnostic imaging is used for the localization of hyperfunctioning parathyroid gland(s) only.

Radionuclide imaging is particularly useful for detecting ectopic parathyroids that cannot be visualized by nUS (e.g., mediastinal topography) or supernumerary gland(s) before a final therapy (i.e., surgery) is planned [14, 32, 39].

Additionally, radionuclide imaging can also be helpful in HPT patients (especially sHPT ones) in whom a revision surgery is required. In such cases, an association between different imaging studies is often necessary, as well as in patients with hyperparathyroidism affected by a genetic syndrome, such as multiple endocrine neoplasia type 1, 2, and 4 (MEN-1, MEN-2, and MEN-4). In these latter, [^{18}F]FCH PET/CT [or positron emission tomography/magnetic resonance imaging (PET/MRI)] or [^{11}C]methionine

($[^{11}C]$MET) PET/CT, or $[^{11}C]$choline ($[^{11}C]$CH) is often preferred to $[^{99m}Tc]$Tc-MIBI SPECT/CT due to their higher spatial resolution [9, 14, 32].

The correct preoperative localization is essential to reduce the duration of surgical approach that nowadays more frequently consists of minimally invasive parathyroidectomy associated with intraoperative PTH determination, especially in pHPT patients having a single lesion [32, 48].

Currently, $[^{99m}Tc]$Tc-MIBI scintigraphy in association with nUS represents the most widespread first-line preoperative imaging procedure used for localizing hyperfunctioning parathyroid gland(s). This combined approach is able to reach an overall sensitivity ranging from 81% to 95% which is especially obtained by $[^{99m}Tc]$Tc-MIBI [30, 32, 38].

In the case of negative first-line imaging approach, second-line imaging procedure can be performed using $[^{18}F]$FCH PET/CT, $[^{11}C]$MET PET/CT, or $[^{11}C]$CH. $[^{18}F]$FCH PET/CT is also considered (whenever possible) as an alternative first-line imaging procedure to reduce the risk of having false-negative results [4, 15, 32].

All in all, $[^{99m}Tc]$Tc-MIBI scintigraphy can be performed by two different methodological approach: dual-tracer parathyroid scintigraphy ($[^{99m}Tc]$Tc-MIBI + Na$[^{99m}Tc]$TcO$_4$ or Na$[^{123}I]$I) or dual-phase parathyroid scintigraphy.

The aim of the present chapter is to describe the radiopharmaceutical characteristics and methodological procedure to obtain $[^{99m}Tc]$Tc-MIBI dual-phase parathyroid scintigraphy. The correct image analysis as well as advantages and possible limits of the procedure will also be highlighted.

5.2 $[^{99m}Tc]$Tc-Hexakis-(2-Methoxy-2-Isobutyl Isonitrile) ($[^{99m}Tc]$Tc-MIBI): Characteristics and Biokinetics

Up to date, $[^{99m}Tc]$Tc-MIBI is the most worldwide used radiotracer for molecular parathyroid scintigraphy. It is a lipophilic cationic complex that, after intravenous administration, is able to accumulate in hyperfunctioning parathyroids due to their increased number of mitochondria, which is mainly related to the number of oxyphil cells. All in all, $[^{99m}Tc]$Tc-MIBI uptake and retention are also related to the phase of the cellular cycle, parathyroid blood supply, permeability of the capillary, serum calcium level, P-glycoprotein expression, and multidrug resistance (MDR) associated protein [2, 12, 32, 35]. $[^{99m}Tc]$Tc-MIBI crosses the cell membrane reversibly penetrating into the cytoplasm through thermodynamic driving forces and then irreversibly moving across mitochondria membrane by a different electrical gradient due to a high negative inner membrane electric potential [10, 32, 33].

$[^{99m}Tc]$Tc-MIBI is accumulated in both thyroid and parathyroid tissue even if its uptake per gram is greater in parathyroid than in thyroid parenchyma [27, 32].

Noteworthy, $[^{99m}Tc]$Tc-MIBI washout is usually faster from thyroid parenchyma than from hyperfunctioning parathyroid gland. Accordingly, the single-tracer dual-phase method is widely used to perform $[^{99m}Tc]$Tc-MIBI parathyroid scintigraphy [32].

Finally, being $[^{99m}Tc]$Tc-MIBI quickly removed from the blood after its administration, it is able to be also concentrated in muscles (e.g., heart), salivary glands, liver, and kidneys [27, 33].

5.3 Single-Tracer ([99mTc] Tc-MIBI) Dual-Phase Parathyroid Scintigraphy: Standard Procedure

$[^{99m}Tc]$Tc-MIBI SPECT/CT scintigraphy is currently considered as a cost-effective standard method for detecting hyperfunctioning parathyroid glands having a reported patient-based and lesion-based pooled detection rate (DR) of 88% in a meta-analysis including 1236 patients with pHPT [29, 41, 44]. However, its sensitivity is significantly lower in patients affected by multiglandular disease compared to those with single-gland disease [23, 26]. Medas and colleagues in a study including more than 200 patients with HPT (8% with MGD, 91.5% with single-gland disease, and 0.5% unknown) reported a sensitivity of [^{99m}Tc]Tc-MIBI for MGD of 26.7% vs. 92.6% for single-gland disease [23].

Dual-phase single-tracer parathyroid scintigraphy is obtained by acquiring planar images at two time points: 10–15 min and 90–150 min after intravenous [^{99m}Tc]Tc-MIBI administration. The administered [^{99m}Tc]Tc-MIBI activity ranges from 400 to 900 MBq, also depending on the patients' body mass. Additionally, nuclear medicine physicians should consider the prescription of tracer activity when SPECT or, ideally, SPECT/CT can be obtained instead of planar imaging.

Parathyroid imaging is performed using a gamma camera with a large field of view, equipped with low-energy, high-resolution (LEHR) parallel-hole collimators. The gamma camera field-of-view should always include the whole neck and the thoracic region, extending to the base of the heart, to avoid/reduce the risk of false-negative results due to ectopic parathyroid tissue.

The energy window should be set at 140 ± 10 keV, associated with both a magnification of 1.0 and a matrix size of 256 × 256 or, alternatively, 128 × 128.

Planar images must be acquired in anterior view, while right and left anterolateral views could be obtained if SPECT or, much better, SPECT/CT imaging cannot be performed. However, nowadays, it is recommended to perform at least a SPECT/CT study (i.e., hybrid imaging) including the body area between the skull base and the heart base since its diagnostic performance (especially in terms of sensitivity, specificity, and accuracy) is significantly superior to planar or stand-alone SPECT imaging, especially in patients with ectopic disease and/or altered neck anatomy [13, 18, 21, 32].

Up to date, there is not definitive evidence on the best timing to perform SPECT/CT imaging in hyperparathyroid patients. However, Wang and colleagues recently published a retrospective study on 17 patients affected by sHPT. Delayed SPECT/CT imaging was reported to have higher diagnostic performance than early-phase SPECT/CT, as it demonstrated a lower washout of [^{99m}Tc]Tc-MIBI from parathyroid lesions compared to the thyroid gland and a better tumor-to-background ratio [47].

Taking into account patients' body mass, nuclear medicine physicians should take care to use the lowest CT dose compatible with the diagnostic purpose whenever hybrid imaging is acquired [32].

5.4 Image Analysis

In dual-phase parathyroid scintigraphy, planar images should always be displayed simultaneously and inspected visually, comparing early and delayed images. A focal area of increased or maintained uptake on the delayed [^{99m}Tc]Tc-MIBI image compared to the early one is considered a positive finding for a hyperfunctioning parathyroid gland (Fig. 5.1) [32]. However, it is essential to consider that not all hyperfunctioning parathyroid glands retain the tracer. Accordingly, [^{99m}Tc]Tc-MIBI washout from parathyroid glands can be faster and might not be clearly identified on delayed images. A faster tracer washout is more common in patients with hyperparathyroidism due to hyperplastic glands (e.g., patients affected by renal failure). Therefore, in such cases, other protocols might be helpful, being reasonable to perform additional images between the standard early (i.e., +10–15 min) and late phase ones (i.e., +90–150 min) [28, 32].

SPECT images may detect hyperfunctioning parathyroid glands that were not seen on planar images (i.e., increased sensitivity). Additionally, CT imaging provides more precise anatomic localization compared with planar images or SPECT images stand-alone (i.e., increased specificity) (Fig. 5.2).

Notably, hybrid imaging should also be analyzed for the presence of different but important findings, even if they are not related to the purpose of the study (Fig. 5.3) [32].

Nuclear medicine physicians evaluating dual-phase single-tracer parathyroid scintigraphy

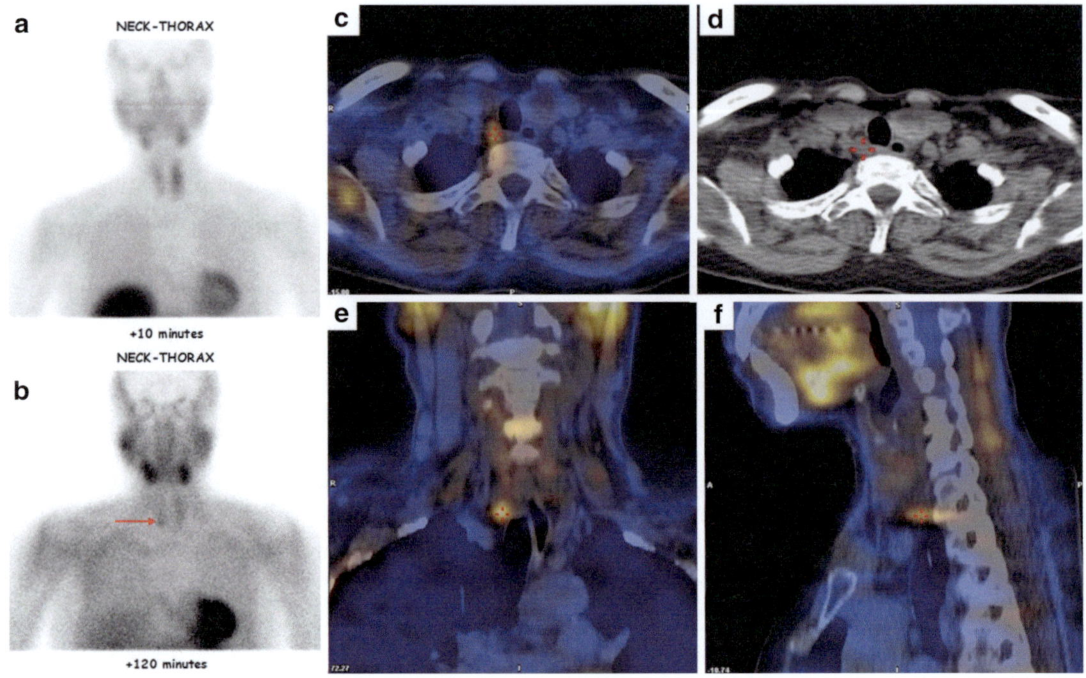

Fig. 5.1 In a female patient (66 years old) affected by moderate-to-severe osteoporosis, laboratory test was consistent with primary hyperparathyroidism (pHPT): intact parathyroid hormone (iPTH) = 134 pg/mL [normal value (n.v.): 15–65]; calcium 11.4 mg/dL (n.v.: 8.2–10.4); phosphorus 2.5 mg/dL (n.v.: 2.5–4.6); vit. D3 = 28 ng/dL (n.v.: 30–100). Neck ultrasound showed a thyroid gland of increased volume and multinodular features. A hypoechoic nodule (18 × 8 × 13 mm) with regular borders was noted just behind the lower pole of the right thyroid lobe. No increased blood flow was noted in such a nodule, as well as no additional suspicious nodules consistent with parathyroid disorders were reported. Dual-phase parathyroid scintigraphy was performed, administering [^{99m}Tc]Tc-MIBI (i.e., molecular imaging) and using a gamma camera equipped with low-energy high-resolution parallel-hole collimators focused on the body area between the skull and the heart base. Planar parathyroid images (panels A and B) were obtained 10 and 120 min after [^{99m}Tc]Tc-MIBI administration (400 MBq). The early (panel A) planar image did not show any abnormal tracer uptake consistent with parathyroid disease, both in typical and ectopic sites. Conversely, a focal area of abnormal but slight ([^{99m}Tc]Tc-MIBI) uptake was noted at the late planar image (panel B) in the correspondence of the lower pole of the right thyroid lobe (red arrow). Panel C, D, E, and F: Single-photon emission computed tomography/computed tomography (SPECT/CT) imaging was acquired 120 min after [^{99m}Tc]Tc-MIBI administration. Axial (panel C), coronal (panel E), and sagittal (panel F) images confirmed an abnormal tracer uptake involving a solid lesion (panel D) located just below and behind with respect to the lower pole of the right thyroid lobe (red cross-marks). The patient underwent parathyroidectomy of the right parathyroid gland. The histopathological report was consistent with a parathyroid adenoma, characterized by a predominant component of oxyphil cells. After parathyroid surgery, serum levels of both iPTH and calcium went back into normal range [49.8 pg/mL (n.v.: 15–65) and 9.2 mg/dL (n.v.: 8.4–10.2), respectively]

should always consider that false-positive or false-negative results can be occasionally encountered. Inflammatory thyroiditis, cervical lymphadenopathy, and thyroid nodules (benign and malignant) represent the most common causes of false-positive results [20, 32].

Conversely, false-negative results usually occur due to small-sized hyperfunctioning glands (e.g., parathyroid hyperplasia due to renal failure), multinodular thyroid disease, lack of oxyphil cells, and high expression of P-glycoprotein [6, 20, 24, 32].

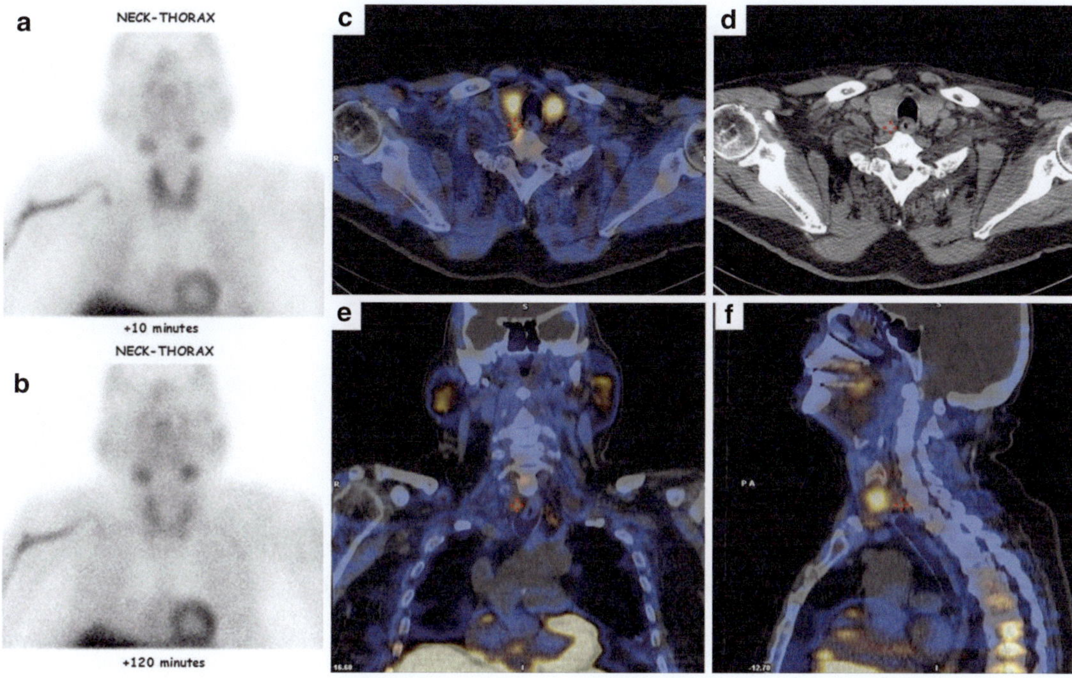

Fig. 5.2 In a male patient (76 years old) affected by renal stones and severe osteoporosis, laboratory test was consistent with primary hyperparathyroidism (pHPT): intact parathyroid hormone (iPTH) = 148 pg/mL [normal value (n.v.): 15–65)]; calcium = 12.8 mg/dL (n.v.: 8.2–10.4); Vit. D3 = 15 ng/dL (n.v.: 30–100). The neck ultrasound revealed an enlarged thyroid gland with multinodular features, particularly affecting the right lobe. Conversely, the neck ultrasound did not reveal any nodular lesions consistent with parathyroid disease. Dual-phase parathyroid scintigraphy was performed, administering [^{99m}Tc]Tc-MIBI) (i.e., molecular imaging and using a gamma camera equipped with low-energy high-resolution parallel-hole collimators focused on the body area between the skull and the heart base. Planar parathyroid images (panels A and B) were obtained 10 and 120 min after [^{99m}Tc]Tc-MIBI administration (400 MBq). Early (panel A) and late (panel B) planar images did not show any abnormal tracer uptake consistent with parathyroid disease, both in typical and ectopic sites. Panel C, D, E, and F: Single-photon emission computed tomography/computed tomography (SPECT/CT) imaging was acquired 120 min after [^{99m}Tc]Tc-MIBI administration. Axial (panel C), coronal (panel E), and sagittal (panel F) images showed an abnormal tracer uptake involving a solid lesion (panel D) located just behind the middle-lower part of the right thyroid lobe (red cross-marks). The patient underwent parathyroidectomy of the right parathyroid gland. The histopathological report was consistent with parathyroid adenoma, characterized by the presence of both typical and oxyphil cells. After parathyroid surgery, serum level of both iPTH and calcium went back into normal range [32.4 pg/mL (n.v.: 15–65) and 9.0 mg/dL (n.v.: 8.4–10.2), respectively]

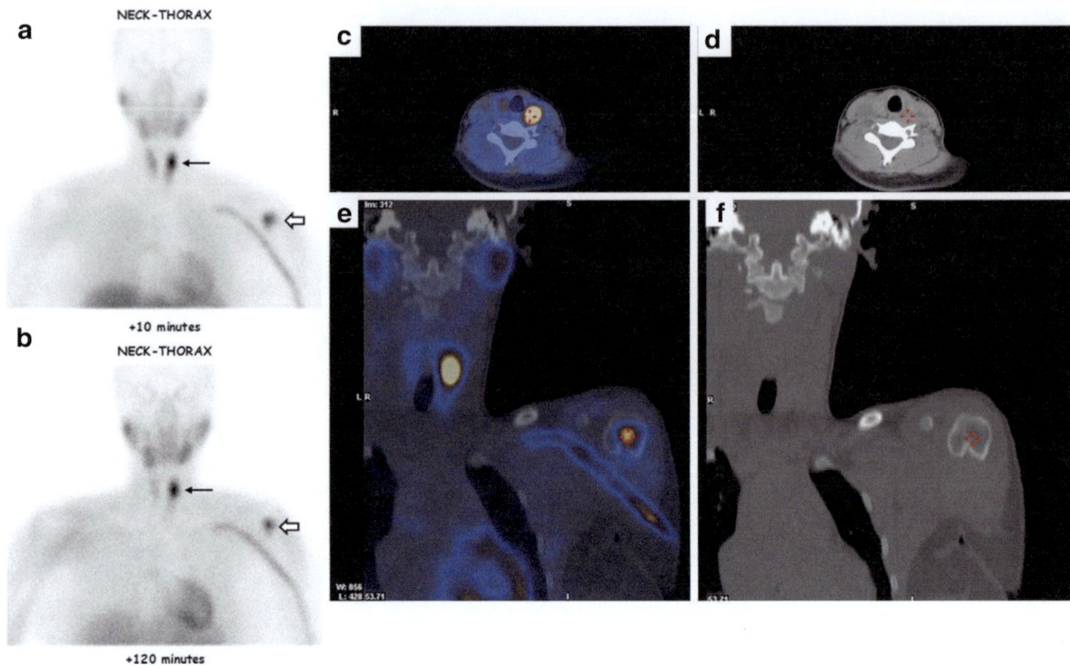

Fig. 5.3 In a young female patient (30 years old) affected by Hashimoto's thyroiditis and nephrolithiasis, nUS showed a hypoechoic and hypervascular nodule suspicious of being a focal parathyroid lesion located behind the upper part of the left thyroid lobe. Laboratory test was consistent with primary hyperparathyroidism (pHPT): intact parathyroid hormone (iPTH) = 300 pg/mL [normal value (n.v.): 15–65]; calcium 11.7 mg/dL (n.v.: 8.2–10.4). Dual-phase parathyroid scintigraphy was performed, administering [^{99m}Tc]Tc-Methoxy-IsoButyl-Isonitrol ([^{99m}Tc]Tc-MIBI) (i.e., molecular imaging) and using a gamma camera equipped with low-energy high-resolution parallel-hole collimators focused on the body area between the skull and the heart base. Planar parathyroid images were obtained 10 and 120 min after [^{99m}Tc]Tc-MIBI administration (400 MBq) (panels A and B, respectively). Abnormal and intense tracer uptake was noted at early (panel A) and late (panel B) planar images in correspondence of the upper part of the left thyroid lobe (black arrows). In addition, an abnormal [^{99m}Tc]Tc-MIBI uptake was noted at the level of the left shoulder. Panel C, D, E, and F: Single-photon emission computed tomography/computed tomography (SPECT/CT) imaging was acquired 120 min after [^{99m}Tc]Tc-MIBI administration. Axial images (panel C) showed an abnormal tracer uptake involving a solid lesion (panel D) located behind the medium-upper part of the left thyroid lobe (red cross-marks). Coronal images (panel E, F) confirmed an abnormal [^{99m}Tc]Tc-MIBI uptake in a hypodense area, with irregular borders, involving the head of the left humerus. The lesion was then confirmed by magnetic resonance (MR) as a brown tumor

5.5 Advantages and Limits

The primary advantage of dual-phase single-tracer parathyroid scintigraphy is its high sensitivity in detecting parathyroid lesions, particularly in patients with pHPT. Additionally, it can be easily performed worldwide with minimal discomfort for patients. Practical limitations include detection of multiglandular disease (i.e., hyperparathyroidism due to hyperplasia), small parathyroids, or focal parathyroid lesions with a reduced number of oxyphil cells. Therefore, PET/CT imaging with tracers such as ^{18}F-labeled choline analogues could be considered, whenever possible, as a potential alternative first-line imaging method. Indeed, the higher resolution of PET/CT imaging and the different mechanism of tracer uptake could improve the detection of the smallest parathyroid lesions, as well as those with a high prevalence of chief cells [32, 42].

On the contrary, the limit related to early washout from parathyroid lesion (i.e., false-negative results) or late tracer washout from thyroid parenchyma (i.e., thyroid "hot" or malignant nodules) producing false-positive results at planar images can be avoided by using hybrid imaging and fine-needle aspiration cytology (FNAC) in selected cases [32].

All in all, dual-phase double-tracer (i.e., [^{99m}Tc]Tc-MIBI + Na[^{99m}Tc]TcO$_4$ or Na[^{123}I]I) parathyroid scintigraphy with subtraction could be considered in patients affected by multinodular thyroid disease since it showed better diagnostic performance [in terms of sensitivity, positive predictive value (PPV), specificity, and negative predictive value (NPV)] than dual-phase single-tracer parathyroid scintigraphy, allowing also to identify associated thyroid disease [19, 49]. Pattou et al. and more recently Kettle et al. suggested using Na[^{123}I]I instead of Na[^{99m}Tc]TcO$_4$ when the subtraction method is used, since there are fewer movement correction issues [16, 31].

However, dual-tracer parathyroid scintigraphy may result in a higher radiation burden to the thyroid gland compared to the dual-phase single-tracer method, although some institutions are reducing the required activities. Additionally, it is more expensive and may require extra time when performed in a dual-day, double-tracer strategy with Na[^{99m}Tc]TcO$_4$ [32].

Notably, in the case of suspicion of intrathyroidal lesion, FNAC with measurement of PTH in the aspirate can be performed [25].

5.6 Conclusion

Dual-phase parathyroid scintigraphy using [^{99m}Tc]Tc-MIBI has established itself as a widely utilized and effective first-line imaging method for localizing hyperfunctioning parathyroid glands. Its clinical utility is particularly valuable in patients with pHPT, where accurate preoperative localization can significantly impact surgical planning and outcomes. The technique leverages the differential washout of the radiopharmaceutical between thyroid and parathyroid tissue, with the latter typically showing increased retention on delayed images.

The method offers several advantages, including worldwide availability, relatively straightforward protocol, and good diagnostic performance, particularly when coupled with SPECT/CT for improved anatomical localization. Modern hybrid imaging substantially enhances diagnostic confidence by providing precise anatomical correlation of functional findings.

Despite its strengths, the technique has recognized limitations, including lower sensitivity in cases of multiglandular disease, hyperplasia, and glands with reduced oxyphil cell content. Additionally, false-positive results may occur due to thyroid pathology such as nodules or thyroiditis. Integrating neck ultrasonography as a complementary modality helps overcome some of these limitations. Dual-tracer [^{99m}Tc]Tc-MIBI, although requires a more complex protocol with higher cost, demonstrates superior performance in challenging cases and is less affected by thyroid abnormalities.

PET imaging with tracers such as ^{18}F-labeled choline analogues shows exceptional performance. Cost-effectiveness studies, such as the one by van Mossel et al., provide valuable insights into the economic implications of different imaging strategies, suggesting that while the one-stop-shop [^{18}F]FCH PET/CT approach provides excellent results, it may require a tariff adjustment to be more cost-effective than conventional approaches.

As imaging technologies continue to evolve, the selection of the optimal imaging protocol should be tailored to patient characteristics, institutional resources, and cost considerations. The primary goal is to enable successful surgical treatment with minimal complications and optimal outcomes for patients with hyperparathyroidism.

Declaration of Competing Interest The authors have no conflict of interest to declare.

Ethical Approval Not applicable.

References

1. Bilezikian JP, Bandeira L, Khan A, Cusano NE. Hyperparathyroidism. Lancet. 2018;391:168–78. https://doi.org/10.1016/S0140-6736(17)31430-7.
2. Carpentier A, Jeannotte S, Verreault J, et al. Preoperative localization of parathyroid lesions in hyperparathyroidism: relationship between

technetium-99mMIBI uptake and oxyphil cell content. J Nucl Med. 1998;39:1441–4. PMID: 9708524
3. Cetani F, Marcocci C. Parathyroid carcinoma. In: Bilezikian JP, Marcus R, Levine MA, Marcocci C, Silverberg SJ, Potts Jr JT, editors. The parathyroids. 3rd ed. USA: Elsevier; 2015. p. 409–22.
4. Chen Y-H, Chen H-T, Lee M-C, et al. Preoperative F-18 fluorocholine PET/CT for the detection of hyperfunctioning parathyroid glands in patients with secondary or tertiary hyperparathyroidism: comparison with Tc-99m sestamibi scan and neck ultrasound. Ann Nucl Med. 2020;1–11 https://doi.org/10.1007/s12149-020-01479-2.25.
5. Dream S, Kuo LE, Kuo JH, et al. The American Association of Endocrine Surgeons Guidelines for the definitive surgical Management of Secondary and Tertiary Renal Hyperparathyroidism. Ann Surg. 2022;276:e141–76. https://doi.org/10.1097/SLA.0000000000005522.
6. Eslamy HK, Ziessman HA. Parathyroid scintigraphy in patients with primary hyperparathyroidism: 99mTc Sestamibi SPECT and SPECT/CT. Radio Graphics. 2008;28:1461–76. https://doi.org/10.1148/rg.285075055.
7. Friedman E, Sakaguchi K, Bale AE, et al. Clonality of parathyroid tumors in familial multiple endocrine neoplasia type 1. N Engl J Med. 1989;321(4):213–8. https://doi.org/10.1056/NEJM198907273210402.
8. Gasser RW. clinical aspects of primary hyperparathyroidism: clinical manifestations, diagnosis, and therapy. Wien Med Wochenschr. 2013;163(17–18):397–402. https://doi.org/10.1007/s10354-013-0235-z.
9. Gauthé M, Dierick-Gallet A, Delbot T, et al. 18F-fluorocholine PET/CT in MEN1 patients with primary hyperparathyroidism. World J Surg. 2020;44(11):3761–9. https://doi.org/10.1007/s00268-020-05695-9.
10. Giovanella L, Trimboli P, Campennì A, et al. Thyroid and parathyroid cancer. In: Multimodality imaging and intervention in oncology. Springer; 2023. https://doi.org/10.1007/978-3-031-28524-0_5.
11. Hedgeman E, Lipworth L, Lowe K, Saran R, Do T, Fryzek J. International burden of chronic kidney disease and secondary hyperparathyroidism: a systematic review of the literature and available data. Int J Nephrol. 2015;2015:184321. https://doi.org/10.1155/2015/184321.
12. Hetrakul N, Civelek AC, Stagg CA, Udelsman R. In vitro accumulation of technetium-99m-sestamibi in human parathyroid mitochondria. Surgery. 2001;130(6):1011–8. https://doi.org/10.1067/msy.2001.118371.
13. Hindié E, Ugur Ö, Fuster D, et al. 2009 EANM parathyroid guidelines. Eur J Nucl Med Mol Imaging. 2009;36(7):1201–16. https://doi.org/10.1007/s00259-009-1131-z.
14. Hindié E, Ureña-Torres PA, Taïeb D. Parathyroid imaging in patients with renal hyperparathyroidism. In: Parathyroid glands in chronic kidney disease. Cham: Springer International Publishing; 2020. p. 35–49. https://doi.org/10.1007/978-3-030-43769-5_3.
15. Huellner MW, Aberle S, Sah B-R, et al. Visualization of parathyroid hyperplasia using 18F-fluorocholine PET/MR in a patient with secondary hyperparathyroidism. Clin Nucl Med. 2016;41(3):e159–61. https://doi.org/10.1097/RLU.0000000000001053.
16. Kettle AG, O'Doherty MJ. Parathyroid imaging: how good is it and how should it be done? Semin Nucl Med. 2006;36(3):206–11. https://doi.org/10.1053/j.semnuclmed.2006.03.003.
17. Kim KJ, Baek S, Yu MH, et al. Secular trends in the incidence and treatment patterns of primary hyperparathyroidism in Korea: a nationwide cohort study. JBMR Plus. 2024;8(7):ziae065. Published 2024 May 13. https://doi.org/10.1093/jbmrpl/ziae065.
18. Krausz Y, Bettman L, Guralnik L, et al. Technetium-99m-MIBI SPECT/CT in primary hyperparathyroidism. World J Surg. 2006;30(1):76–83. https://doi.org/10.1007/s00268-005-7849-2.
19. Krakauer M, Wieslander B, Myschetzky PS, et al. A prospective comparative study of parathyroid dual-phase scintigraphy, dual-isotope subtraction scintigraphy, 4D-CT, and ultrasonography in primary hyperparathyroidism. Clin Nucl Med. 2016;41(2):93–100. https://doi.org/10.1097/RLU.0000000000000988.
20. Kunstman JW, Kirsch JD, Mahajan A, Udelsman R. Parathyroid localization and implications for clinical management. J Clin Endocrinol Metab. 2013;98(3):902–12. https://doi.org/10.1210/jc.2012-3168.
21. Lavely WC, Goetze S, Friedman KP, et al. Comparison of SPECT/CT, SPECT, and planar imaging with single- and dual-phase (99m)Tc-sestamibi parathyroid scintigraphy. J Nucl Med. 2007;48(7):1084–9. https://doi.org/10.2967/jnumed.107.040428.
22. Marx SJ. Hyperparathyroid and hypoparathyroid disorders. N Engl J Med. 2000;343(25):1863–75. https://doi.org/10.1056/NEJM200012213432508.
23. Medas F, Erdas E, Longheu A, et al. Retrospective evaluation of the pre- and postoperative factors influencing the sensitivity of localization studies in primary hyperparathyroidism. Int J Surg. 2016;25:82–7. https://doi.org/10.1016/j.ijsu.2015.11.045.
24. Melloul M, Paz A, Koren R, Cytron S, Feinmesser R, Gal R. 99mTc-MIBI scintigraphy of parathyroid adenomas and its relation to tumour size and oxyphil cell abundance. Eur J Nucl Med. 2001;28(2):209–13. https://doi.org/10.1007/s002590000406.
25. Morris MA, Saboury B, Ahlman M, et al. Parathyroid imaging: past, present, and future. Front Endocrinol (Lausanne). 2022;12:760419. https://doi.org/10.3389/fendo.2021.760419.
26. Nichols KJ, Tomas MB, Tronco GG, Palestro CJ. Sestamibi parathyroid scintigraphy in multigland disease. Nucl Med Commun. 2012;33(1):43–50. https://doi.org/10.1097/MNM.0b013e32834bfeb1.
27. O'Doherty MJ, Kettle AG, Wells P, Collins REC, Coakley AJ. Parathyroid imaging with technetium-

99m-sestamibi: preoperative localization and tissue uptake studies. J Nucl Med. 1992;33(3):313–8.
28. Palestro CJ, Tomas MB, Tronco GG. Radionuclide imaging of the parathyroid glands. Semin Nucl Med. 2005;35(4):266–76. https://doi.org/10.1053/j.semnuclmed.2005.06.001.
29. Pata G, Casella C, Magri GC, et al. Financial and clinical implications of low-energy CT combined with 99mtechnetium-sestamibi SPECT for primary hyperparathyroidism. Ann Surg Oncol. 2011;18:2555–63. https://doi.org/10.1245/s10434-011-1641-3.
30. Patel CN, Salahudeen HM, Lansdown M, Scarsbrook AF. Clinical utility of ultrasound and 99mTc sestamibi SPECT/CT for preoperative localization of parathyroid adenoma in patients with primary hyperparathyroidism. Clin Radiol. 2010;65(4):278–87. https://doi.org/10.1016/j.crad.2009.12.005.
31. Pattou F, Huglo D, Proye C. Radionuclide scanning in parathyroid diseases. Br J Surg. 1998;85(12):1605–16. https://doi.org/10.1046/j.1365-2168.1998.00942.x.
32. Petranović Ovčariček P, Giovanella L, Carrió Gasset I, et al. The EANM practice guidelines for parathyroid imaging. Eur J Nucl Med Mol Imaging. 2021;48:2801–22. https://doi.org/10.1007/s00259-021-05334-y.
33. Petranović Ovčariček P, Calderoni L, Campenni A, Fanti S, Giovanella L. Molecular imaging of thyroid and parathyroid diseases. Expert Rev Endocrinol Metab. 2024;19:317–33. https://doi.org/10.1080/17446651.2024.2365776.
34. Pitt SC, Sippel RS, Chen H. Secondary and tertiary hyperparathyroidism, state of the art surgical management. Surg Clin North Am. 2009;89:1227–39. https://doi.org/10.1016/j.suc.2009.06.011.
35. Pons F, Torregrosa JV, Fuster D. Biological factors influencing parathyroid localization. Nucl Med Commun. 2003;24(2):121–4. https://doi.org/10.1097/00006231-200302000-00003.
36. Ruggeri RM, Benevento E, De Cicco F, et al. Multiple endocrine neoplasia type 4 (MEN4): a thorough update on the latest and least known MEN syndrome. Endocrine. 2023;82:480–90. https://doi.org/10.1007/s12020-023-03497-2.
37. Silva BC, Cusano NE, Bilezikian JP. Primary hyperparathyroidism. Best Pract Res Clin Endocrinol Metab. 2024;38(1):101247. https://doi.org/10.1016/j.beem.2018.09.013.
38. Sukan A, Reyhan M, Aydin M, et al. Preoperative evaluation of hyperparathyroidism: the role of dual-phase parathyroid scintigraphy and ultrasound imaging. Ann Nucl Med. 2008;22(2):123–31. https://doi.org/10.1007/s12149-007-0086-z.
39. Taïeb D, Ureña-Torres P, Zanotti-Fregonara P, et al. Parathyroid scintigraphy in renal hyperparathyroidism: the added diagnostic value of SPECT and SPECT/CT. Clin Nucl Med. 2013;38(8):630–5. https://doi.org/10.1097/RLU.0b013e31829af5bf.
40. Thakker RV, Bouloux P, Wooding C, et al. Association of parathyroid tumors in multiple endocrine neoplasia type 1 with loss of alleles on chromosome 11. N Engl J Med. 1989;321(4):218–24. https://doi.org/10.1056/NEJM198907273210403.
41. Treglia G, Sadeghi R, Schalin-Jäntti C, et al. Detection rate of 99m Tc-MIBI single photon emission computed tomography (SPECT)/CT in preoperative planning for patients with primary hyperparathyroidism: a metaanalysis. Head Neck. 2016;38(S1):E2159–72. https://doi.org/10.1002/hed.2402757.
42. Treglia G, Piccardo A, Imperiale A, et al. Diagnostic performance of choline PET for detection of hyperfunctioning parathyroid glands in hyperparathyroidism: a systematic review and meta-analysis. Eur J Nucl Med Mol Imaging. 2019;46(3):751–65. https://doi.org/10.1007/s00259-018-4123-z.
43. Van der Plas WY, Noltes ME, van Ginhoven TM, Kruijff S. Secondary and tertiary hyperparathyroidism: a narrative review. Scand J Surg. 2020;109(4):271–8. https://doi.org/10.1177/1457496919866015.
44. Van Mossel S, Saing S, Appelman-Dijkstra N, et al. Cost-effectiveness of one-stop-shop [18F] Fluorocholine PET/CT to localise parathyroid adenomas in patients suffering from primary hyperparathyroidism. Eur J Nucl Med Mol Imaging. 2024;51(12):3585–95. https://doi.org/10.1007/s00259-024-06771-1.
45. Yeh MW, Ituarte PH, Zhou HC, et al. Incidence and prevalence of primary hyperparathyroidism in a racially mixed population. J Clin Endocrinol Metab. 2013;98(3):1122–9. https://doi.org/10.1210/jc.2012-4022.
46. Yu N, Donnan PT, Murphy MJ, Leese GP. Epidemiology of primary hyperparathyroidism in Tayside, Scotland, UK. Clin Endocrinol (Oxf). 2009;71(4):485–93. https://doi.org/10.1111/j.1365-2265.2008.03520.x.
47. Wang Y, Liu Y, Li N, Xu K, Zhang W. Quantitative application of dual-phase 99mTc-sestamibi SPECT/CT imaging of parathyroid lesions: identification of optimal timing in secondary hyperparathyroidism. EJNMMI Phys. 2023;10(1):29. https://doi.org/10.1186/s40658-023-00548-5.
48. Wilhelm SM, Wang TS, Ruan DT, et al. The American Association of Endocrine Surgeons guidelines for definitive management of primary hyperparathyroidism. JAMA Surg. 2016;151(10):959–68. https://doi.org/10.1001/jamasurg.2016.2310.
49. Woods AM, Bolster AA, Han S, et al. Dual-isotope subtraction SPECT-CT in parathyroid localization. Nucl Med Commun. 2017;38(12):1047–54. https://doi.org/10.1097/MNM.0000000000000765.
50. Zhang JLH, Appelman-Dijkstra NM, Fu EL, et al. Practice variation in the treatment of patients with renal hyperparathyroidism: a survey-based study in The Netherlands. BMC Nephrol. 2021;22(1):150. Published 2021 Apr 23. https://doi.org/10.1186/s12882-021-02361-7.

6 Dual-Tracer Parathyroid Scintigraphy in the Era of 18F-Fluorocholine PET

David Taïeb and Elif Hindié

▶ **Definition** *Parathyroid scintigraphy* is a nuclear medicine imaging technique used to localize hyperfunctioning parathyroid tissue(s) in the context of primary and renal hyperparathyroidism. It may rely on the differential uptake and washout characteristics of 99mTc-MIBI between thyroid and parathyroid tissue or on eliminating background thyroid activity by using a second thyroid-specific agent such as iodine-123 (123I)—the latter offering higher sensitivity. The purpose of these techniques is not to establish the diagnosis of hyperparathyroidism, but to guide surgical strategy, facilitating minimally invasive approaches and avoiding unnecessary exploration.

Learning Objectives

- Understand why imaging should not precede the diagnosis of primary hyperparathyroidism (PHPT).
- Clarify the specific role of imaging in preoperative planning.
- Know the principles of parathyroid scintigraphy and the superiority of the iodine-123I/99mTc-MIBI subtraction technique over the dual-phase method.
- Recognize that the systematic use of choline PET as a first-line approach can be justified when the parathyroid scintigraphy protocol is suboptimal.
- Be aware that normocalcemic PHPT remains a diagnostic challenge for all imaging modalities.

Disclosure summary: DT is a cofounder, stakeholder, and the chief medical officer (CMO) of SILON Therapeutics.

D. Taïeb (✉)
Department of Nuclear Medicine, La Timone Hospital, Aix-Marseille University, Marseille, France
e-mail: david.taieb@ap-hm.fr

E. Hindié
Department of Nuclear Medicine, Bordeaux University Hospital, Bordeaux, France
e-mail: Elif.hindie@chu-bordeaux.fr

6.1 Why Should the Diagnostic Step Come Before Imaging?

Primary hyperparathyroidism (PHPT) affects about 1 in 1000 individuals, with prevalence rising to around 2% in postmenopausal women. It is caused by the autonomous overproduction of parathyroid hormone (PTH) from one or more abnormal glands. In more than 80% of cases, the culprit is a single parathyroid adenoma—a monoclonal tumor often linked to mutations in genes

© The Author(s), under exclusive license to Springer Nature Switzerland AG 2026

P. Petranović Ovčariček et al. (eds.), *Parathyroid Imaging*,
https://doi.org/10.1007/978-3-032-14178-1_6

controlling parathyroid cell growth. Multiple gland disease, present in up to 15–20% of cases, may result from multiple adenomas—either sporadic or related to prior neck irradiation—or from parathyroid hyperplasia [1–3]. PHPT can be observed in hereditary diseases such as *MEN 1* (menin gene *MEN1* mutation), *MEN 2A* (*RET* oncogene mutation), MEN 4 (*CDKN1B* mutation), and hyperparathyroidism-jaw tumor (*HRPT2/CDC73* mutation; risk of parathyroid carcinoma) syndromes [4]. Hyperplasia can occur sporadically or as part of Multiple Endocrine Neoplasia type 1 (MEN1), in which case genetic screening is essential.

The cornerstone of management is a secure biochemical diagnosis before any imaging is performed. PHPT is defined by elevated serum calcium in association with increased or inappropriately normal PTH levels. PHPT should only be diagnosed after excluding secondary causes of hypercalcemia or elevated PTH [5]. Crucially, familial hypocalciuric hypercalcemia (FHH) must be distinguished from PHPT to avoid unnecessary surgery [6]. FHH is an autosomal dominant condition producing lifelong mild to moderate asymptomatic hypercalcemia, with inappropriately normal or elevated PTH and low urinary calcium excretion—most often a calcium-to-creatinine clearance ratio (CCCR) <0.01. Genetic testing can confirm the diagnosis.

By establishing the biochemical and differential diagnosis first, clinicians ensure that subsequent imaging is both justified and accurately interpreted, avoiding inappropriate interventions.

6.2 Why Does Preoperative Imaging Matter?

In humans, the parathyroid glands originate from the third and fourth pharyngeal pouches. The third pouch gives rise to the thymus and the inferior parathyroid glands (PIII-derived), while the fourth pouch forms the superior parathyroid glands (PIV-derived). During development, the PIII-derived glands migrate along with the thymus, and the PIV-derived glands follow the ultimobranchial bodies. Anatomically, inferior parathyroid glands are typically located at the posterolateral aspect of the lower thyroid poles or along the thyrothymic tract. In contrast, the superior glands are usually found posterior to the recurrent laryngeal nerve and above the inferior thyroid artery, on the posteromedial surface of the thyroid lobes. Normal parathyroid glands are approximately lentil-sized, with an individual weight ranging from 35 to 50 mg. Parathyroid lesions can develop from glands located in their normal anatomical position (eutopic) or from ectopic glands due to abnormal migration during embryogenesis (mainly for PIII-derived lesions) or be displaced by gravity (acquired ectopia mainly observed for PIV-derived lesions). Multiglandular disease is observed as previously stated in approximately 15% of cases.

Primary hyperparathyroidism can be cured by removal of the involved parathyroid gland or glands. For decades, the gold standard surgical approach for primary hyperparathyroidism has been bilateral neck exploration, involving the identification of all four parathyroid glands before removing the affected one(s). In expert hands, this approach achieves cure rates of about 95%, even without imaging, since ectopic glands inaccessible via the cervical route are rare (<2%). Nevertheless, preoperative imaging plays an important role and offers distinct advantages:

1. *Avoiding inappropriate surgical approaches*—Positive localization can reveal major ectopia, particularly in glands located deep within the mediastinum (e.g., in the aortopulmonary window) that require a thoracic rather than a cervical approach.
2. *Guiding and limiting surgical dissection*—Targeted localization helps the surgeon focus exploration, reducing the extent of dissection, minimizing complications, and shortening operative time.
3. *Flagging complex or atypical cases*—Multiple uptake foci are indicative of multigland disease (MGD). A negative scan can suggest MGD, small adenoma, or even the absence of true primary hyperparathyroidism. Such patients benefit from referral to high-volume tertiary centers for repeat or expanded biochemical, genetic, and imaging work-up [7].

4. *Providing ancillary thyroid assessment*—Beyond parathyroid localization, sestamibi imaging can help characterize thyroid nodules, offering a high negative predictive value for malignancy.
5. *Identify any additional lesions* that may appear as incidental findings or diagnostic caveats (e.g., brown tumors, thymoma, or thymic neuroendocrine tumors).

In short, while successful surgery is possible without preoperative imaging, its strategic use can refine the surgical plan, prevent inappropriate procedures, and optimize patient outcomes.

6.3 What Are the Principles of Parathyroid Scintigraphy?

SestaMIBI (methoxyisobutylisonitrile) labeled with technetium-99 m (99mTc-MIBI) is routinely used in all parathyroid scintigraphy protocols. Although SestaMIBI is not specific to parathyroid tissue and can be taken up by the thyroid, the challenge of the imaging protocols is to eliminate the thyroid signal using two approaches: performing delayed imaging (single-tracer–dual-phase protocol) or subtracting the thyroid image (dual-tracer–subtraction protocol).

Single-Tracer–Dual-Phase Protocol Delayed image acquisition highlights prolonged SestaMIBI retention in hyperfunctioning parathyroid glands compared to normal thyroid tissue. In this method, two planar images are obtained: an early scan (~15 min post-injection) and a late scan (2–3 h) [8, 9]. Parathyroid lesions typically retain the tracer longer, while thyroid tissue shows faster washout. Lesions with rapid clearance may be missed, possibly due to factors such as increased expression of efflux proteins, a reduced number of mitochondrial-rich oxyphil cells, or a low active growth phase.

Dual-Tracer–Subtraction Protocol Thyroid activity is imaged with a specific tracer and digitally subtracted from the 99mTc-MIBI image. The optimal protocol uses 99mTc-MIBI (^{99m}Tc half-life 6 h, 140 keV) and iodine-123 (half-life 13.2 h, 159 keV). Administering 123I 2 h before 99mTc-MIBI allows simultaneous dual-energy acquisition (e.g., 130–150 keV for 99mTc-MIBI, 152–175 keV for 123I) [10, 11]. Pinhole imaging begins 2–3 min after MIBI injection, and subtraction yields images showing only hyperfunctioning parathyroid tissue. This method provides high sensitivity for both single and multiple eutopic glands.

When 99mTc-pertechnetate (99mTcO4–) is used instead of 123I as a thyroid tracer, thyroid and parathyroid acquisitions are performed sequentially, but patient movement between scans may create subtraction artifacts.

Imaging Coverage and Additional Acquisition Regardless of protocol, imaging should extend from the mandibular angle to the upper myocardium, as ectopic adenomas can occur in a wide range of locations. A cervico-mediastinal SPECT/CT—preferably with dual-tracer acquisition—should follow pinhole imaging. While less sensitive than pinhole views, SPECT/CT provides precise anatomical localization, gland size estimation, increased diagnostic confidence in equivocal cases, and occasionally detection of lesions missed on pinhole images.

Reporting On planar pinhole images, a positive finding is defined as residual 99mTc-MIBI activity after normalization and subtraction. On SPECT/CT, a positive eutopic finding is characterized by focal extrathyroidal uptake located posterior or inferior to the thyroid lobe. Lesions are classified as superior (PIV-derived) if they appear posteriorly within the upper two-thirds of the thyroid lobe (in the tracheoesophageal groove close to the recurrent laryngeal nerve). Lesions are classified as PIII if they are anterior and located at the tip of the inferior pole of the thyroid lobe or along the thyrothymic tract. Other possible (ectopia) locations include the posterior mediastinum—often in the close contact to the esophagus (PIV-derived)—within the carotid sheath (usually in the posterior dihedral angle between IJV/CCA) or aortopulmonary window due to supernumerary glands associated with the vagus nerve, within the thyroid gland itself, or near the submandibular glands or anterolateral thyroid region due to undescended glands (mostly PIII-derived due to abnormal migration of the parathymic complex) [12].

Although a single parathyroid adenoma is the most frequent occurrence on imaging, multiglandular disease that includes multiple adenomas (most commonly bilateral PIV-derived) and multiglandular hyperplasia is observed in the remaining cases.

6.4 Tips for Interpretation

- *Use appropriate imaging tools:*
  Employ pinhole collimator imaging for lesion detection and SPECT/CT for accurate anatomical localization.
- *Unilateral PIV adenoma detected:*
  Always assess for contralateral PIV gland involvement, as bilateral disease may be present.
- *Right-sided PIV adenoma identified:*
  Look for the presence of an arteria lusoria (aberrant right subclavian artery), and document it if found, as it may have surgical implications.
- *Involvement of both PIV and PIII glands:*
  Consider the possibility of four-gland hyperplasia and screen for Multiple Endocrine Neoplasia type 1 (MEN1) syndrome.
- *No focal uptake detected:*
  Evaluate for calcium-sensing receptor (CaSR) mutations. In cases with confirmed mutations, surgical intervention should be avoided.
- *Lateral neck uptake focus present:*
  Examine the great vessels. This may indicate an adenoma arising from an undescended gland or one associated with the vagus nerve within the carotid sheath.
- *Intrathyroidal uptake focus observed:*
  This could represent either a major ectopic parathyroid adenoma or a thyroid nodule. In uncertain cases, perform in situ parathyroid hormone (PTH) assay for clarification.
- *Mediastinal uptake focus seen:*
  Differentiate between:
  - *Middle mediastinum lesions* (often vagus nerve-related).
  - *Anterior mediastinum lesions*, typically associated with *PIII-derived adenomas* or *supernumerary glands located in the thymus.*

6.5 Is 123I/99mTc-MIBI Subtraction Scintigraphy Superior to Other Scintigraphic Protocols?

Several prospective comparative studies [13–16] have demonstrated a preference for dual-tracer imaging, showing at least a 20% improvement in sensitivity compared to dual-phase parathyroid scintigraphy [17]. This method exhibits high sensitivity for detecting multigland disease (MGD) [18]. However, careful image interpretation is essential because tracer uptake may vary among glands in cases of MGD [18]. Therefore, incorporating a pinhole view is critical to achieving optimal sensitivity [14, 19, 20]. The contribution of single-photon emission computed tomography (SPECT) systems equipped with cadmium-zinc-telluride (CZT) detectors, which offer high contrast resolution, warrants further investigation in this context (Table 6.1, Fig. 6.1).

The main false positives observed on sestamibi scintigraphy are thyroid nodules and thymomas. Unlike 18F-fluorocholine PET/CT, there is minimal to no uptake observed in the inflammatory lymph nodes.

Table 6.1 Comparative analysis of parathyroid scintigraphy techniques

	Detection	Localization
Dual phase	++	+
Subtraction 99mTcMIBI/99mTcO4 with pinhole	++	++/+++
Subtraction 99mTcMIBI/123I with pinhole	++++	++/+++
SPECT/CT	++	++++ (CZT)

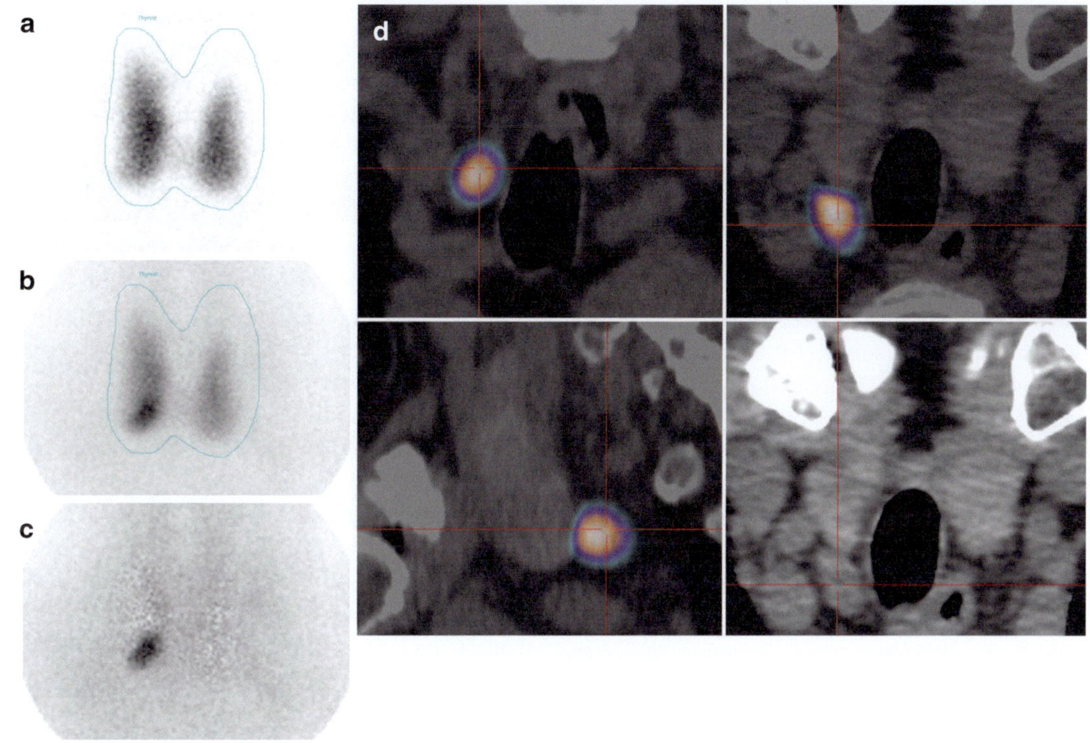

Fig. 6.1 A panel of medical imaging scans showing different views of a typical right PIV-derived parathyroid adenoma. Subfigures (**a**), and (**b**), display grayscale images labeled as 123I and 99mTc-MIBI planar pinhole images respectivement. Subfigure (**c**), shows a similar grayscale image of subtraction with a darker central region corresponding to the parathyroid adenoma. Subfigure (**d**), consists of three subtraction SPECT/CT sections and an unenhanced CT scan image, each with crosshairs indicating the adenoma

6.6 Should Scintigraphy be Abandoned Considering the Growing Evidence on 18F-Fluorocholine PET/CT?

Many authors have proposed 18F-fluorocholine PET/CT as the first-line imaging modality in PHPT [17] and the abandonment of parathyroid scintigraphy. However, caution is warranted. Beyond its higher cost, no study has demonstrated improved surgical outcomes with a 18F-fluorocholine PET strategy [21, 22]. As previously stated, first-line imaging must reliably detect multigland disease (MGD), found in ~15% of patients, and ectopic glands [23]. In the APACHE2 trial, no MGD cases were detected in the 18F-fluorocholine-first group [21]. Furthermore, many groups advocating the abandonment of 99mTc-MIBI use the less sensitive double-phase protocol rather than dual isotope subtraction method, for which FCH PET/CT has not proven superiority [23]. Parathyroid scintigraphy also shows excellent sensitivity and positive predictive value (PPV) for ectopic glands [24], with a PPV of 100% in APACHE2 compared to 92% for FCH [21]. In one study, dual-tracer PS and 11C-choline have similar results [25]. Nuclear physicians should be aware of several causes of false-positive or false-negative results, incidental finding, and pitfalls [26, 27], and arterial-phase CT may be needed to recognize these false positives. Thus, adopting FCH PET/CT as first-line should be tempered by the principle that "seeing more" is not always "seeing better."

6.7 What Issues Do the New Presentations of HPT Raise for All Types of Imaging?

Primary hyperparathyroidism (PHPT) is a heterogeneous disorder with a broad clinico-biological spectrum. In PHPT, the median weight of the parathyroid glands at diagnosis is approximately 650 mg, highlighting the delayed detection typically associated with this condition. Considering that the diagnostic sensitivity of the pinhole collimator is optimal for glands exceeding 300 mg in weight, this examination provides clinically relevant information in over 80% of cases. In recent years, normocalcemic primary hyperparathyroidism (NPHPT) has been recognized as a newly described subtype. While it remains uncertain whether NPHPT represents an early stage of hypercalcemic PHPT or a distinct entity, it may be associated with osteoporosis, fractures, or kidney stones, as well as abnormalities detected on dual-energy X-ray absorptiometry (DEXA) scans or renal ultrasounds [28, 29]. Elevated blood pressure, neuropsychiatric symptoms, and decreased QoL have also been reported [30]. Although the direct causal relationship is unclear, parathyroidectomy has been shown to improve certain clinical features and bone metabolism. This situation is challenging for imaging, regardless of the modality, because it is associated with small-sized lesions that are often multiglandular with higher risk of recurrence [31–33]. In this situation, 18F-fluorocholine PET/CT outperforms PS but can also underestimate the number of involved glands and lead to inappropriate surgical approach. This could need to be evaluated in the context of clinical trials. In a study examining the role of 18F-fluorocholine PET/CT in normocalcemic patients with negative or discordant results on 99mTc-MIBI scintigraphy and ultrasound, 18F-fluorocholine PET/CT was positive in less than 50% of cases and was associated with high but reduced cure rate as compared to classical presentations [34] (Figs. 6.2 and 6.3).

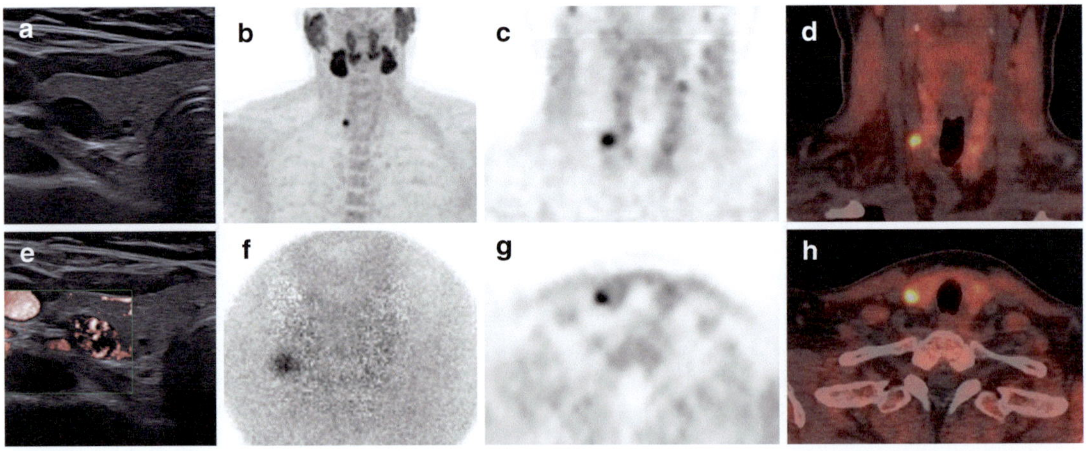

Fig. 6.2 A panel of medical imaging scans labeled a to h. Images a and e show ultrasound scans with an homogeneous hypoechoic (**a**), and hypervascular (**e**), intrathyroidal nodule. Images (**b–d**, **g**, and **h**), and h display 18F-Fluorocholine PET scans (PET/CT fusion scans on d and h) highlighting a right intrathyroidal uptake foci. Images f is subtraction planar pinhole scan with a concordant imaging finding. Each subfigure presents distinct anatomical views of an ectopic intrathyroidal parathyroid adenoma

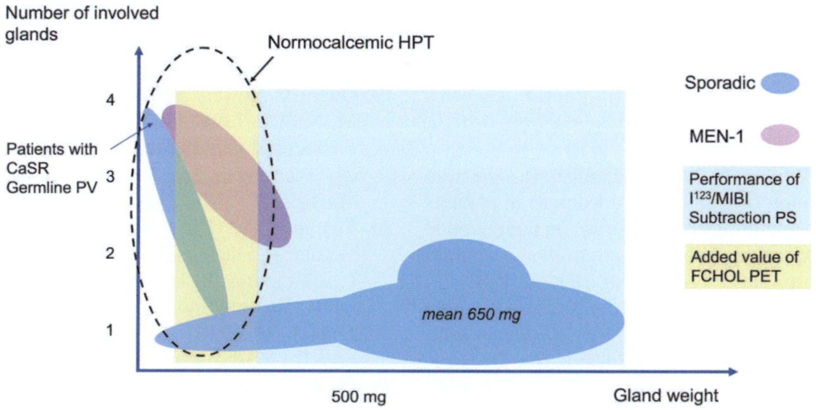

Fig. 6.3 Bubble chart illustrating the relationship between the number of involved glands and gland weight (author's view). The x-axis represents gland weight in milligrams, with a notable point at 500 mg, and the y-axis shows the number of involved glands, ranging from 1 to 4. The chart includes colored bubbles representing different conditions: blue for sporadic, purple for MEN-1, and green for patients with CaSR germline PV. A dashed oval highlights the area labeled "Normocalcemic HPT." Annotations indicate the performance of I-123/MIBI subtraction PS and the added value of FCHOL PET. The mean gland weight at diagnosis is noted as 650 mg

6.8 Conclusion

Nuclear medicine physicians should have a thorough understanding of the anatomy/embryology and genetics of the parathyroid disorders. Advances in parathyroid imaging and adoption of MIP methods have prompted a reassessment of their role in managing patients with primary hyperparathyroidism (PHPT). An optimized parathyroid scintigraphy (PS) protocol—combining 123I/99mTc-MIBI planar pinhole imaging centered on the thyroid region with subsequent cervico-mediastinal SPECT/CT acquisition—yields clinically relevant results in classical forms of PHPT. 18F-fluorocholine (FCH) PET/CT serves as a valuable imaging modality for primary hyperparathyroidism (PHPT) patients with negative/inconclusive/discordant imaging results, reducing unnecessary bilateral neck exploration [35–37]. New clinico-biological presentations characterized by normocalcemic profiles pose a challenge for all imaging modalities, and their characterization and management will need to incorporate additional parameters in the future.

References

1. al Zahrani A, Levine MA. Primary hyperparathyroidism. Lancet. 1997;349:1233–8.
2. Russell CF, Edis AJ. Surgery for primary hyperparathyroidism: experience with 500 consecutive cases and evaluation of the role of surgery in the asymptomatic patient. Br J Surg. 1982;69:244–7.
3. Duan K, Gomez Hernandez K, Mete O. Clinicopathological correlates of hyperparathyroidism. J Clin Pathol. 2015;68:771–87. https://doi.org/10.1136/jclinpath-2015-203186.
4. Udelsman R, Akerstrom G, Biagini C, Duh QY, Miccoli P, Niederle B, et al. The surgical management of asymptomatic primary hyperparathyroidism: proceedings of the fourth international workshop. J Clin Endocrinol Metab. 2014;99:3595–606. https://doi.org/10.1210/jc.2014-2000.
5. Bollerslev J, Rejnmark L, Zahn A, Heck A, Appelman-Dijkstra NM, Cardoso L, et al. European expert consensus on practical management of specific aspects of parathyroid disorders in adults and in pregnancy: recommendations of the ESE educational program of parathyroid disorders. Eur J Endocrinol. 2022;186:R33–63. https://doi.org/10.1530/EJE-21-1044.
6. Lasbleiz A, Paladino NC, Romanet P, Castinetti F, Cuny T, Sebag F, et al. Familial hypocalciuric hypercalcemia: the challenge of diagnosis. Endocrine. 2022;75:646–9. https://doi.org/10.1007/s12020-021-02909-5.

7. English KA, Pieterman CRC, Marini F, Lines KE, Cuny T, Saulle R, et al. Treatments for MEN1-associated endocrine tumours: three systematic reviews and a meta-analysis. Lancet Diabetes Endocrinol. 2025;13:685–98. https://doi.org/10.1016/S2213-8587(25)00118-4.
8. Taillefer R, Boucher Y, Potvin C, Lambert R. Detection and localization of parathyroid adenomas in patients with hyperparathyroidism using a single radionuclide imaging procedure with technetium-99m-sestamibi (double-phase study). J Nucl Med. 1992;33:1801–7.
9. Martin D, Rosen IB, Ichise M. Evaluation of single isotope technetium 99M-sestamibi in localization efficiency for hyperparathyroidism. Am J Surg. 1996;172:633–6.
10. Hindie E, Melliere D, Jeanguillaume C, Chéhadé F, Galle P. Acquisition double-fenêtre 99mTcMIBI/123I vs 99mTc-MIBI seul dans l'hyperparathyroïdie primitive. XXXVe Colloque de Médecine Nucléaire; 1996.
11. Hindie E, Melliere D, Jeanguillaume C, Perlemuter L, Chehade F, Galle P. Parathyroid imaging using simultaneous double-window recording of technetium-99m-sestamibi and iodine-123. J Nucl Med. 1998;39:1100–5.
12. Henry JF, Iacobone M. Ectopic parathyroid glands. Heidelberg/New York/Dordrecht/London: Springer; 2012.
13. Caveny SA, Klingensmith WC 3rd, Martin WE, Sage-El A, McIntyre RC Jr, Raeburn C, et al. Parathyroid imaging: the importance of dual-radiopharmaceutical simultaneous acquisition with 99mTc-sestamibi and 123I. J Nucl Med Technol. 2012;40:104–10. https://doi.org/10.2967/jnmt.111.098400.
14. Klingensmith WC 3rd, Koo PJ, Summerlin A, Fehrenbach BW, Karki R, Shulman BC, et al. Parathyroid imaging: the importance of pinhole collimation with both single- and dual-tracer acquisition. J Nucl Med Technol. 2013;41:99–104. https://doi.org/10.2967/jnmt.112.118208.
15. Krakauer M, Wieslander B, Myschetzky PS, Lundstrom A, Bacher T, Sorensen CH, et al. A prospective comparative study of parathyroid dual-phase scintigraphy, dual-isotope subtraction scintigraphy, 4D-CT, and ultrasonography in primary hyperparathyroidism. Clin Nucl Med. 2016;41:93–100. https://doi.org/10.1097/RLU.0000000000000988.
16. Tunninen V, Varjo P, Schildt J, Ahonen A, Kauppinen T, Lisinen I, et al. Comparison of five parathyroid scintigraphic protocols. Int J Mol Imaging. 2013;2013:921260. https://doi.org/10.1155/2013/921260.
17. Petranovic Ovcaricek P, Giovanella L, Carrio Gasset I, Hindie E, Huellner MW, Luster M, et al. The EANM practice guidelines for parathyroid imaging. Eur J Nucl Med Mol Imaging. 2021;48:2801–22. https://doi.org/10.1007/s00259-021-05334-y.
18. Hindie E, Melliere D, Jeanguillaume C, Urena P, deLabriolle-Vaylet C, Perlemuter L. Unilateral surgery for primary hyperparathyroidism on the basis of technetium Tc 99m sestamibi and iodine 123 subtraction scanning. Arch Surg. 2000;135:1461–8.
19. Guerin C, Lowery A, Gabriel S, Castinetti F, Philippon M, Vaillant-Lombard J, et al. Preoperative imaging for focused parathyroidectomy: making a good strategy even better. Eur J Endocrinol. 2015; https://doi.org/10.1530/EJE-14-0964.
20. Tunninen V, Varjo P, Kauppinen T, Holm A, Eskola H, Seppanen M. (99m)Tc-Sestamibi/(123)I subtraction SPECT/CT in parathyroid scintigraphy: is additional pinhole imaging useful? Int J Mol Imaging. 2017;2017:2712018. https://doi.org/10.1155/2017/2712018.
21. Quak E, Lasne-Cardon A, Cavarec M, Lireux B, Bastit V, Roudaut N, et al. F18-Choline PET/CT or MIBI SPECT/CT in the surgical management of primary hyperparathyroidism: a diagnostic randomized clinical trial. JAMA Otolaryngol Head Neck Surg. 2024;150:658–65. https://doi.org/10.1001/jamaoto.2024.1421.
22. Cuderman A, Senica K, Rep S, Hocevar M, Kocjan T, Sever MJ, et al. (18)F-Fluorocholine PET/CT in primary hyperparathyroidism: superior diagnostic performance to conventional scintigraphic imaging for localization of hyperfunctioning parathyroid glands. J Nucl Med. 2020;61:577–83. https://doi.org/10.2967/jnumed.119.229914.
23. Hindie E, Schwartz P, Avram AM, Imperiale A, Sebag F, Taieb D. Primary hyperparathyroidism: defining the appropriate preoperative imaging algorithm. J Nucl Med. 2021;62:3S–12S. https://doi.org/10.2967/jnumed.120.245993.
24. Phitayakorn R, McHenry CR. Incidence and location of ectopic abnormal parathyroid glands. Am J Surg. 2006;191:418–23. https://doi.org/10.1016/j.amjsurg.2005.10.049.
25. Ismail A, Christensen JW, Krakauer M, Sondergaard SB, Zerahn B, Nygaard B, et al. (11)C-choline PET/CT vs. (99m)Tc-MIBI/(123)iodide subtraction SPECT/CT for preoperative detection of abnormal parathyroid glands in primary hyperparathyroidism: a prospective, single-centre clinical trial in 60 patients. Diagnostics (Basel). 2020;10 https://doi.org/10.3390/diagnostics10110975.
26. Noskovicova L, Balogova S, Aveline C, Tassart M, Zhang-Yin J, Kerrou K, et al. (18)F-Fluorocholine-positron emission tomography/computerized tomography (FCH PET/CT) imaging for detecting abnormal parathyroid glands: indication, practice, interpretation and diagnostic performance. Semin Nucl Med. 2024;54:875–95. https://doi.org/10.1053/j.semnuclmed.2024.08.002.
27. Talbot JN, Zhang-Yin J, Kerrou K, Aveline C, Vagne B, Belissant O, et al. Multiple endocrine neoplasia type 1 or 4: detection of hyperfunctioning parathyroid glands with 18F-fluorocholine PET/CT. Illustrative cases and pitfalls. Q J Nucl Med Mol Imaging. 2022;66:130–40. https://doi.org/10.23736/S1824-4785.22.03440-9.

28. Rubin MR, Bilezikian JP, McMahon DJ, Jacobs T, Shane E, Siris E, et al. The natural history of primary hyperparathyroidism with or without parathyroid surgery after 15 years. J Clin Endocrinol Metab. 2008;93:3462–70. https://doi.org/10.1210/jc.2007-1215.
29. Wu C, Gillis A, Lindeman B, Chen H, Fazendin J. Normocalcemic primary hyperparathyroidism: from pathophysiology to clinical management. Am J Surg. 2024;235:115812. https://doi.org/10.1016/j.amjsurg.2024.115812.
30. Ryhanen EM, Heiskanen I, Sintonen H, Valimaki MJ, Roine RP, Schalin-Jantti C. Health-related quality of life is impaired in primary hyperparathyroidism and significantly improves after surgery: a prospective study using the 15D instrument. Endocr Connect. 2015;4:179–86. https://doi.org/10.1530/EC-15-0053.
31. Hellums RN, Pichardo PFA, Lesh RW, Wivell M, Qatanani A, Guo T, et al. Biochemical profile of and factors associated with recurrence in primary hyperparathyroidism. JAMA Otolaryngol Head Neck Surg. 2025; https://doi.org/10.1001/jamaoto.2025.1346.
32. Liu Y, Sinha Gregory N, Andreopoulou P, Kashyap S, Cusano N. Approach to the patient: normocalcemic primary hyperparathyroidism. J Clin Endocrinol Metab. 2025;110:e868–e77. https://doi.org/10.1210/clinem/dgae659.
33. Trebouet E, Bannani S, Wargny M, Leux C, Caillard C, Kraeber-Bodere F, et al. Mild sporadic primary hyperparathyroidism: high rate of multiglandular disease is associated with lower surgical cure rate. Langenbeck's Arch Surg. 2019;404:431–8. https://doi.org/10.1007/s00423-019-01782-1.
34. Koumakis E, Gauthe M, Martinino A, Sindayigaya R, Delbot T, Wartski M, et al. FCH-PET/CT in primary hyperparathyroidism with discordant/negative MIBI scintigraphy and ultrasonography. J Clin Endocrinol Metab. 2023;108:1958–67. https://doi.org/10.1210/clinem/dgad073.
35. Tlili G, Mesguich C, Gaye D, Tabarin A, Haissaguerre M, Hindie E. Dual-tracer 99mTc-sestamibi/123I imaging in primary hyperparathyroidism. Q J Nucl Med Mol Imaging. 2023;67:114–21. https://doi.org/10.23736/S1824-4785.23.03509-4.
36. Carrillo Lizarazo JL, Cecchin D, Camozzi V, Crimi F, Torresan F, Iacobone M. Impact of 18F-choline PET-CT or PET-MRI on surgical strategy in patients with primary hyperparathyroidism. BJS Open. 2025;9 https://doi.org/10.1093/bjsopen/zraf069.
37. Lee SW, Shim SR, Jeong SY, Kim SJ. Direct comparison of preoperative imaging modalities for localization of primary hyperparathyroidism: a systematic review and network meta-analysis. JAMA Otolaryngol Head Neck Surg. 2021;147:692–706. https://doi.org/10.1001/jamaoto.2021.0915.

11C-Methionine PET/CT in Parathyroid Imaging

7

Elena Romano Gargarella, Flaminia Vocaturo, and Désirée Deandreis

▶ **Definitions** PET/CT: positron emission tomography

Methionine: essential α-amino acid, used in the biosynthesis of proteins

Carbon-11: radioactive isotope of carbon

PTH: parathyroid hormone

Learning Objectives

1. Understand the role of 11C-methionine in localizing hyperfunctioning parathyroid glands
2. Compare the diagnostic performance of 11C-methionine with other imaging modalities in different clinical settings
3. Understand strengths and limitations of 11C-methionine PET/CT

E. R. Gargarella · F. Vocaturo
Department of Radiological Sciences and Haematology, Section of Nuclear Medicine, Università Cattolica del Sacro Cuore, Rome, Italy
e-mail: elena.romanogargarella01@icatt.it; flaminia.vocaturo01@icatt.it

D. Deandreis (✉)
Gustave Roussy, Nuclear Medicine Division, Department of Medical Imaging, Villejuif, France
e-mail: Desiree.DEANDREIS@gustaveroussy.fr

7.1 Rationale and Technical Principles for 11C-Methionine Use in Parathyroid Imaging

Methionine is an essential exogenous amino acid (molar mass: 142.91 g/mol) composed of a five-carbon chain containing a sulfur atom. It is recognized as the initiating amino acid residue in protein synthesis across all nuclear organisms. Owing to its central role in the synthesis of most proteins and its involvement in cellular energy metabolism, methionine is a critical component of numerous biological processes [1].

11C-methionine uptake in hyperfunctioning parathyroid tissue reflects the incorporation of this amino acid into newly synthesized proteins. In parathyroid cells, methionine is specifically incorporated into pre-pro-parathyroid hormone (pre-pro-PTH), the early precursor of PTH. L-[methyl-11C] methionine enters cells through passive diffusion and active transport via several neutral amino acid transporters, predominantly L-Type Amino Acid Transporter 1 (LAT1) and L-Type Amino Acid Transporter 2 (LAT2), which are located on the cell surface. The overexpression of these transporters, particularly LAT1 (SLC7A5), in hyperfunctioning parathyroid tissue accounts for the high target-to-background ratio observed on 11C-methionine PET/CT imaging [1, 2].

© The Author(s), under exclusive license to Springer Nature Switzerland AG 2026
P. Petranović Ovčariček et al. (eds.), *Parathyroid Imaging*,
https://doi.org/10.1007/978-3-032-14178-1_7

Carbon-11 (11C) is produced in the cyclotron by bombardment of nitrogen-14 with protons. The radiochemical synthesis of 11C-methionine is relatively simple and efficient, allowing for rapid production with high radiochemical yield and purity without requiring complex purification procedures [3]. However, the short half-life of carbon-11 (20.4 min) may pose some challenges, since it has to be produced on-site, restricting its use to specialized centers equipped with a cyclotron and limiting its widespread availability.

The injected activity ranges from 400 to 800 MBq (10–20 mCi) even if in some studies up to 1100 MBq have been administered, and images are normally performed at 5–10 min post-injection (dual-phase sometimes used with late acquisition at 40 min) [4, 5].

The radiation exposure is relatively modest with an effective dose per procedure ranging from 1.9 to 5.2 mSv, with low exposure especially to organs such as the kidneys and liver [1]. Shorter acquisition times, higher PET imaging accuracy, as well as a lower uptake in the thyroid gland give this methodology some advantages in diagnostic accuracy compared to 99mTc-sestamibi scintigraphy when detecting hyperfunctioning parathyroids [6].

In the literature, many articles investigated the impact of 11C-methionine in the evaluation of HPT, and it emerged as a valuable functional imaging modality for localizing hyperfunctioning parathyroid tissue, especially in cases of negative standard imaging (neck ultrasound and 99Tc-sestamibi scintigraphy). It has demonstrated the ability to distinguish orthotopic and ectopic lesions, facilitate precise preoperative planning, support focused surgical management of parathyroid disease, and detect post-treatment recurrence.

7.2 Role of 11C-Methionine in Primary Hyperparathyroidism

The leading cause of primary HPT is usually represented in 80% of cases by a solitary adenoma, although multiglandular disease and carcinoma can play a role as well [7]. PET/CT constitutes an effective second-line imaging modality, especially when first-line imaging (ultrasound, 99mTc-sestamibi scintigraphy) ends up negative or equivocal.

The first prominent meta-analysis was published in 2013, and it included 9 studies (5 retrospective and 4 prospective) and a total of 258 patients who underwent 11C-methionine in the presurgical setting. It reported a pooled sensitivity of 81% (95% CI 74–86%) and a detection rate of 70% (95% CI 62–77%) on a patient-based analysis, endorsing the use of 11C-methionine PET as a reliable imaging modality when first-line imaging fails [4]. It should be noticed that six of the nine studies evaluated included PET without combined CT. The heterogeneity among studies was high concerning different technical aspects (combined or not combined CT, administered activity, delay from injection to imaging).

A second meta-analysis published 3 years later analyzed 24 studies: 14 on 11C-methionine, 6 on 18-FDG, 1 on 18F-DOPA, and 3 on 11C/18F-choline. The 14 studies investigating 11C-methionine included a total of 327 patients with 364 lesions. The sensitivity of 11C-methionine for the detection of a lesion in the correct quadrant ranged from 44% to 91%, with a pooled estimate of 77% (95% CI 71–84%) and a pooled positive predictive value of 98% (95% CI 96–100%), compared to 80–100% and 89–100% for choline tracers, respectively [8]. There was no difference in sensitivity between patients with previous negative or inconclusive standard imaging (81% vs. 78%, respectively).

Another more recent meta-analysis by Bioletto analyzed the diagnostic accuracy of 11C-methionine (n = 8 studies) and that of 18F-fluorocholine (n = 14). No study directly comparing the two tracers was reported. The pooled sensitivity of 18F-fluorocholine was higher than that of 11C-methionine (92% vs 80%, $P < 0.01$), while the positive predictive value was similar (94% vs 95%, $P = 0.99$), confirming previous findings [9].

According to this and previous results, 18F-fluorocholine should be considered the preferred PET tracer method. However, 11C-methionine, due to its very good diagnostic accuracy, should be viewed as a valuable choice if available.

Many single works have demonstrated the additional value of 11C-methionine PET/CT in cases where ultrasound or scintigraphy is negative or discordant, thereby guiding surgeons to lesions otherwise undetectable, even though the detection rate was variable [10–12].

The retrospective study by Noltes et al. directly compared 11C-methionine, 11C-choline, and 4DCT as second-line imaging in 32 patients. Of these, 30 patients underwent surgery, and 32 parathyroid lesions were histologically confirmed as parathyroid adenomas. With blind evaluation, 11C-choline PET/CT was positive in 28 patients (88%), 11C-methionine PET/CT in 23 (72%), and 4D-CT in 15 patients (47%), respectively. 11C-methionine PET/CT was able to identify parathyroid lesions on the correct side in only 64% (18/28) of patients after prior negative 99mTc-sestamibi SPECT/CT and/or cervical ultrasonography, a detection rate lower compared to previous studies. Based on blinded evaluation, lesion-based sensitivity of 11C-choline PET/CT, 11C-methionine PET/CT, and 4D-CT was 85%, 67%, and 39%, respectively. The sensitivity of 11C-choline PET/CT differed significantly from that of 11C-methionine PET/CT and 4D-CT ($p = 0.031$ and $p < 0.0005$, respectively) [12]. Interestingly, the sensitivity for 11C-methionine PET/CT imaging decreased when the scans were interpreted non-blindly, as compared to the blinded interpretation.

In a cohort of 38 patients with primary HPT and inconclusive standard preoperative imaging (ultrasound, 99mTc-sestamibi scintigraphy), Maccora and colleagues demonstrated a sensitivity of 79% and specificity of 75% for lateralizing the hyperfunctioning parathyroid gland (right/left side) and a sensitivity of 75% and specificity of 50% for exact localization (superior/inferior position) [13]. This indicates that 11C-methionine PET/CT is a valuable second-line imaging modality for uncovering abnormal parathyroid tissue when conventional imaging is non-diagnostic. The study also assessed semi-quantitative PET parameters, including standardized uptake value (SUV), functional lesion volume (FLV), and total lesion activity (TLA), and found that these metrics were significantly higher in patients with elevated preoperative PTH levels and in glands with greater size and weight on histology. Thus, higher SUV, FLV, and TLA values correlated with both biochemical severity and glandular pathology, supporting the use of semi-quantitative analysis to help predict the functional and morphological characteristics of the hyperfunctioning gland (Fig. 7.1).

A multicenter registry study including 776 patients from 53 hospitals who underwent parathyroid surgery after 18F-fluorocholine or 11C-methionine PET/CT reported in 50 patients studied with 11C-methionine a sensitivity of 83.2% (vs 87.9% for 18F-fluorocholine) and a positive predictive value of 85.6% (vs 88.5% for 18F-fluorocholine) [14]. Beyond raw performance metrics, 11C-methionine PET/CT translated into tangible surgical benefits: reduced operative times, higher cure rates, and facilitation of minimally invasive approaches.

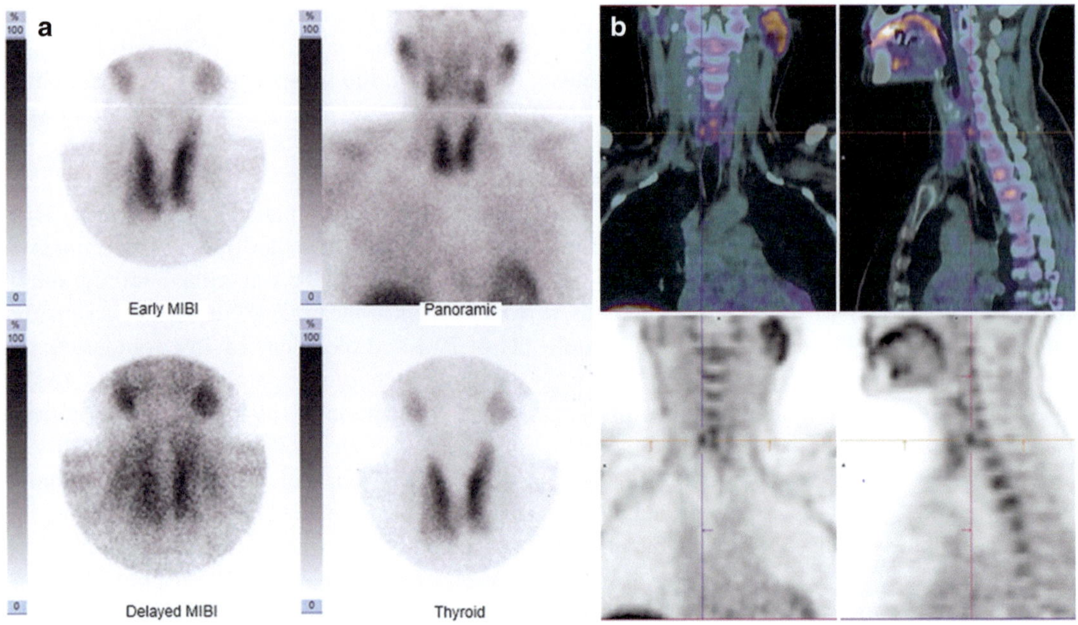

Fig. 7.1 A 53-year-old woman with serum calcium 12.7 mg/dl (normal range: 8.5–10.5) and PTH 211.4 pg/ml (normal range: 10.0–65.0). Early and delayed 99mTc-sestamibi images do not show any focal abnormal uptake in the neck and upper chest scan (**a**); (**b**) 11C-MET (fused and PET only) shows abnormal uptake posterior to the superior-medium third of the right thyroid lobe. (Images obtained with permission by Maccora et al. [13])

We should take into account that some false-positive results can occur, even if rare, in case of benign and malignant tumors (including head and neck tumors and thyroid adenomas), while false-negative results may occur in case of multiglandular hyperplasia, small parathyroid adenomas, and diffuse thyroid disease [2, 15].

7.3 11C-Methionine in Persistent and Recurrent Hyperparathyroidism

A particularly clinically challenging scenario is persistent or recurrent HPT after previous neck surgery. Altered anatomy and scarring often render ultrasound and scintigraphy unreliable. In this setting, methionine PET/CT has shown meaningful utility.

A recent cohort and registry studies demonstrate that 11C-methionine PET/CT achieves sensitivities ranging from 70% to 74% for the detection of hyperfunctioning parathyroids in patients with persistent primary HPT following previous neck surgery [11, 14]. Nevertheless, in the Weber et al. study, a subgroup analysis revealed more positive results for 18F-fluorocholine PET/CT in patients with previous neck surgery (89.0%) than for 11C-methionine PET/CT (74.2%, $P = 0.0411$). One of the key impacts of PET in this context was its capacity to optimize and guide surgical interventions. Positive PET/CT results significantly reduced surgery times, decreasing from 93 min (±56.54) to 71 min (±43.48, $P < 0.0001$).

7.4 11C-Methionine in Secondary-Tertiary Hyperparathyroidism

In secondary or tertiary HPT, often seen in dialysis patients, the disease is usually multiglandular, and it might involve ectopic glands. One of the first studies, conducted by Otto et al., demonstrated that in 12 patients with secondary or tertiary HPT, 36 hyperplastic parathyroid glands were histologically identified [5]. Twenty-five of

36 lesions (69%) were detected with 11C-methionine PET and only 17 (47%) with 99mTc-sestamibi scintigraphy. In 10/11 patients with recurrent HPT and non-diagnostic scintigraphy/SPECT, hyperfunctional parathyroid tissue was identified by 11C-methionine PET. Of note, the highest SUV(parathyroid)/SUV(cervical soft tissue) ratio was found at 10 min acquisition time, and the highest SUV(parathyroid tissue)/SUV(thyroid tissue) ratio was 40 min post-injection.

11C-methionine PET/CT demonstrates high sensitivity for localizing multiple and ectopic lesions, facilitating targeted surgical intervention when conventional modalities fail [16, 17].

In the study of Rubello et al., PET/CT with 11C-methionine was performed in 18 patients hemodialyzed for renal failure (11 women and 7 men). Parathyroid adenomas were not localized by other conventional nuclear medicine modalities. In 3/10 of patients with normo- or hypocalcemia, increased 11C-methionine accumulation was detected in one gland. In 7/8 patients with HPT and hypercalcemia PET showed increased uptake in one or more glands [16].

In a group of 19 patients with severe tertiary HPT, 11C-methionine PET/CT was positive in 89.5% of the patients (17/19). Parathyroidectomy was performed in 52.9% of the patients (9/17), and PET results were fully consistent with the results of the histopathological examinations of the removed parathyroid glands. On this basis, the sensitivity of PET/CT with 11C-methionine in the preoperative localization diagnosis of patients with tHPT was found to be 100%. Multiple lesions were visualized in 57.9% of the patients (11/19), and ectopic lesions were visualized in 21.1% of the patients (4/19) [17].

7.5 Parathyroid Carcinoma: Rare but Detectable

Parathyroid carcinoma remains a rare cause of HPT (<1% of cases) [18]. Evidence for 11C-methionine PET/CT is based on a few clinical reports and is therefore limited. However, Mathey et al. documented the successful detection of carcinoma lesions alongside adenomas and hyperplasia [19], while Weber et al. identified carcinoma in their large registry and included these cases within the high overall detection [14]. Damien et al. also reported a case of positive 11C-methionine PET in a bifocal intrathyroidal parathyroid carcinoma [20], and Omi et al. reported, as well, the capability of 11C-methionine to detect multifocal relapse after surgery [21]. Although histopathology remains the gold standard, 11C-methionine uptake seems to be present in malignant disease as well.

7.6 Strengths and Limitations

The strengths of 11C-methionine PET/CT include its high sensitivity in detecting hyperfunctioning parathyroid in all clinical settings, especially when first-line imaging is inconclusive, correlating also with biochemical activity [4, 13, 16]. Limitations revolve primarily around logistics: the short half-life demands on-site cyclotron production, which limits availability, and a lack of reimbursement [2, 6]. Additionally, 11C-methionine seems generally less sensitive than 18F-fluorocholine, particularly for small adenomas or multiglandular disease [9, 12, 18].

7.7 Future Perspectives

The future role of 11C-methionine PET/CT will likely be specialized rather than universal. Its utility in tertiary HPT and in complex re-operative cases is already established, and further studies may refine its value as part of hybrid PET/MRI protocols [2]. Research into novel amino acid tracers with longer half-lives may also extend the molecular approach pioneered by 11C-methionine. Meanwhile, cost-effectiveness analyses comparing 11C-methionine and 18F-fluorocholine PET/CT will be essential to guide policy and practice.

7.8 Conclusions

11C-methionine PET/CT, owing to its high sensitivity, low radiation burden, and close correlation with disease biology, has emerged as a valuable diagnostic modality in parathyroid imaging—particularly in centers equipped with an on-site cyclotron or lacking access to 18F-fluorocholine. Its use has been shown to increase the success rate of focused parathyroidectomy and postoperative evaluation in patients with inconclusive conventional imaging. Accordingly, 11C-methionine PET/CT can therefore be recommended as an evaluable tool in the diagnostic work-up of parathyroid disease.

References

1. Durma AD, Saracyn M, Kołodziej M, et al. The use of [11C]C-methionine in diagnostics of endocrine disorders with focus on pituitary and parathyroid glands. Pharmaceuticals (Basel). 2025;18(2):229. https://doi.org/10.3390/ph18020229.
2. Habener JF, Maunus R, Dee PC, Potts JT Jr. Early events in the cellular formation of proparathyroid hormone. J Cell Biol. 1980;85:292–8.
3. Jager PL, Vaalburg W, Pruim J, de Vries EGE, Langen K-J, Piers DA. Radiolabeled amino acids: basic aspects and clinical applications in oncology. J Nucl Med. 2001;42:432–45.
4. Caldarella C, Treglia G, Isgrò MA, et al. Diagnostic performance of positron emission tomography using ^{11}C-methionine in patients with suspected parathyroid adenoma: a meta-analysis. Endocrine. 2013;43(1):78–83. https://doi.org/10.1007/s12020-012-9746-4.
5. Otto D, Boerner AR, Hofmann M, Brunkhorst T, Meyer GJ, Petrich T, et al. Pre-operative localisation of hyperfunctional parathyroid tissue with 11C-methionine PET. Eur J Nucl Med Mol Imaging. 2004 Oct 29 [cited 2019 Aug 27];31(10):1405–12.
6. Petranović Ovčariček P, Giovanella L, Carrió Gasset I, Hindié E, Huellner MW, Luster M, Piccardo A, Weber T, Talbot JN, Verburg FA. The EANM practice guidelines for parathyroid imaging. Eur J Nucl Med Mol Imaging. 2021;48(9):2801–22. https://doi.org/10.1007/s00259-021-05334-y.
7. Silverberg SJ, Lewiecki EM, Mosekilde L, Peacock M, Rubin MR. Presentation of asymptomatic primary hyperparathyroidism: proceedings of the third international workshop. J Clin Endocrinol Metab. 2009;94(2):351–65.
8. Kluijfhout WP, Pasternak JD, Drake FT, et al. Use of PET tracers for parathyroid localization: a systematic review and meta-analysis. Langenbecks Arch Surg. 2016;401:925–35. https://doi.org/10.1007/s00423-016-1425-0.
9. Bioletto F, Barale M, Parasiliti-Caprino M, et al. Comparison of the diagnostic accuracy of 18F-Fluorocholine PET and 11C-methionine PET for parathyroid localization in primary hyperparathyroidism: a systematic review and meta-analysis. Eur J Endocrinol. 2021;185(1):109–20. https://doi.org/10.1530/EJE-21-0038.
10. Saerens J, Velkeniers B, Keyaerts M, et al. Value of [11C]-methionine PET/CT in preoperative localization of parathyroid adenomas. Horm Metab Res. 2021;53(7):444–52. https://doi.org/10.1055/a-1475-4600.
11. Huynh KA, MacFarlane J, Newman C, et al. Diagnostic utility of (11) C-methionine PET/CT in primary hyperparathyroidism in a UK cohort: a single-centre experience and literature review. Clin Endocrinol. 2023;99(3):233–45. https://doi.org/10.1111/cen.14933.
12. Noltes ME, Kruijff S, Appelman APA, et al. Head-to-head comparison of [(11)C]methionine PET, [(11)C]choline PET, and 4-dimensional CT as second-line scans for detection of parathyroid adenomas in primary hyperparathyroidism. Eur J Nucl Med Mol Imaging. 2024;51(4):1050–9. https://doi.org/10.1007/s00259-023-06488-713.
13. Maccora D, Caldarella C, Calcagni ML. 11C-methionine PET/CT in patients with primary hyperparathyroidism and inconclusive preoperative imaging work-up: diagnostic accuracy and role of semi-quantitative analysis. Ann Nucl Med. 2021;35(4):469–78. https://doi.org/10.1007/s12149-021-01584-w.
14. Weber T, Smaxwil C, Hermann M, et al. Results of (18)F-choline and (11)C-methionine positron emission tomography/computed tomography for the preoperative localization of hyperfunctional parathyroid glands in primary hyperparathyroidism. Surgery. 2025;180:109056. https://doi.org/10.1016/j.surg.2024.109056.
15. Cook GJR, Maisey MN, Fogelman I. Normal variants, artefacts and interpretative pitfalls in PET imaging with 18-fluoro-2-deoxyglucose and carbon-11 methionine. Eur J Nucl Med. 1999;26:1363–78. https://doi.org/10.1007/s002590050597.
16. Rubello D, Fanti S, Nanni C, et al. 11C-methionine PET/CT in 99mTc-sestamibi-negative hyperparathyroidism in patients with renal failure on chronic haemodialysis. Eur J Nucl Med Mol Imaging. 2006;33:453–9. https://doi.org/10.1007/s00259-005-0008-z.
17. Kołodziej M, Saracyn M, Lubas A, et al. Usefulness of PET/CT with Carbon-11-labeled methionine in the diagnosis of tertiary hyperparathyroidism. Nutrients. 2022;15(1):188. https://doi.org/10.3390/nu15010188.
18. Cetani F, Pardi E, Marcocci C. Parathyroid carcinoma. Front Horm Res. 2019;51:63–76. https://doi.org/10.1159/000491039.

19. Mathey C, Keyzer C, Blocklet D, et al. (18) F-fluorocholine PET/CT is more sensitive than (11) C-methionine PET/CT for the localization of hyperfunctioning parathyroid tissue in primary hyperparathyroidism. J Nucl Med. 2022;63(5):785–91. https://doi.org/10.2967/jnumed.121.262395.
20. Damien M, Rodriguez A, Bouland C. An unusual case of primary hyperparathyroidism: case report of a bifocal Intrathyroidal parathyroid carcinoma. Ear Nose Throat J. 2023;102(1):NP5–7. https://doi.org/10.1177/0145561320977466.
21. Omi Y, Yamamoto T, Nagashima Y, et al. Parathyroid carcinoma in a 13-year-old girl with a long-term survival. Surg Case Rep. 2020;6:145. https://doi.org/10.1186/s40792-020-00914-w.

$[^{18}F]$Fluorocholine PET/CT and $[^{11}C]$ Choline PET/CT in Parathyroid Imaging

8

Ujwal Bhure, Klaus Strobel, and Hannes Grünig

▶ **Definitions**

- Primary hyperparathyroidism: An endocrine disorder characterized by the overproduction of parathyroid hormone (PTH), most often caused by solitary parathyroid adenoma.
- Secondary hyperparathyroidism: Parathyroid hyperplasia with overproduction of PTH, "secondary" to hypocalcemia, due to a chronic stimulus, such as chronic kidney disease (CKD) or vitamin D deficiency.
- Tertiary hyperparathyroidism: Autonomous (unregulated) overproduction of PTH associated with hypercalcemia, after long-standing secondary hyperparathyroidism, typically occurring in patients with CKD who have been on dialysis.
- Orthotopic parathyroid gland: It refers to a parathyroid gland that is located in its normal anatomical position situated in the neck behind the thyroid gland.
- Ectopic parathyroid gland: It refers to a parathyroid gland that is located outside the usual anatomic location, for example, in the mediastinum or around the carotid sheath.
- Hybrid imaging: The combination of functional (PET) and anatomical (MR, CT) imaging into a single examination for improved localization and characterization of lesions.
- PET/CT: Positron emission tomography/computed tomography.
- $[^{18}F]$fluorocholine (FCH): A PET radiotracer, which is a structural analogue of choline and closely follows its metabolic pathways, taken up by cells with increased phospholipid-dependent choline kinase activity, a cellular mechanism prevalent in hyperfunctioning parathyroid adenomas.
- Brown tumor: It is a non-neoplastic bone lesion that occurs as a result of hyperparathyroidism, caused by excessive activity of osteoclasts, leading to bone resorption, consisting of fibrous tissue and hemosiderin deposits.
- Parathyroid carcinoma: a rare malignant tumor of the parathyroid glands, also associated with excessive production of PTH, and has the potential to metastasize to other parts of the body.

U. Bhure · K. Strobel (✉) · H. Grünig
Department of Nuclear Medicine and Radiology, Luzerner Kantonsspital, University Teaching and Research Hospital, University of Lucerne, Lucerne, Switzerland
e-mail: bnujwal@yahoo.com; klaus.strobel@luks.ch; hannes.gruenig@luks.ch

© The Author(s), under exclusive license to Springer Nature Switzerland AG 2026
P. Petranović Ovčariček et al. (eds.), *Parathyroid Imaging*,
https://doi.org/10.1007/978-3-032-14178-1_8

Learning Objectives

- To learn the role and performance of choline PET/CT in hyperparathyroidism.
- Pre-requisites, protocol, and interpretation of choline PET/CT in hyperparathyroidism.
- Performance of choline PET/CT as first- and second-line imaging in the localization of hyperfunctioning parathyroid glands.
- Role of choline PET/CT in secondary and tertiary hyperparathyroidism, in the localization of ectopic parathyroid glands, parathyroid carcinoma, and brown tumors.
- Pitfalls in choline PET/CT.
- Cost-effectiveness.

8.1 Introduction

The curative treatment for symptomatic patients with pHPT is surgical removal of hyperfunctioning parathyroid glands. While bilateral neck exploration has historically been the standard surgical approach, the advent of minimally invasive parathyroidectomy has shifted the emphasis toward precise preoperative anatomical localization of the hyperfunctioning glands, including the identification of ectopic parathyroid adenomas, to guide targeted surgery. Among the available imaging modalities, including US, [^{99m}Tc]Tc-Sestamibi subtraction scintigraphy, dual-timepoint scintigraphy with or without SPECT/CT, 4D-CT, and MRI, choline PET/CT has emerged as a first-line imaging technique, where available. Its superior diagnostic accuracy and high sensitivity in both routine and complex cases are supported by extensive data from multiple centers, positioning it as a key tool in the preoperative evaluation and surgical planning for pHPT.

8.2 Radiotracers

The various radiotracers utilized for parathyroid imaging have been described in the previous chapters extensively and are summarized in the following table (Table 8.1):

Table 8.1 Radiotracers used for the preoperative localization of parathyroid adenomas

	^{201}Thallium	^{99m}Tc-pertechnetate	^{99m}Tc-Sestamibi	123Iodine	11C-methionine	11C-choline	18F-fluorocholine
Half-life time	73 h	6.01 h	6.01 h	13.2 h	20 min	20 min	109.8 min
Photon energy (keV)	69–81	140.5	140.5	159	511	511	511
Approximate effective radiation dose per examination (mSv)	15	2.4	6.3	1.6	6.0	2.9	6.0
Availability and reimbursement	Limited	Widely	Widely	Limited	Limited	Limited	Limited
Cost	Expensive	Inexpensive	Inexpensive	Expensive	Expensive	Expensive	Expensive

8.3 What Is Choline?

Choline is a quaternary ammonium compound consisting of a nitrogen atom bonded to three methyl (CH_3) groups and one ethyl (CH_2CH_2OH) group, resulting in the molecular structure $(CH_3)_3N^+CH_2CH_2OH$. It is an essential component of phospholipids in the cell membranes, playing a crucial role in both animals and plants. After entering the cell via a carrier-mediated transport mechanism, choline is phosphorylated by choline kinase and subsequently incorporated into phosphatidylcholine, a major component of cellular membranes. Phosphatidylcholine is crucial for maintaining membrane structural integrity and fluidity, and it participates in various biological processes, including cell signalling, membrane trafficking, and lipid metabolism.

8.4 [^{18}F]Fluorocholine PET/CT

Fluorocholine is a structural analogue of choline that closely follows its metabolic pathways. It was initially introduced as an oncologic radiotracer after increased choline kinase activity was observed in malignant cells, resulting in enhanced uptake and accumulation of radiolabeled choline derivatives within neoplasms. Fluorocholine has since been widely applied in clinical practice for the diagnostic imaging of various cancers, most notably prostate and hepatocellular carcinomas. Interestingly, a similar mechanism has been identified in parathyroid adenomas, where increased phospholipid-dependent choline kinase activity occurs due to the translocation of the enzyme from the cytosol to the cell membrane. This phenomenon, driven by the hypersecretion of parathyroid hormone (PTH), results in elevated fluorocholine uptake, providing a reliable imaging target for detecting hyperfunctioning parathyroid tissue [1].

8.5 [^{11}C]Choline PET/CT

[^{11}C]choline ([11C]2-hydroxy-N,N,N-trimethylethanamium) contains the same chemical structure as "choline" and follows the same biological principle as [^{18}F]fluorocholine, accumulating in hyperfunctioning parathyroid glands. The key difference lies in the radioisotope: Carbon-11 is used instead of Fluorine-18 [2]. While Carbon-11 offers advantages for radiolabelling, as it can be incorporated into organic molecules without significantly altering their structure, its short physical half-life necessitates on-site production and rapid synthesis. This restricts the use of [^{11}C]choline to facilities with an in-house cyclotron. In contrast, [^{18}F]fluorocholine, despite requiring more complex labelling chemistry, has become the more widely adopted radiotracer due to its longer half-life and broader commercial availability.

8.6 Imaging Protocol for [^{18}F]Fluorocholine PET/CT

- Pre-imaging.
  - Fasting is not required for [^{18}F]fluorocholine PET scan (in contrast to [^{18}F]FDG).
  - No restriction based on blood sugar level or diabetes status.
  - Patients should be advised to avoid vigorous physical activity before the scan, as this may increase muscular uptake of [^{18}F]fluorocholine.
  - If the protocol includes a diagnostic CT scan with intravenous iodinated contrast medium, the following should be confirmed:
    - No known allergy to iodinated contrast agents.
    - Adequate renal function, typically assessed by serum creatinine levels.
    - Normal thyroid function, to minimize the risk of contrast-induced thyroid dysfunction.

- Scan acquisition.
  - The PET/CT scan is typically acquired 45–60 min after intravenous administration of [^{18}F]fluorocholine (activity dose: 1.5–3.2 MBq/kg).
  - Optional early-phase imaging can be performed, starting with a dynamic acquisition immediately after the intravenous administration of the radiotracer, followed by static imaging approximately 5 min later. However, this approach may not be feasible in high-throughput clinical settings.
  - A diagnostic CT scan with an intravenous contrast agent can be incorporated to enhance soft tissue contrast and provide more anatomical detail. The optimal phase is the late arterial phase, approximately 30 s after injection. Many surgeons prefer to have this additional information for preoperative planning.
  - The recommended scan range extends from the base of the skull to the base of the diaphragm, striking a balance between diagnostic utility and radiation exposure. In selected cases, such as suspected or known parathyroid carcinoma or the presence of brown tumors, a whole-body PET/CT is indicated to assess for distant disease.

8.7 Image Analysis

Focal radiotracer accumulation in a nodule in the typical (orthotopic) location around the thyroid gland is highly suggestive of a hyperfunctioning parathyroid adenoma. These lesions typically demonstrate an SUVmax exceeding that of the thyroid gland parenchyma, while appearing hypodense compared to the thyroid gland on corresponding non-enhanced CT images (Figs. 8.1, 8.2, 8.3, 8.4, 8.5, 8.6 and 8.7). In a study by Quak et al., choline uptake in parathyroid adenomas was reported to be approximately 5.5 times higher than the background muscle activity and three times higher than the uptake of the thyroid gland, allowing for confident interpretation of PET images in the majority of cases [3]. However, differentiation between parathyroid adenomas and parathyroid hyperplasia based solely on SUVmax remains challenging, and that is when the accompanying structural imaging (CT or MRI) provides helpful information about the presence of a nodule, which would favor adenoma over hyperplasia. In a study by Beheshti et al., wherein histopathology was used as a standard of reference, although the choline-positive adenomas exhibited higher SUVmax (6.80 ± 3.78) compared to hyperplastic glands (4.53 ± 0.40), this difference was not statistically significant, with considerable overlap [4]. The timing of image acquisition also appears to have a limited influence on lesion detectability. A study by Uslu-Besli et al. involving 105 patients with hyperparathyroidism found no significant difference in mean SUVmax between early imaging (SUVmax: 7.1 ± 3.5, acquired at 15 min post-injection) and late imaging (7.3 ± 3.6, acquired at 45 min post-injection), without missing any adenoma on imaging at either time point [5]. Nevertheless, the EANM guidelines recommend including an early-phase acquisition, as supported by a study by Rep et al., in which a parathyroid adenoma was visualized exclusively on early-phase images in one patient [6, 7].

The SUVmax of a parathyroid adenoma or hyperplastic gland on choline PET/CT has been shown to correlate with disease severity, particularly in relation to serum PTH levels and bone mineral densitometry (BMD) scores. In a study by Araz et al., patients with an SUVmax exceeding 4.4 demonstrated significantly higher serum PTH levels and significantly lower femoral and lumbar T-scores on BMD assessment, reflecting more severe disease and advanced bone involvement [8]. The relationship between serum PTH levels and choline uptake in parathyroid lesions is likely attributable to the upregulation of phospholipid/Ca^{2+}-dependent choline kinase activity, an enzyme responsible for cellular choline uptake. Notably, choline kinase activity is increased in hypersecreting parathyroid adenomas compared to normal parathyroid glands [1].

Fig. 8.1 Parathyroid glands: orthotopic and ectopic locations

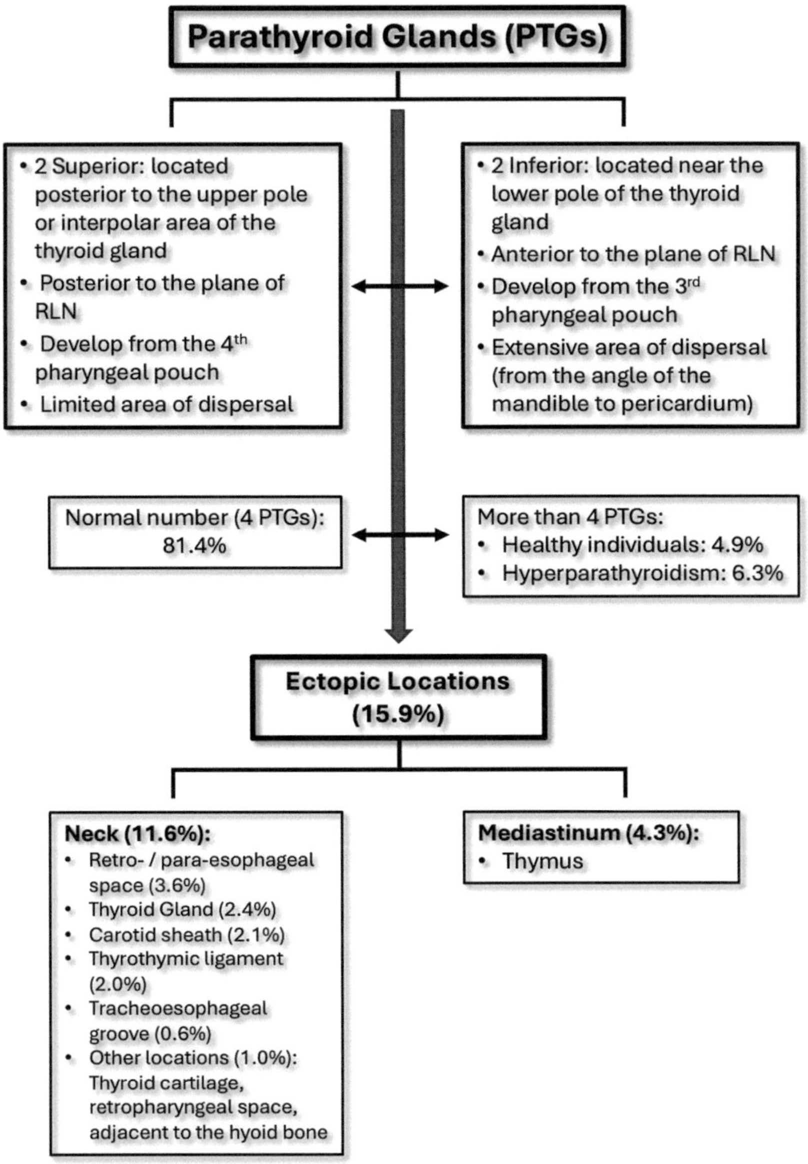

Furthermore, a marked shift in the cellular localization of this enzyme has been observed, with translocation from the cytosol to the cell membranes in parathyroid adenomas, likely contributing to the increased radiotracer accumulation detectable on PET imaging [1].

Ectopic parathyroid adenomas can be located anywhere along the migration pathway of the parathyroid glands from the angle of the mandible to the mediastinum (Fig. 8.1). When evaluating CT images, it is essential to systematically review all available window settings, including lung, soft tissue, and bone windows, to identify not only the target lesions but also any relevant incidental findings. It should be noted that choline uptake within the thyroid gland may be higher than expected in the presence of underlying thyroid pathologies, such as thyroiditis or Graves' disease, which must be considered to avoid potential misinterpretation of the PET/CT findings.

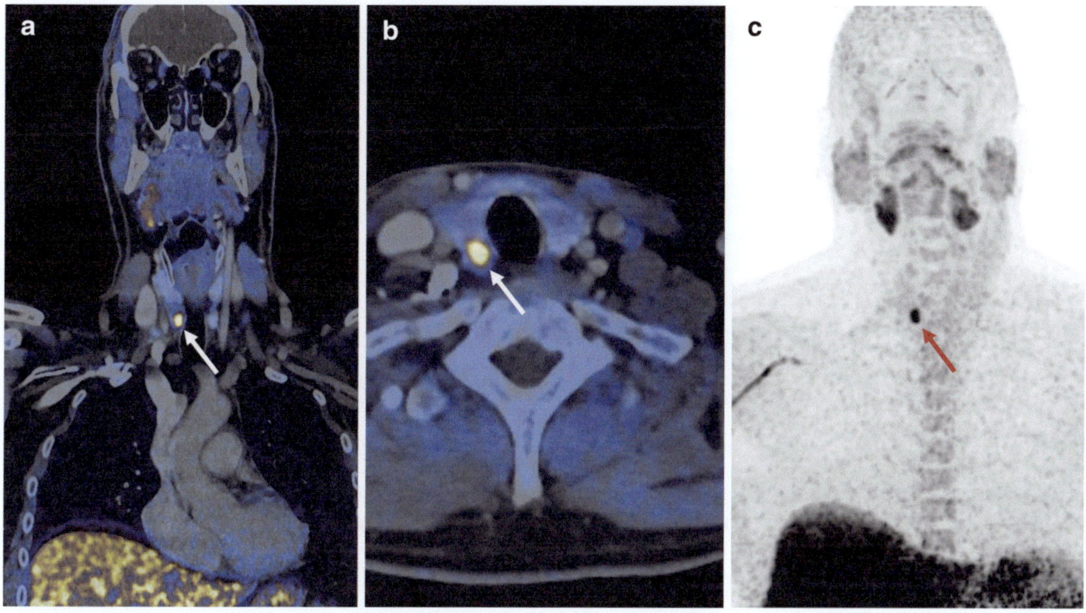

Fig. 8.2 A 45-year-old male patient with primary hyperparathyroidism and elevated parathyroid hormone level (78.9 pg/mL). [^{18}F]fluorocholine PET/CT (**a**: coronal fused PET/CT, **b**: axial fused, **c**: MIP) demonstrates a singular orthotopic small parathyroid adenoma (arrows), located posterior to the lower pole of the right lobe of the thyroid gland, showing high uptake of the radiotracer

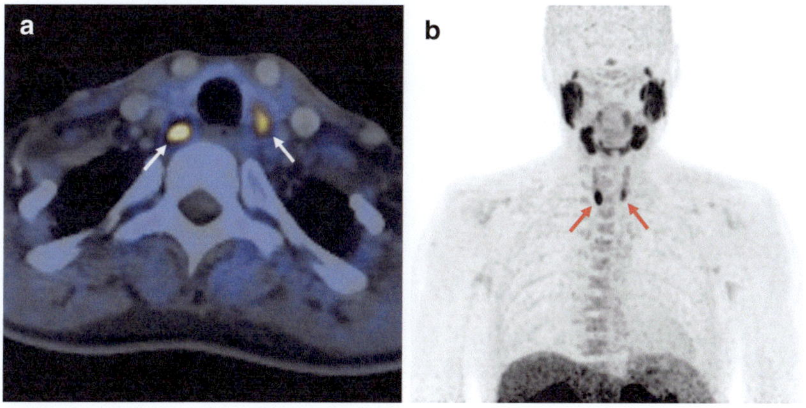

Fig. 8.3 A 48-year-old female patient with primary hyperparathyroidism. [^{18}F]fluorocholine PET/CT (**a**: fused axial, **b**: MIP) demonstrates two small orthotopic parathyroid adenomas with high uptake (arrows) posterior to the lower poles of both lobes of the thyroid gland

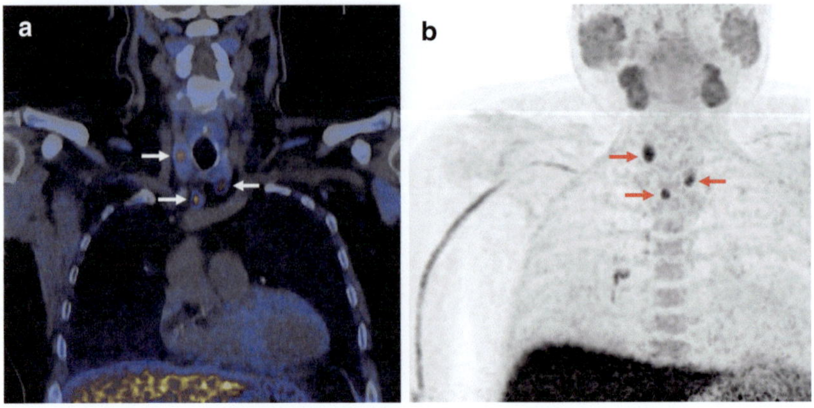

Fig. 8.4 A 68-year-old male patient, following two kidney transplantations, developed tertiary hyperparathyroidism with an elevated parathyroid hormone level (353 pg/mL). [^{18}F]fluorocholine PET/CT (**a**: coronal fused, **b**: MIP) demonstrates three small orthotopic hyperfunctioning parathyroid glands (arrows) with high uptake located posterior to the right upper and bilateral lower poles of the thyroid gland

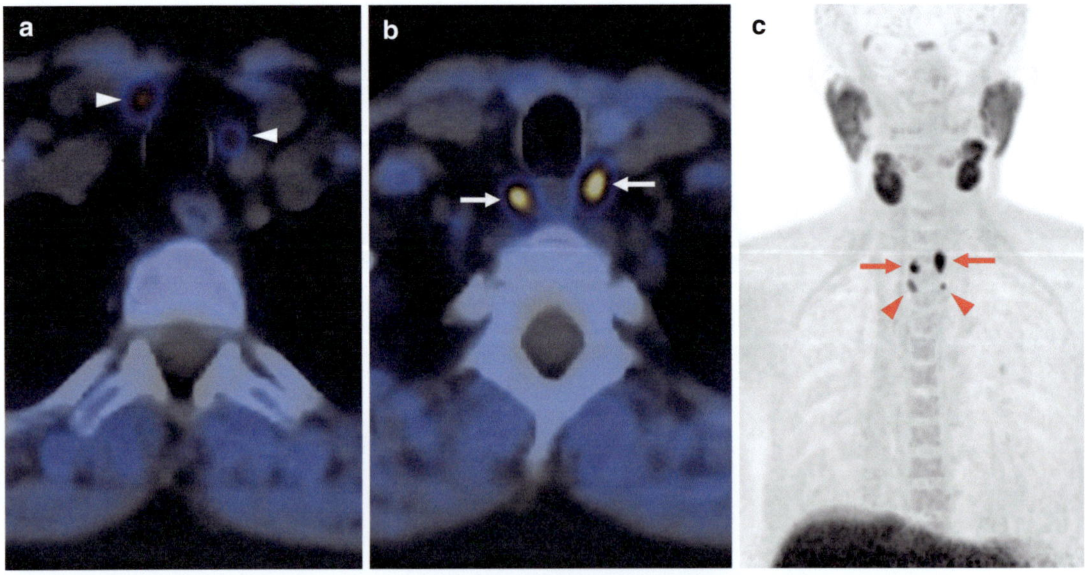

Fig. 8.5 A 61-year-old female patient with IgA nephritis, who underwent kidney transplantation, developed tertiary hyperparathyroidism. [^{18}F]fluorocholine PET/CT demonstrates four small orthotopic hyperfunctioning parathyroid glands (arrows) (**a**, **b**: axial fused, **c**: MIP)

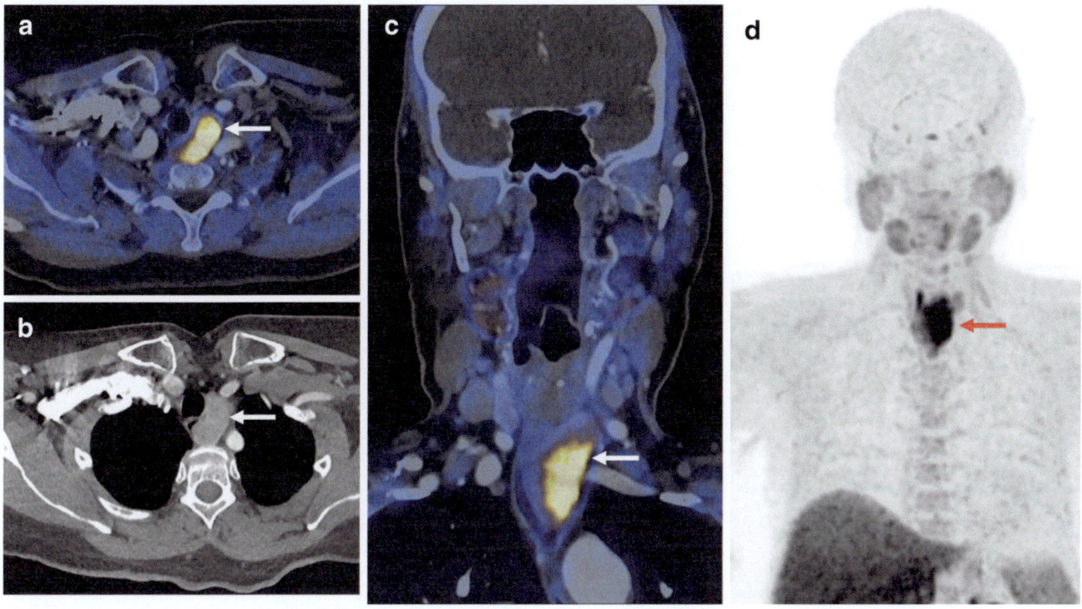

Fig. 8.6 A 74-year-old female patient with primary hyperparathyroidism with elevated parathyroid hormone level (211 pg/mL). PET/CT (**a**: axial fused, **b**: axial CT, **c**: coronal fused, **d**: MIP) demonstrates a large orthotopic enhancing parathyroid adenoma (arrows) with high [^{18}F] fluorocholine uptake, posterior to the lower pole of the left lobe of the thyroid gland, extending into the superior mediastinum, displacing the trachea and esophagus, and causing rightward deviation of the trachea

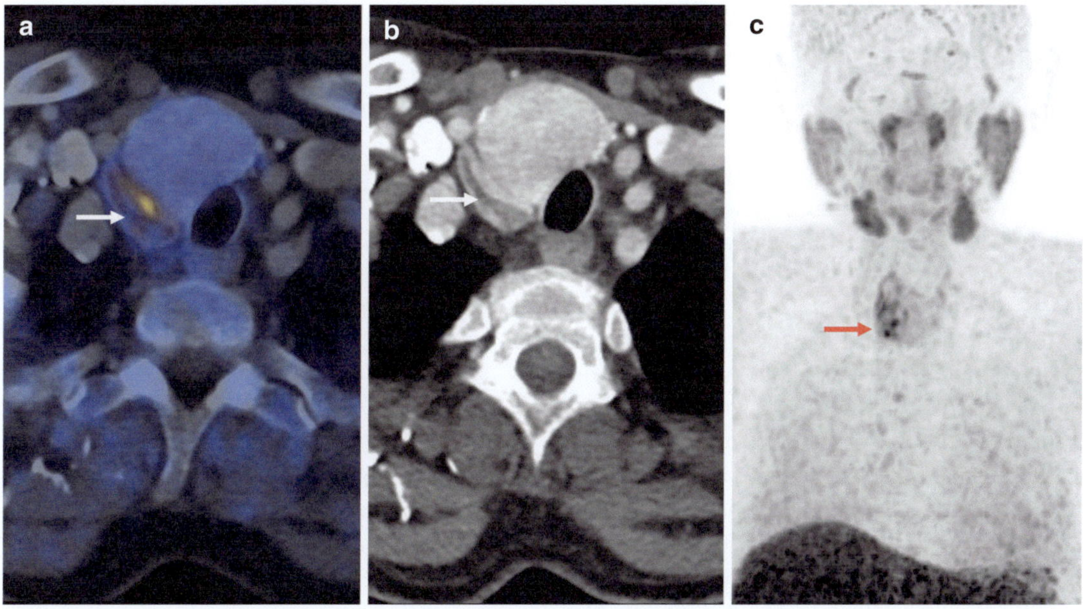

Fig. 8.7 A 49-year-old female patient with primary hyperparathyroidism with elevated parathyroid hormone level (312 pg/mL). [^{18}F]fluorocholine PET/CT demonstrates a large cystic parathyroid adenoma with peripheral uptake, posterior to the enlarged right thyroid lobe (arrows)

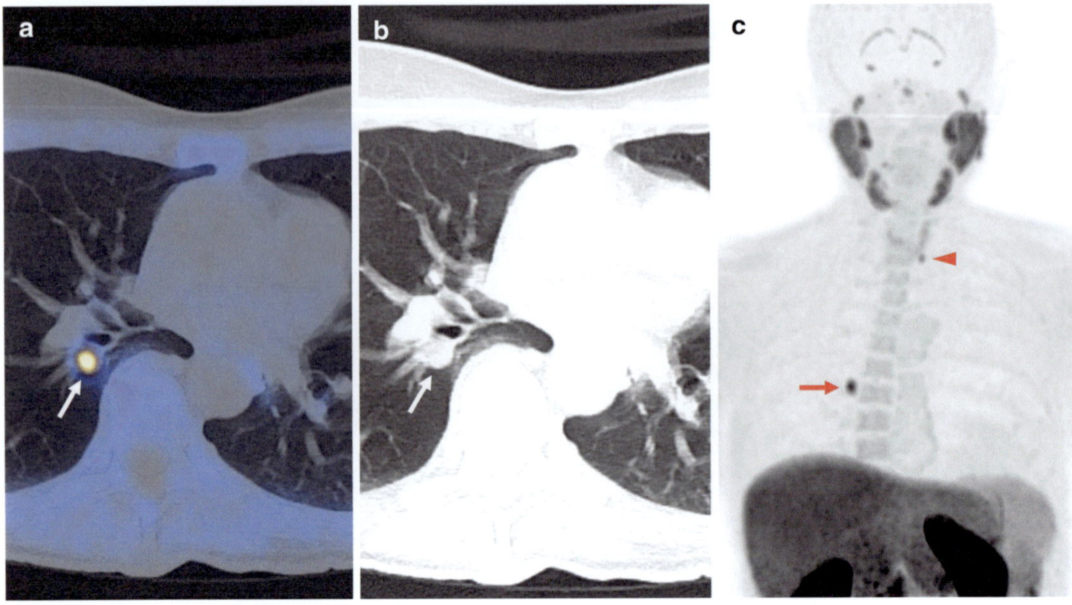

Fig. 8.8 A 59-year-old female patient with primary hyperparathyroidism. [^{18}F]fluorocholine PET/CT demonstrates a small orthotopic left inferior parathyroid adenoma with moderate uptake (arrowhead **c**). Additionally, a focal lesion with high uptake is observed in the right lower lung lobe (arrows **a**, **b**, **c**). Bronchoscopic biopsy revealed a typical lung carcinoid

8.8 False-Positive Findings on Choline PET/CT

Not all that glitters is an adenoma. Similarly, focal radiotracer accumulation on choline PET/CT is not always indicative of a hyperfunctioning parathyroid gland but may instead be associated with other benign, inflammatory, or malignant pathologies.

- Focal radiotracer uptake within the thyroid gland may be attributable to benign or malignant thyroid nodules or, in some cases, may represent an intrathyroidal parathyroid gland [9]. Residual thyroid tissue following partial or total thyroidectomy may also demonstrate choline uptake.
- Reactive or inflammatory lymph nodes in the cervical, mediastinal, or axillary regions may show choline uptake. Careful interpretation of corresponding CT (or MR) images, combined with clinical history and laboratory parameters, is essential to avoid misdiagnosis. Additionally, dynamic imaging may aid in differentiating hyperfunctioning parathyroid tissue from active lymph nodes [10, 11].
- Focal choline uptake in the forearm may indicate an implanted hyperfunctioning parathyroid gland following autotransplantation [12, 13].
- Incidental focal choline uptake in the breast [14], lung [15], or other locations may raise suspicion of a secondary malignancy, warranting further diagnostic workup, including biopsy confirmation (Fig. 8.8).

8.9 False-Negative Findings

Despite its high diagnostic accuracy, choline PET/CT is not entirely immune to false-negative results. Several factors may contribute to missed lesions:

- Patients with only mild to moderate hypercalcemia and non-elevated serum PTH levels may present with inconspicuous findings on choline PET/CT, leading to false-negative results.

- Very small adenomas or cystic parathyroid lesions may exhibit insufficient choline uptake, rendering them undetectable with this imaging modality.
- In cases of secondary HPT (sHPT) or MEN syndromes with multiglandular parathyroid disease (MGD), one or more hyperplastic glands may remain undetected, even with the use of choline PET/CT.

8.10 First-Line Imaging

[^{18}F]fluorocholine (FCH) PET/CT has now been established as the first-line imaging modality for the detection of hyperfunctioning parathyroid tissue, with the following advantages and disadvantages compared to conventional imaging [6, 16–22] (Table 8.2).

Preoperative choline PET/CT demonstrates high sensitivity and positive predictive value (PPV) for detecting hyperfunctioning parathyroid adenomas in patients with pHPT. This facilitates accurate anatomical localization, enabling precise surgical planning and promoting minimally invasive parathyroidectomy procedures. As a result, operative time, morbidity, and complication rates are significantly reduced. In clinical practice, growing experience has shown that endocrine surgeons increasingly prefer choline PET/CT over conventional imaging due to its superior diagnostic performance and reliability.

Table 8.2 Advantages and disadvantages of [^{18}F]fluorocholine (FCH) PET/CT

Advantages	Disadvantages
Higher spatial resolution	False-positive uptake by inflammatory lesions/nodes, thyroid nodules
Detection of smaller lesions (<10 mm)	Higher costs
Superior image quality	Availability
More straightforward image interpretation	Reimbursement and licensing issues, if any
Shorter acquisition time	
Extendable to whole-body acquisition	
Lower radiation exposure	
Sensitivity, 95%; PPV, 97%	

In 2014, Orevi et al. conducted a study involving 40 patients with pHPT, demonstrating that [^{11}C]choline PET/CT achieved a sensitivity of 92.3% for localizing histopathologically confirmed parathyroid adenomas, compared to 88.5% for [^{99m}Tc]Tc-Sestamibi [23]. In a comparative study by Noltes et al., [^{11}C]choline PET/CT demonstrated a positive detection rate of 88%, outperforming [^{11}C]methionine PET/CT (72%) and 4D-CT (47%) for localizing parathyroid adenomas [24].

Three recent meta-analyses have highlighted the high diagnostic performance of choline PET/CT in detecting hyperfunctioning parathyroid tissue in patients with pHPT (Tables 8.3 and 8.4). Treglia et al. analyzed 14 studies with 517 patients, reporting a per-patient sensitivity of 95% and a PPV of 97%, with per-lesion sensitivity and PPV reaching 92% [19]. Similarly, Quak et al., in a systematic review of 23 studies with 1716 patients, demonstrated a sensitivity of 93.8% and a positive predictive value (PPV) of 97%, accompanied by a surgical cure rate of 92.8% [25]. In a comprehensive meta-analysis by Ferrari et al., evaluating 32 studies with 1520 patients, choline PET/CT significantly outperformed [^{99m}Tc]Tc-Sestamibi scintigraphy, with reported sensitivity and accuracy rates of 96.4% and 96.2%, respectively, compared to 62.9% and 85.3% for [^{99m}Tc]Tc-Sestamibi [26] (Table 8.3). These results confirm the superior diagnostic accuracy and clinical utility of choline PET/CT, particularly in cases that are complex or inconclusive.

Choline PET/CT significantly reduces the need for bilateral neck exploration, avoiding this invasive procedure in approximately 75% of cases, as shown in the APACH1 study [3]. In addition, it also reliably detects parathyroid hyperplasia, which is frequently missed by US and [^{99m}Tc]Tc-Sestamibi, with reported sensitivities of 72% for choline PET/CT, compared to 39% for US and 25% for [^{99m}Tc]Tc-Sestamibi [27]. For parathyroid adenomas, choline PET/

Table 8.3 Performance of [^{18}F]fluorocholine (FCH) PET/CT when used as a first-line imaging modality in the localization of hyperfunctioning parathyroid glands

Study/authors	RP/PP	Tracer/modality	No. of pts	Sensitivity (patient-based)	Sensitivity (gland/lesion-based)	Specificity	PR/DR/Acc	Detection of MGD
Lezaic et al. [31]	PP	FCH	24	92%		100%	Acc: 98%	In 7 pts., 20/22 lesions
		Sestamibi		64%		100%	Acc: 88%	7/22 lesions
Thanseer et al. [32]	PP	FCH	54	100%	100%		Acc: 96.3%	
		Sestamibi		80.7%	76.4%		Acc: 79.6%	
		US		69.3%	69.3%		Acc: 62.9%	
Beheshti et al. [4]	PP	FCH	82		93.7%	96%	DR: 93%	In 9 pts
		Sestamibi/Tetrofosmin			60.8%	98.5%	DR: 61%	
Rep et al. [18]	PP	FCH	36		97%	99%		In 3 pts
		Sestamibi			64%	96%		
Araz et al. [8]	PP	FCH	35		96%	100%	Acc: 97%	
		Sestamibi			78%	100%	Acc: 86%	
Bossert et al. [33]	PP	FCH	34	88%			DR: 71%	
		Sestamibi		17%			DR: 15%	
		US		82%			DR: 68%	
Talbot et al. [27]	RP	FCH	392	91%	91%	89%	67%	59%
		US/Sestamibi	346/178	54%/42%	45%/30%	78%/100%	47%/37%	32%/15%
Broos et al. [16]	RP	FCH	271	96%	90%	–	75%	In 10 pts
Seyedinia et al. [34]	RP	FCH	321	99%		91%	93%	In 24 pts
		US	50	41%		66%	37%	
Quak et al. [35]	PP	FCH	29		82%		83%	
		Sestamibi	28		63%		64%	
Cuderman et al. [20]	PP	FCH	103	92%	95.5%	99.7%		Sen: 88%
		CI (Sestamibi)		65%	76%	100%		Sen: 44%
Imperiale et al. [36]	RP	FCH	64		93%	99%		In 5 pts
		Sestamibi			82%	95%		

Boudousq et al. [37]	RP	FCH	144		99.3%	97%	Acc: 98%	In 6 pts
		Sestamibi			65.1%	97.8%	Acc: 81%	
		US			75.2%	94%	Acc: 84%	
		Sestamibi+US			89.9%	92.5%	Acc: 91%	
Manyalich-Blasi et al. [38]	PP	FCH	37		92.1%	98.0%	Acc: 96.4%	In 4 pts
		Sestamibi			57.9%	96.1%	Acc: 85.7%	0
		US			32.4%	96.7%	Acc: 79.0%	0
Dudoignon et al. [39]	PP	FCH	51	76%	60%	97%	Acc: 76%	9/15
		Sestamibi		33%	26%	100%	Acc: 33%	4/15
		US		71%	56%	96%	Acc: 71%	11/15
		All 3 combined		94%	77%	95%	Acc: 94%	14/15
Latge et al. [40]	RP	FCH	42		91.3%		DR: 87.5%	
		4D-CT	37		65.2%		DR: 62.5%	
		Sestamibi	14		46.1%		DR: 46.7%	
		US	16		50%		DR: 57.1%	
Kaseb et al. [41]	RP	FCH	166	83%		97%	Acc: 93%	
		4D-CT	166	53%		84%	Acc: 75%	
		FCH + 4D-CT	166	88%		98%	Acc: 95%	
		FCH-, 4D-CT	44	80%		97%	Acc: 92%	
Patranovic et al. [42]	RP	FCH PET/CT	14	100%		100%	Acc: 100%	
		FCH PET/MRI	109	94.8%		84.6%	Acc: 93.6%	

FCH, [18F]fluorocholine PET/CT; Sestamibi, [99mTc]Tc-Sestamibi scintigraphy; *US*, ultrasound; *4D-CT*, four-dimensional computed tomography; *PET/MRI*, positron emission tomography/magnetic resonance imaging; *RP*, retrospective; *PP*, prospective; *MGD*, multiglandular disease; *HP*, histopathology; *CI*, conventional imaging; *DR*, detection rate; *PR*, positivity rate; *Acc*, accuracy

Table 8.4 Performance of [^{18}F]fluorocholine (FCH) PET/CT when used as a second-line imaging modality in the localization of hyperfunctioning parathyroid glands

Study	RP/PP	Tracer/modality	No. of Pts	Sensitivity (patient-based)	Sensitivity (gland/lesion-based)	Specificity	PR/DR/Acc	Detection of MGD
Michaud et al. [43]	PP	FCH	17	94%	96%	56%	Acc: 85%	
		Sestamibi		94%	83%	56%	Acc: 76%	
		US		50%	50%	33%	Acc: 46%	
Grimaldi et al. [44]	PP	FCH	27	81%	76%	91%	PR: 89%	In 6 pts
Quak et al. [3]	PP	FCH	25	90.5%	91.3%		PR: 76%	In 1 pt
Kluijfhout et al. [45]	RP	FCH	44		94.3%		PR: 77.3%, PPV: 97.1%	In 3 pts
		Sestamibi	29	30%			PPV: 69.2%	
		US	19	14.3%			PPV: 60%	
Uslu-Besli et al. [5]	RP	FCH	105	94.1%			Acc: 92.4%	
		Sestamibi		45.1%			Acc: 45.7%	
		US		44.1%			Acc: 42.9%	
Zajíčková et al. [46]	RP	FCH	13	92%	93%		PPV: 100% (PP) PPV: 81% (PL)	
Fischli et al. [29]	RP	FCH	23	95.5%	87.5%		PR: 95.6%	
Dekorsy et al. [47]	RP	FCH	33	TPR: 100%		TNR: 100%	PR: 72.7%	
Ferrari et al. [30]	RP	FCH	68	97.1%			FP: 1.47%	
		Sestamibi/tetrofosmin	138	56.5%			FP: 5.1%	
		US	138	47.1%			FP: 17.4%	
Garnier et al. [28]	RP	FCH	156	97.95%		40%	Acc: 94.2%	In 7 pts
		Sestamibi	142	46.21%		50%	Acc: 46%	
		US	155	60.14%		35.29%	Acc: 57%	
		Sestamibi+US	142	80.1%		78.8%	Acc: 79.5%	
Amadou et al. [48]	RP	FCH	27	85.2%	95.8%	12.5%	NPV: 50.0%	
		4DCT	19	63.2%	75.0%	40.0%	NPV: 33.3%	
		Sestamibi	26	48.0%	50.0%	75.0%	NPV: 33.3%	
		US	25	46.2%	54.2%	75.0%	NPV: 35.3%	
Piccardo et al. [49]	PP	FCH	44	81%			DR: 56.8%	
		4DCT		74%			DR: 54.5%	
		FCH + 4DCT		100%			DR: 72.7%	

Pretet et al. [50]	RP	FCH	50	93%	88%		DR: 82%	
		4DCT		80%	66%		DR: 68%	
		FCH + 4DCT		95%	92%		DR: 84%	
Patranovic et al. [42]	RP	FCH PET/CT	44	97.3%		85.7%	Acc: 95.5%	
		FCH PET/MRI	155	97.9%		77.8%	Acc: 96.8%	

FCH, [18F]fluorocholine PET/CT; *Sestamibi*, [99mTc]Tc-Sestamibi scintigraphy; *US*, ultrasound; *4DCT*, four-dimensional computed tomography; *PET/MRI*, positron emission tomography/magnetic resonance imaging; *RP*, retrospective study; *PP*, prospective study; *DR*, detection rate; *PR*, positivity rate; *Acc*, accuracy; *MGD*: multiglandular disease; *PPV*, positive predictive value; *PP*, per patient; *PL*, per lesion; *FP*, false-positive rate; *TPR*, true positive detection rate; *TNR*, true negative detection rate; *NPV*, negative predictive value

CT achieves a sensitivity of 86%, compared to 51% for US and 37% for [^{99m}Tc]Tc-Sestamibi. Notably, in cases of MGD, choline PET/CT achieves a sensitivity of 100%, markedly surpassing the diagnostic capabilities of other modalities [20, 28]. It also shows superior performance in challenging clinical scenarios, such as patients with prior neck surgery, obesity, or multinodular goiter [29]. Known predictors of poor [^{99m}Tc]Tc-Sestamibi performance, including low PTH levels, concomitant structural thyroid disease, and negative sonography, further support the role of choline PET/CT as the preferred first-line imaging modality in these patients [30].

Choline PET/CT is particularly recommended as a first-line imaging tool in clinical settings of hyperparathyroidism when there is a high suspicion of parathyroid hyperplasia, in cases of persistent or recurrent pHPT, with MGD disease, during the initial imaging workup of renal hyperparathyroidism (rHPT), and in patients with HPT persisting after surgery.

8.11 Secondary and Tertiary Hyperparathyroidism

Patients with chronic kidney disease (CKD) of prolonged duration may develop secondary (sHPT) or tertiary (tHPT) hyperparathyroidism, due to progressive parathyroid gland hyperplasia, resulting in excessive PTH secretion. While sHPT and tHPT are pathophysiologically related, they represent distinct clinical entities. sHPT typically presents with hypocalcemia, whereas tHPT is characterized by hypercalcemia that follows a prolonged phase of sHPT, during which the parathyroid glands may become autonomous. Spontaneous resolution of HPT occurs in up to 60% of patients after successful kidney transplantation. However, persistent HPT develops in approximately 20–30% of cases, often due to autonomous hyperfunctioning of one or more parathyroid glands. MGD is more frequent in sHPT or tHPT compared to pHPT.

The primary objective of parathyroid imaging in the setting of sHPT or tHPT is to precisely localize all hyperfunctioning parathyroid glands, including both orthotopic and ectopic glands, as part of the preoperative assessment. Choline PET/CT has demonstrated high diagnostic performance in both sHPT and tHPT and can be effectively utilized for this purpose. In a study by Aymard et al., the diagnostic performance of [^{18}F]fluorocholine PET/CT, neck US, [^{99m}Tc]Tc-Sestamibi scintigraphy, and 4D-CT was evaluated in 30 patients with CKD and HPT (18 with sHPT and 12 with tHPT), involving 65 hyperplastic parathyroid glands and six adenomas. [^{18}F]fluorocholine PET/CT outperformed all other imaging modalities, with reported sensitivities of 72% for [^{18}F]fluorocholine PET/CT, 25% for neck US, 35% for [^{99m}Tc]Tc-Sestamibi scintigraphy, and 40% for 4D-CT [51]. Similarly, [^{18}F]fluorocholine PET/CT demonstrated the highest diagnostic accuracy at 71%, compared to 43% for US, 47% for [^{99m}Tc]Tc-MIBI scintigraphy, and 47% for 4D-CT. Notably, the sensitivity of [^{18}F]fluorocholine PET/CT was significantly higher in patients with tHPT (88%) compared to those with sHPT (66%).

8.12 Ectopic Localization

The anatomy of the parathyroid glands exhibits considerable variability in the general population, both in terms of number and location. Although typically four parathyroid glands are present, variations can occur, with some individuals having fewer glands and others possessing up to 12 glands in rare cases [52]. The superior parathyroid glands, derived embryologically from the fourth pharyngeal pouch, have a relatively short migration pathway and are usually located posterior to the upper poles to midportions of the thyroid gland. Consequently, they exhibit less anatomical variability in their final location. However, a considerable proportion of superior glands are found in an overly descended position, located at the level of the lower pole of the thyroid or even below this level. Some experts regard this as a form of minor ectopia, although these glands remain within the expected surgical field of view. In contrast, the inferior parathyroid glands originate from the third pharyngeal pouch and descend during embryological development in association with the thymus. Their longer migratory path results in a broader spectrum of possible ectopic locations. While their normal position is next to the thyroid, at the level of anterior half of the trachea, or inferior to the lower pole of the thyroid gland, their ectopic locations can range from high in the neck at the angle of the mandible (due to incomplete descent) to the upper or anterior mediastinum, including within or adjacent to the thymus or even as far as the pericardium [53, 54] (Figs. 8.9, 8.10, and 8.11).

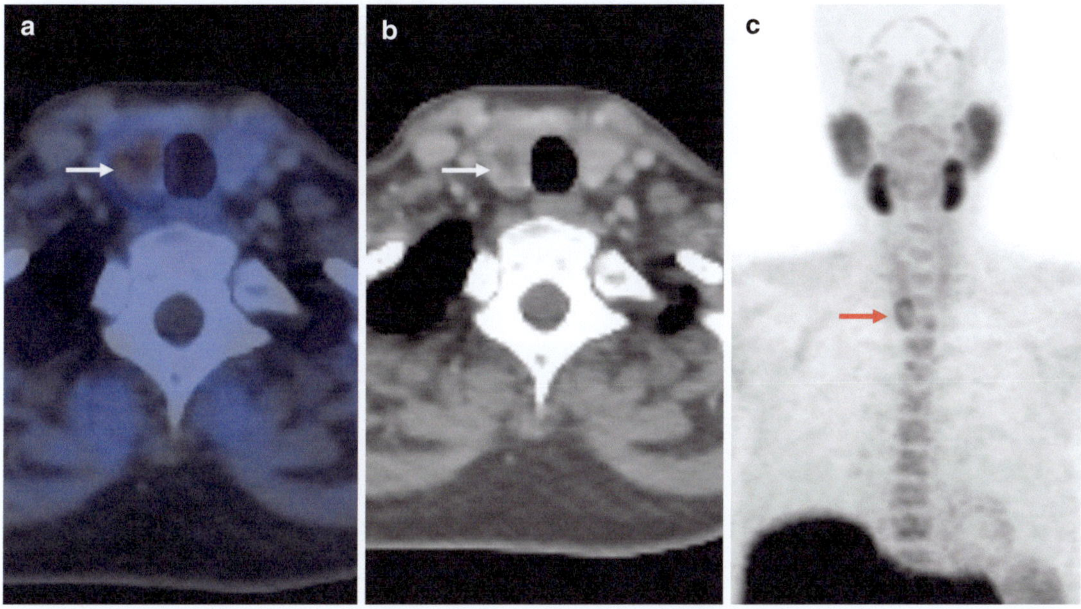

Fig. 8.9 A 46-year-old female patient with primary hyperparathyroidism with elevated parathyroid hormone (128 pg/mL). [18F]fluorocholine PET/CT demonstrates a well-defined hypodense ovoid lesion with moderately increased uptake in the right thyroid lobe (arrows). Hemithyroidectomy confirmed an ectopic intrathyroidal parathyroid adenoma

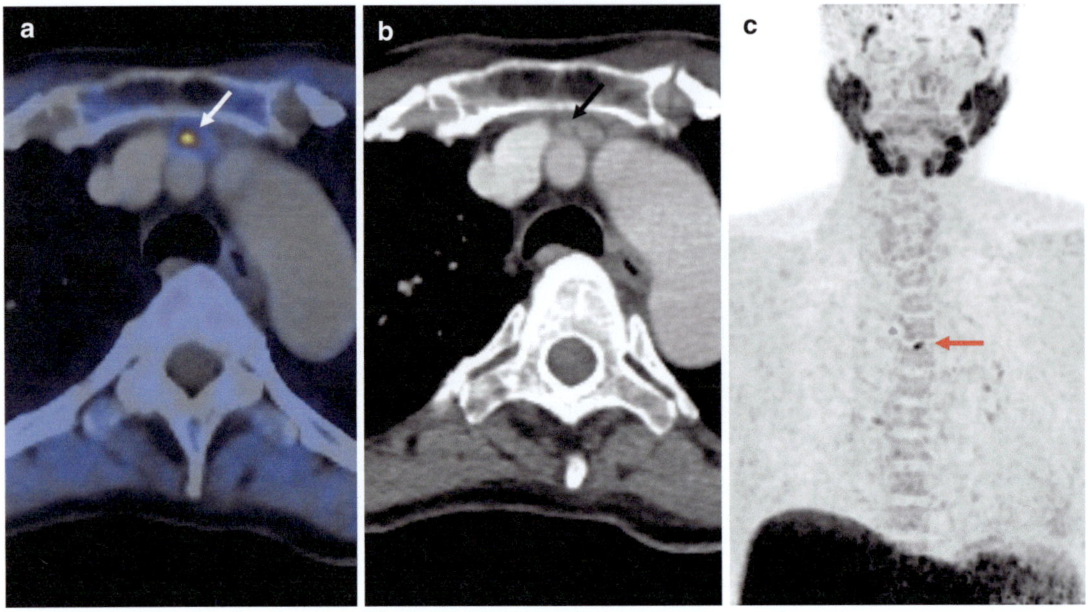

Fig. 8.10 A 65-year-old female patient with primary hyperparathyroidism. [^{18}F]fluorocholine PET/CT demonstrates a small ectopic parathyroid adenoma in the anterior mediastinum (arrows, **a**, **b**, **c**)

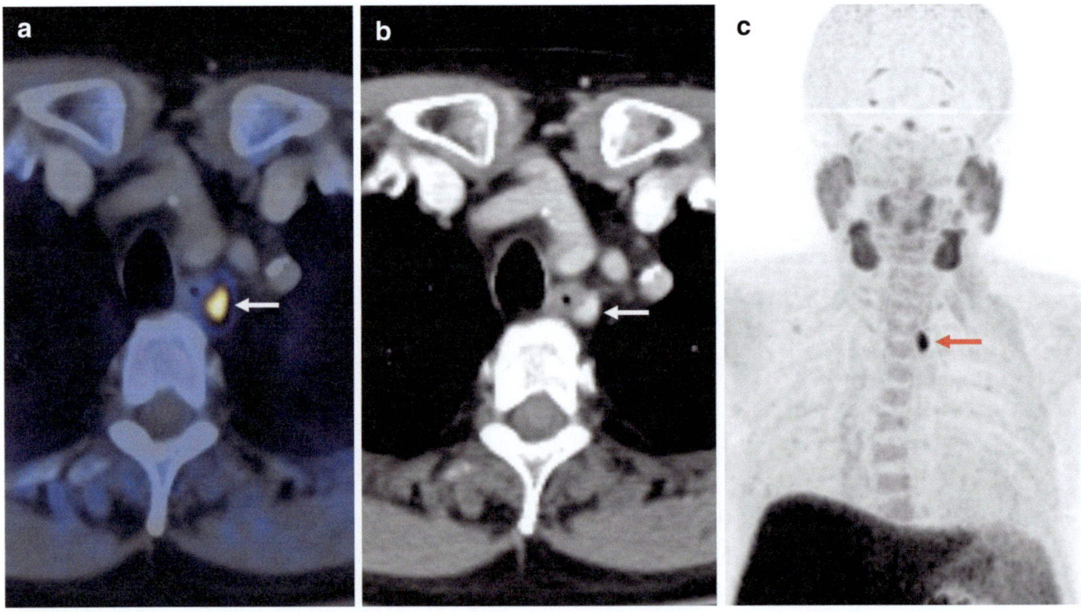

Fig. 8.11 A 65-year-old female patient with primary hyperparathyroidism with elevated parathyroid hormone level (116 pg/mL). [^{18}F]fluorocholine PET/CT demonstrates a small ectopic paraesophageal parathyroid adenoma with high uptake (arrows)

8.13 Parathyroid Carcinoma

Parathyroid carcinoma is a rare but potentially aggressive malignant tumor of the parathyroid glands, accounting for approximately 1% of primary hyperparathyroidism cases and 0.005% of all malignancies. When detected early and completely resected, the prognosis can be relatively favorable. However, parathyroid carcinoma carries a considerable risk of local recurrence and has the potential to metastasize to the lungs, liver, and bones. Due to its rarity and the significant overlap of clinical and biochemical features with more common benign parathyroid disorders, the diagnosis of parathyroid carcinoma remains a considerable challenge.

Suspicion of malignancy should be raised in patients presenting with markedly elevated biochemical parameters, particularly when serum PTH levels are 3–10 times above the upper normal limit and serum calcium levels exceed 3 mmol/L, often accompanied by a palpable neck mass larger than 3 cm, a practical diagnostic aid referred to as the "rule of 3 + 3" [55]. In the US, suspicious neck lesions typically appear hypoechoic, inhomogeneous, and lobulated. These cases are frequently associated with exacerbated skeletal disease, such as brown tumors, and renal complications, including nephrolithiasis or nephrocalcinosis. Choline PET/CT has demonstrated a valuable role in the detection of both primary parathyroid lesions and metastatic disease, showing a higher detection rate than [^{18}F]FDG PET/CT or other conventional radionuclide imaging modalities [56, 57]. Supporting this, a study by Uslu-Besi et al. found that four patients with parathyroid neoplasia had significantly higher SUVmax values compared to the broader patient cohort with parathyroid adenoma or hyperplasia [5]. Specifically, early-phase imaging revealed an SUVmax of 10.8 ± 5.0, and late-phase imaging an SUVmax of 11.8 ± 5.8, while the mean SUVmax for the entire group was 7.1 ± 3.5 (early) and 7.3 ± 3.6 (late).

Metastatic liver lesions may demonstrate reduced choline avidity and can therefore be missed on choline PET imaging. However, the diagnostic CT component of the PET/CT protocol plays a crucial role in such cases, as it can reliably detect these lesions based on morphological criteria, even when PET findings are negative [58].

8.14 Bone and Brown Tumors

Bone-specific complications of hyperparathyroidism commonly present as focal osteolytic or multilobular cystic lesions known as osteitis fibrosa cystica or brown tumors, which are benign, non-neoplastic bone lesions. These arise due to chronic disturbances in bone remodelling caused by persistently elevated PTH levels. Excess PTH stimulates osteoclastic bone resorption, leading to the breakdown of bone tissue and release of calcium into the bloodstream. The resorbed bone is replaced by fibrous tissue, resulting in the formation of cyst-like brown tumors. Intralesional hemorrhage and breakdown of red blood cells lead to hemosiderin deposition, which imparts the characteristic brown coloration to these lesions. Brown tumors can develop in any bone but are most frequently observed in the ribs, pelvis, clavicles, and long bones of the extremities (Fig. 8.12). Clinically, they may present with bone pain, swelling, or pathological fractures due to the underlying weakening of the bone. These lesions are typically negative on [^{99m}Tc]Tc-Sestamibi but can be detected using choline PET/CT, which offers improved sensitivity [6, 59, 60]. It is important to consider differential diagnoses for focal bone uptake on choline PET/CT, including primary or secondary bone neoplasms, such as multiple myeloma or bone metastases, particularly from prostate cancer. Additionally, diffuse increased choline uptake in the mandible may indicate Paget's disease [61] or hyperparathyroidism-jaw tumor (HPT-JT) syndrome, a rare autosomal dominant condition associated with pHPT and an increased risk of jaw tumors.

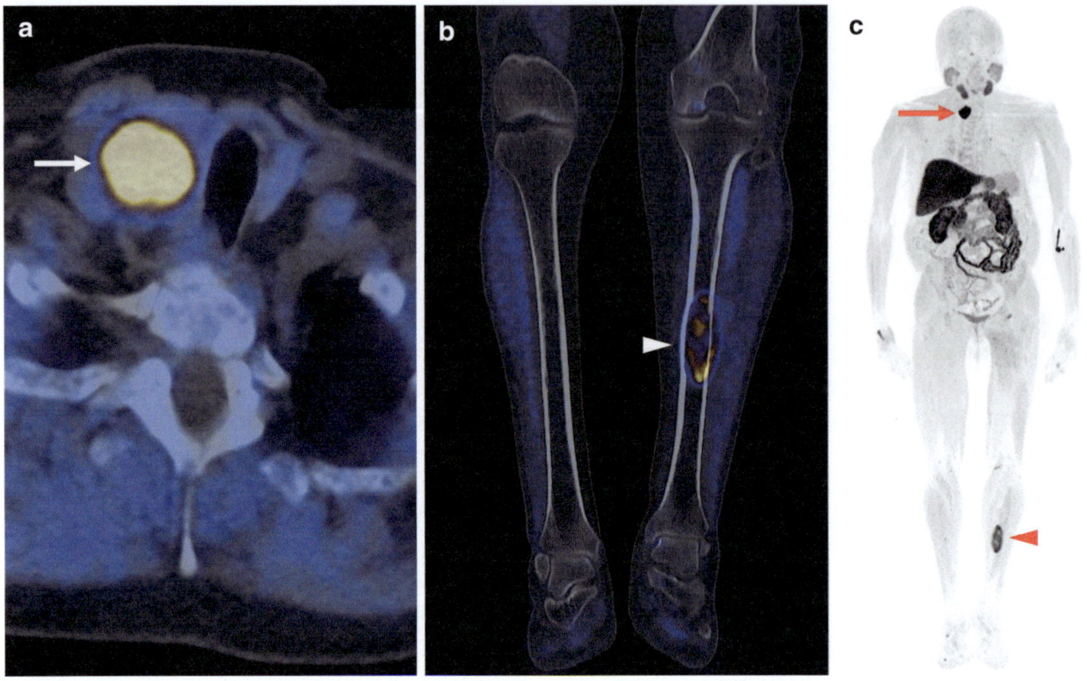

Fig. 8.12 A 68-year-old female patient with primary hyperparathyroidism with elevated parathyroid hormone level (916 pg/mL). [^{18}F]fluorocholine PET/CT demonstrates a large orthotopic right-sided parathyroid adenoma (arrows, **a**, **c**) with high uptake. Additionally, a focal expansive osteolytic lesion is seen in the diaphysis of the left tibia (arrowheads **b**, **c**) with moderate uptake. Biopsy of the tibial lesion confirmed a brown tumor

8.15 Thyroid Cancer and Thyroiditis on CH PET/CT

Incidental focal and diffuse thyroid uptake on choline PET is a relevant finding that may provide additional clinically useful information beyond parathyroid imaging. In a retrospective study involving 195 patients with hyperparathyroidism, Grunig et al. reported that 25 patients (13%) demonstrated incidental [^{18}F]fluorocholine uptake in the thyroid gland [9]. Diffuse choline uptake in the thyroid gland is most commonly associated with multinodular goiter or Hashimoto's thyroiditis, probably reflecting diffuse metabolic activity within the gland. In contrast, focal thyroid uptake may indicate the presence of a thyroid nodule, which can be either benign or malignant. Such findings warrant further evaluation with neck ultrasound, followed by fine-needle aspiration cytology (FNAC) if clinically indicated (Figs. 8.13 and 8.14). It is important to note that a choline-avid thyroid nodule may also represent an intrathyroidal parathyroid adenoma. In such cases, histopathological differentiation from a thyroid adenoma can be challenging, particularly when based solely on FNAC, which may not provide definitive discrimination between these entities. However, FNAC in combination with measurement of PTH in the aspirate usually provides a diagnosis of parathyroid lesion [62].

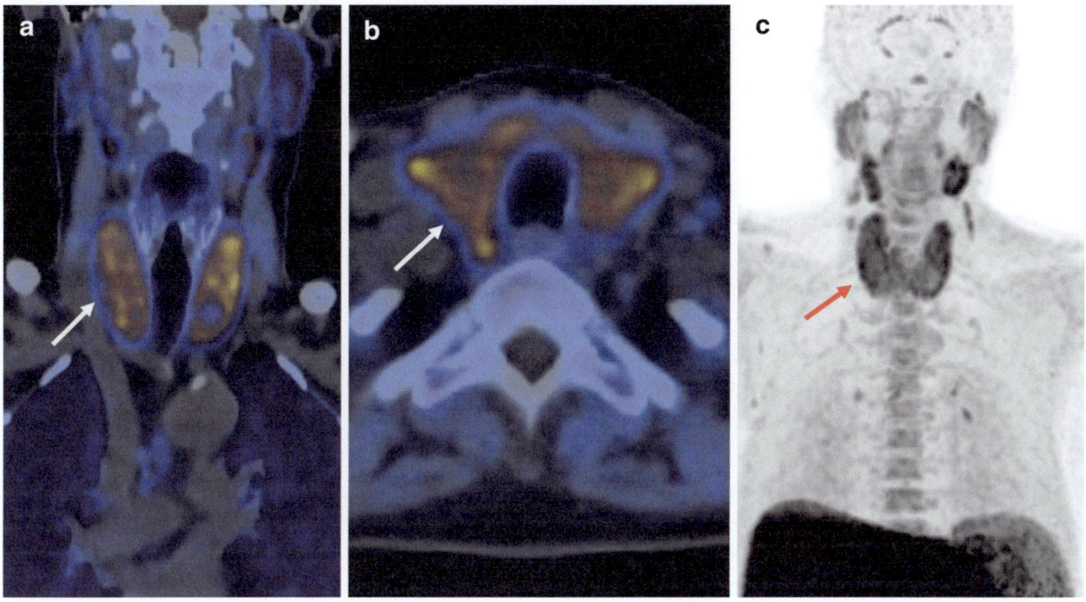

Fig. 8.13 A 55-year-old female patient with primary hyperparathyroidism with elevated parathyroid hormone level (188 pg/mL). [18F]fluorocholine PET/CT demonstrates diffuse, heterogeneous, moderately increased uptake in the enlarged thyroid gland (arrows), compatible with Basedow's/Graves' disease. No hyperfunctioning parathyroid gland or adenoma was detected

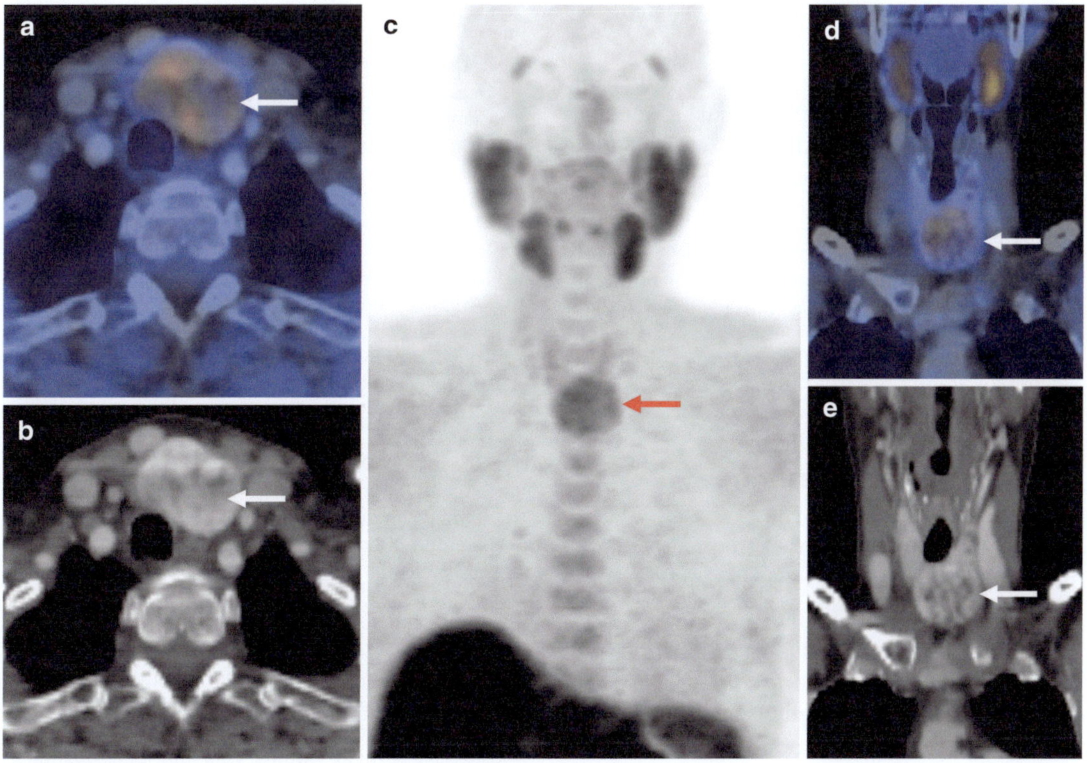

Fig. 8.14 A 74-year-old female patient with primary hyperparathyroidism with elevated parathyroid hormone level (75 pg/mL). [18F]fluorocholine PET/CT demonstrates a thyroid nodule with moderate uptake. Total thyroidectomy showed a papillary thyroid carcinoma (arrows **a**, **b**, **c**, **d**, **e**)

8.16 Cost-Effectiveness

Cost-effectiveness and economic evaluation studies across various healthcare systems have shown that [^{18}F]fluorocholine PET/CT is a cost-effective alternative to conventional imaging modalities [63–65]. Enhanced detection and precise localization of hyperfunctioning parathyroid tissue result in reduced operative risks, fewer complications, shorter surgery durations and hospital stays, as well as decreased need for repeat imaging and reoperations. In the United States, Yap et al. reported that [^{18}F]fluorocholine PET/CT achieved the highest number of quality-adjusted life years (QALYs) at 23.9 and was deemed cost-effective despite its higher upfront cost of $2096 [64]. Similarly, van Mossel et al., in the Netherlands, found comparable health outcomes and overall costs when [^{18}F]fluorocholine was used as a first-line versus a second-line imaging modality, recommending its routine adoption depending on local resource availability [63]. In France, Mamou et al. concluded that [^{18}F]fluorocholine PET/CT was cost-effective, with an incremental cost-effectiveness ratio of €12,650 per QALY, advocating for its use as a first-line imaging option [65]. Operational advantages include substantial reductions in imaging time (83%), radiopharmaceutical preparation (89%), and quality control time (75%) when compared with conventional [^{99m}Tc]Tc-Sestamibi scintigraphy [66]. Additionally, the ability to omit intraoperative PTH testing in selected cases further shortens surgical time.

8.17 Artificial Intelligence and Deep Learning

Parathyroid adenomas are frequently small (often <8 mm) and can be elusive, making their localization on imaging particularly challenging. The EANM guidelines for parathyroid imaging recommend the use of a PET/CT scanner with the highest available sensitivity, alongside reconstruction protocols optimized for small lesion detection, to maximize diagnostic accuracy [6]. In this context, emerging technologies such as artificial intelligence (AI) and deep learning show significant promise. Recently, Bradley et al. demonstrated that deep learning algorithms enhanced the visualization of a small 6 mm parathyroid adenoma on [^{18}F]fluorocholine PET/CT in a patient with persistent pHPT, following both negative [^{99m}Tc]Tc-Sestamibi and 4D-CT scans, as well as a failed surgical neck exploration [67]. These developments highlight how AI-driven image enhancement is posited to further improve the detection and localization of small or atypically located parathyroid lesions, particularly in complex clinical scenarios.

References

1. Ishizuka T, Kajita K, Kamikubo K, Komaki T, Miura K, Nagao S, et al. Phospholipid/Ca2+-dependent protein kinase activity in human parathyroid adenoma. Endocrinol Jpn. 1987;34(6):965–8.
2. Parvinian A, Martin-Macintosh EL, Goenka AH, Durski JM, Mullan BP, Kemp BJ, et al. (11) C-choline PET/CT for detection and localization of parathyroid adenomas. AJR Am J Roentgenol. 2018;210(2):418–22.
3. Quak E, Blanchard D, Houdu B, Le Roux Y, Ciappuccini R, Lireux B, et al. F18-choline PET/CT guided surgery in primary hyperparathyroidism when ultrasound and MIBI SPECT/CT are negative or inconclusive: the APACH1 study. Eur J Nucl Med Mol Imaging. 2018;45(4):658–66.
4. Beheshti M, Hehenwarter L, Paymani Z, Rendl G, Imamovic L, Rettenbacher R, et al. (18) F-Fluorocholine PET/CT in the assessment of primary hyperparathyroidism compared with (99m) Tc-MIBI or (99m)Tc-tetrofosmin SPECT/CT: a prospective dual-Centre study in 100 patients. Eur J Nucl Med Mol Imaging. 2018;45(10):1762–71.
5. Uslu-Besli L, Sonmezoglu K, Teksoz S, Akgun E, Karayel E, Pehlivanoglu H, et al. Performance of F-18 fluorocholine PET/CT for detection of hyperfunctioning parathyroid tissue in patients with elevated parathyroid hormone levels and negative or discrepant results in conventional imaging. Korean J Radiol. 2020;21(2):236–47.
6. Petranovic Ovcaricek P, Giovanella L, Carrio Gasset I, Hindie E, Huellner MW, Luster M, et al. The EANM practice guidelines for parathyroid imaging. Eur J Nucl Med Mol Imaging. 2021;48(9):2801–22.
7. Rep S, Lezaic L, Kocjan T, Pfeifer M, Sever MJ, Simoncic U, et al. Optimal scan time for evaluation of parathyroid adenoma with [(18)F]-fluorocholine PET/CT. Radiol Oncol. 2015;49(4):327–33.

8. Araz M, Soydal C, Ozkan E, Kir MK, Ibis E, Gullu S, et al. The efficacy of fluorine-18-choline PET/CT in comparison with 99mTc-MIBI SPECT/CT in the localization of a hyperfunctioning parathyroid gland in primary hyperparathyroidism. Nucl Med Commun. 2018;39(11):989–94.
9. Grunig H, Strobel K, Zander A, Perez Lago MDS, Lima T, Wicke C, et al. Significance of incidental thyroid 18 F-fluorocholine uptake in patients with hyperparathyroidism imaged for localizing hyperfunctioning parathyroid glands. Nucl Med Commun. 2024;45(11):938–46.
10. Broos WAM, Wondergem M, van der Zant FM, Schaper NC, Knol RJJ. Dynamic 18F-fluorocholine PET/CT for parathyroid imaging in patients with primary hyperparathyroidism. Nucl Med Commun. 2020;41(8):776–82.
11. Prabhu M, Kumari G, Damle NA, Arora G, Kumar P, Kumar R, et al. Assessment of the role of early dynamic PET/CT with 18F-fluorocholine in detection of parathyroid lesions in patients with primary hyperparathyroidism. Nucl Med Commun. 2018;39(12):1190–6.
12. Ardito G, Revelli L, Giustozzi E, Giordano A. Radioguided parathyroidectomy in forearm graft for recurrent hyperparathyroidism. Br J Radiol. 2012;85(1009):e1–3.
13. Garrou F, Rizzo A, Rosso D, Bondi S, Racca M. 18F-fluorocholine PET/CT in the detection of hyperfunctioning transplanted parathyroid tissue. Clin Nucl Med. 2023;48(12):e580–e2.
14. Jozanovic V, Huic D. Incidental detection of breast cancer by 18F-fluorocholine PET/CT performed for primary hyperparathyroidism. Nucl Med Rev Cent East Eur. 2022;25(1):66–7.
15. Jacquet-Francillon N, Granjon D, Casteillo F, Prevot N, Habouzit V. Incidental detection of a small cell lung cancer by 18F-choline PET/CT performed for recurrent hyperparathyroidism after parathyroidectomy. Clin Nucl Med. 2021;46(2):e109–e11.
16. Broos WAM, Wondergem M, Knol RJJ, van der Zant FM. Parathyroid imaging with (18)F-fluorocholine PET/CT as a first-line imaging modality in primary hyperparathyroidism: a retrospective cohort study. EJNMMI Res. 2019;9(1):72.
17. Giovanella L, Bacigalupo L, Treglia G, Piccardo A. Will (18)F-fluorocholine PET/CT replace other methods of preoperative parathyroid imaging? Endocrine. 2021;71(2):285–97.
18. Rep S, Hocevar M, Vaupotic J, Zdesar U, Zaletel K, Lezaic L. (18)F-choline PET/CT for parathyroid scintigraphy: significantly lower radiation exposure of patients in comparison to conventional nuclear medicine imaging approaches. J Radiol Prot. 2018;38(1):343–56.
19. Treglia G, Piccardo A, Imperiale A, Strobel K, Kaufmann PA, Prior JO, et al. Diagnostic performance of choline PET for detection of hyperfunctioning parathyroid glands in hyperparathyroidism: a systematic review and meta-analysis. Eur J Nucl Med Mol Imaging. 2019;46(3):751–65.
20. Cuderman A, Senica K, Rep S, Hocevar M, Kocjan T, Sever MJ, et al. (18)F-fluorocholine PET/CT in primary hyperparathyroidism: superior diagnostic performance to conventional scintigraphic imaging for localization of hyperfunctioning parathyroid glands. J Nucl Med. 2020;61(4):577–83.
21. Hocevar M, Lezaic L, Rep S, Zaletel K, Kocjan T, Sever MJ, et al. Focused parathyroidectomy without intraoperative parathormone testing is safe after preoperative localization with (18)F-fluorocholine PET/CT. Eur J Surg Oncol. 2017;43(1):133–7.
22. Lopez-Mora DA, Sizova M, Estorch M, Flotats A, Camacho V, Fernandez A, et al. Superior performance of 18F-fluorocholine digital PET/CT in the detection of parathyroid adenomas. Eur J Nucl Med Mol Imaging. 2020;47(3):572–8.
23. Orevi M, Freedman N, Mishani E, Bocher M, Jacobson O, Krausz Y. Localization of parathyroid adenoma by (1)(1)C-choline PET/CT: preliminary results. Clin Nucl Med. 2014;39(12):1033–8.
24. Noltes ME, Kruijff S, Appelman APA, Jansen L, Zandee WT, Links TP, et al. Head-to-head comparison of [(11)C]methionine PET, [(11)C]choline PET, and 4-dimensional CT as second-line scans for detection of parathyroid adenomas in primary hyperparathyroidism. Eur J Nucl Med Mol Imaging. 2024;51(4):1050–9.
25. Quak E, Cavarec M, Ciappuccini R, Girault G, Rouzier R, Lequesne J. Detection, resection and cure: a systematic review and meta-analysis of 18F-choline PET in primary hyperparathyroidism. Q J Nucl Med Mol Imaging. 2023;67(2):122–9.
26. Ferrari C, Santo G, Mammucci P, Pisani AR, Sardaro A, Rubini G. Diagnostic value of choline PET in the preoperative localization of hyperfunctioning parathyroid gland(s): a comprehensive overview. Biomedicine. 2021;9(3)
27. Talbot JN, Perie S, Tassart M, Delbot T, Aveline C, Zhang-Yin J, et al. 18F-fluorocholine PET/CT detects parathyroid gland hyperplasia as well as adenoma: 401 PET/CTs in one center. Q J Nucl Med Mol Imaging. 2023;67(2):96–113.
28. Garnier S, Maheo C, Potard G, Cavarec MB, Roudaut N, Thuillier P, et al. Contribution of 18 F-fluorocholine PET-CT to the preoperative localisation of parathyroid adenoma for the treatment of primary hyperparathyroidism. Sci Rep. 2025;15(1):10018.
29. Fischli S, Suter-Widmer I, Nguyen BT, Muller W, Metzger J, Strobel K, et al. The significance of 18F-fluorocholine-PET/CT as localizing imaging technique in patients with primary hyperparathyroidism and negative conventional imaging. Front Endocrinol (Lausanne). 2017;8:380.
30. Ferrari SB, Morand GB, Rupp NJ, Krutzfeldt J, Vetter D, Hullner MW, et al. Clinical predictors of negative/equivocal SPECT imaging outcomes in primary hyperparathyroidism: factors calling for (18)F-choline-PET. Am J Otolaryngol. 2024;45(4):104315.

31. Lezaic L, Rep S, Sever MJ, Kocjan T, Hocevar M, Fettich J. (1)(8)F-fluorocholine PET/CT for localization of hyperfunctioning parathyroid tissue in primary hyperparathyroidism: a pilot study. Eur J Nucl Med Mol Imaging. 2014;41(11):2083–9.
32. Thanseer N, Bhadada SK, Sood A, Mittal BR, Behera A, Gorla AKR, et al. Comparative effectiveness of ultrasonography, 99mTc-Sestamibi, and 18F-fluorocholine PET/CT in detecting parathyroid adenomas in patients with primary hyperparathyroidism. Clin Nucl Med. 2017;42(12):e491–e7.
33. Bossert I, Chytiris S, Hodolic M, Croce L, Mansi L, Chiovato L, et al. PETC/CT with (18)F-choline localizes hyperfunctioning parathyroid adenomas equally well in normocalcemic hyperparathyroidism as in overt hyperparathyroidism. J Endocrinol Investig. 2019;42(4):419–26.
34. Seyedinia SS, Mirshahvalad SA, Schweighofer-Zwink G, Hehenwarter L, Rendl G, Pirich C, et al. Evolving role of [(18)F]fluorocholine PET/CT in assessing primary hyperparathyroidism: can it be considered the first-line functional imaging approach? J Clin Med. 2023;12(3)
35. Quak E, Lasne-Cardon A, Cavarec M, Lireux B, Bastit V, Roudaut N, et al. F18-choline PET/CT or MIBI SPECT/CT in the surgical management of primary hyperparathyroidism: a diagnostic randomized clinical trial. JAMA Otolaryngol Head Neck Surg. 2024;150(8):658–65.
36. Imperiale A, Bani J, Bottoni G, Latge A, Heimburger C, Catrambone U, et al. Does (18)F-fluorocholine PET/CT add value to positive parathyroid scintigraphy in the presurgical assessment of primary hyperparathyroidism? Front Med (Lausanne). 2023;10:1148287.
37. Boudousq V, Guignard N, Gilly O, Chambert B, Mamou A, Moranne O, et al. Diagnostic performance of cervical ultrasound, (99m)Tc-sestamibi scintigraphy, and contrast-enhanced (18)F-fluorocholine PET in primary hyperparathyroidism. J Nucl Med. 2022;63(7):1081–6.
38. Manyalich-Blasi M, Dominguez-Garijo P, Saavedra-Perez D, Sanchez-Izquierdo N, Casanueva Eliceiry S, Perissinotti A, et al. Comparison of [(18)F]fluorocholine PET/CT with [(99)mTc]sestamibi and ultrasonography to detect parathyroid lesions in primary hyperparathyroidism: a prospective study. Gland Surg. 2022;11(11):1764–71.
39. Dudoignon D, Delbot T, Cottereau AS, Dechmi A, Bienvenu M, Koumakis E, et al. 18F-fluorocholine PET/CT and conventional imaging in primary hyperparathyroidism. Diagn Interv Imaging. 2022;103(5):258–65.
40. Latge A, Riehm S, Vix M, Bani J, Ignat M, Pretet V, et al. (18)F-fluorocholine PET and 4D-CT in patients with persistent and recurrent primary hyperparathyroidism. Diagnostics (Basel). 2021;11(12)
41. Kaseb A, Benider H, Treglia G, Cusumano C, Bessac D, Trimboli P, et al. Refining the role of presurgical PET/4D-CT in a large series of patients with primary hyperparathyroidism undergoing [(18)F]fluorocholine PET/CT. Eur J Clin Investig. 2025;55(2):e14336.
42. Petranovic Ovcaricek P, Schaab J, Beintner-Skawran S, Maurer A, Rupp NJ, Ikenberg K, et al. [(18)F]Fluorocholine PET/MRI and [(18)F]Fluorocholine PET/CT as first- and second-line imaging in primary hyperparathyroidism—who takes the lead? Eur J Nucl Med Mol Imaging. 2025;52:5165.
43. Michaud L, Balogova S, Burgess A, Ohnona J, Huchet V, Kerrou K, et al. A pilot comparison of 18F-fluorocholine PET/CT, ultrasonography and 123I/99mTc-sestaMIBI dual-phase dual-isotope scintigraphy in the preoperative localization of hyperfunctioning parathyroid glands in primary or secondary hyperparathyroidism: influence of thyroid anomalies. Medicine (Baltimore). 2015;94(41):e1701.
44. Grimaldi S, Young J, Kamenicky P, Hartl D, Terroir M, Leboulleux S, et al. Challenging pre-surgical localization of hyperfunctioning parathyroid glands in primary hyperparathyroidism: the added value of (18)F-Fluorocholine PET/CT. Eur J Nucl Med Mol Imaging. 2018;45(10):1772–80.
45. Kluijfhout WP, Vorselaars WM, van den Berk SA, Vriens MR, Borel Rinkes IH, Valk GD, et al. Fluorine-18 fluorocholine PET-CT localizes hyperparathyroidism in patients with inconclusive conventional imaging: a multicenter study from The Netherlands. Nucl Med Commun. 2016;37(12):1246–52.
46. Zajickova K, Zogala D, Kubinyi J. Parathyroid imaging by (18)F-fluorocholine PET/CT in patients with primary hyperparathyroidism and inconclusive conventional methods: clinico-pathological correlations. Physiol Res. 2018;67(Suppl 3):S551–S7.
47. Dekorsy FJ, Beyer L, Spitzweg C, Schmidmaier R, Todica A, Trupka A, et al. Preoperative imaging with [(18)F]-Fluorocholine PET/CT in primary hyperparathyroidism. J Clin Med. 2022;11(10)
48. Amadou C, Bera G, Ezziane M, Chami L, Delbot T, Rouxel A, et al. 18F-Fluorocholine PET/CT and parathyroid 4D computed tomography for primary hyperparathyroidism: the challenge of reoperative patients. World J Surg. 2019;43(5):1232–42.
49. Piccardo A, Trimboli P, Rutigliani M, Puntoni M, Foppiani L, Bacigalupo L, et al. Additional value of integrated (18)F-choline PET/4D contrast-enhanced CT in the localization of hyperfunctioning parathyroid glands and correlation with molecular profile. Eur J Nucl Med Mol Imaging. 2019;46(3):766–75.
50. Pretet V, Rotania M, Helali M, Ignat M, Vix M, Imperiale A. (18)F-Fluorocholine PET and multiphase CT integrated in dual modality PET/4D-CT for preoperative evaluation of primary hyperparathyroidism. J Clin Med. 2020;9(6)
51. Aymard S, Leroy-Freschini B, Kaseb A, Marx D, Helali M, Averous G, et al. (18)F-Fluorocholine PET/CT compared with current imaging procedures for preoperative localization of hyperfunctioning para-

thyroids in patients with chronic kidney disease. Diagnostics (Basel). 2023;13(8)
52. Taterra D, Wong LM, Vikse J, Sanna B, Pekala P, Walocha J, et al. The prevalence and anatomy of parathyroid glands: a meta-analysis with implications for parathyroid surgery. Langenbeck's Arch Surg. 2019;404(1):63–70.
53. Akerstrom G, Malmaeus J, Bergstrom R. Surgical anatomy of human parathyroid glands. Surgery. 1984;95(1):14–21.
54. Policeni BA, Smoker WR, Reede DL. Anatomy and embryology of the thyroid and parathyroid glands. Semin Ultrasound CT MR. 2012;33(2):104–14.
55. Schulte KM, Talat N. Diagnosis and management of parathyroid cancer. Nat Rev Endocrinol. 2012;8(10):612–22.
56. Deandreis D, Terroir M, Al Ghuzlan A, Berdelou A, Lacroix L, Bidault F, et al. (1)(8)Fluorocholine PET/CT in parathyroid carcinoma: a new tool for disease staging? Eur J Nucl Med Mol Imaging. 2015;42(12):1941–2.
57. Morand GB, Helmchen BM, Steinert HC, Schmid C, Broglie MA. 18F-choline-PET in parathyroid carcinoma. Oral Oncol. 2018;86:314–5.
58. Su C, Zhang J, Yang H, Xu Y, Lu X. Diagnosis and treatment of liver metastases of parathyroid carcinoma. Front Endocrinol (Lausanne). 2022;13:982972.
59. Zhang-Yin J, Gaujoux S, Delbot T, Gauthe M, Talbot JN. 18F-fluorocholine PET/CT imaging of brown tumors in a patient with severe primary hyperparathyroidism. Clin Nucl Med. 2019;44(12):971–4.
60. Werner J, Grunig H, Loher H, Fischli S, Strobel K, Wicke C. Localization of brown tumors with 18 F-fluorocholine PET/CT imaging in severe primary hyperparathyroidism. Clin Nucl Med. 2023;48(8):e387–e9.
61. Prakash S, Damle NA, Kumar P, Dharmashaktu Y, Bal CS. Lincoln sign in a case of primary hyperparathyroidism on 18 F-fluorocholine PET/CT. Clin Nucl Med. 2023;48(7):e343–e4.
62. Trimboli P, D'Aurizio F, Tozzoli R, Giovanella L. Measurement of thyroglobulin, calcitonin, and PTH in FNA washout fluids. Clin Chem Lab Med. 2017;55(7):914–25.
63. van Mossel S, Saing S, Appelman-Dijkstra N, Quak E, Schepers A, Smit F, et al. Cost-effectiveness of one-stop-shop [(18)F]Fluorocholine PET/CT to localise parathyroid adenomas in patients suffering from primary hyperparathyroidism. Eur J Nucl Med Mol Imaging. 2024;51(12):3585–95.
64. Yap A, Hope TA, Graves CE, Kluijfhout W, Shen WT, Gosnell JE, et al. A cost-utility analysis of 18F-fluorocholine-positron emission tomography imaging for localizing primary hyperparathyroidism in the United States. Surgery. 2022;171(1):55–62.
65. Mamou A, Chkair S, Gilly O, Maimoun L, Mamou Y, Sheppard SC, et al. Economic evaluation of [(18)F] fluorocholine PET/CT in preoperative assessment of hyperfunctional parathyroids in primary hyperparathyroidism: a cost effectiveness analysis. EJNMMI Rep. 2025;9(1):11.
66. Rep S, Sirca K, Lezaic EM, Zaletel K, Hocevar M, Lezaic L. [(18)F]fluorocholine PET vs. [(99m)Tc]sestamibi scintigraphy for detection and localization of hyperfunctioning parathyroid glands in patients with primary hyperparathyroidism: outcomes and resource efficiency. Radiol Oncol. 2024;58(4):486–93.
67. Bradley KM, McGowan DR, Bartley L, Scott-Coombes D, Rees JI. Ectopic, intra-thyroid parathyroid adenoma better visualised by deep learning enhanced choline PET/CT. QJM. 2025;

4D-CT and (4D)-MRI in Parathyroid Imaging

9

Nicolin Hainc and Eugene Yu

► **Definitions**

4DCT: Four-dimensional computed tomography
4DMRI: Four-dimensional magnetic resonance imaging
BNE: Bilateral neck exploration
DECT: Dual energy computed tomography
MIP: Minimally invasive parathyroidectomy
mSv: Millisievert
PHPT: Primary hyperparathyroidism
RLN: Recurrent laryngeal nerve
SPECT: Single-photon emission computed tomography
US: Ultrasound
VNC: Virtual noncontrast

Learning Objectives

1. Understand the fundamental principles of 4DCT and 4DMRI in the evaluation of parathyroid adenomas.
2. Compare the advantages and limitations of 4DCT and 4DMRI with those of ultrasound and nuclear medicine imaging.
3. Describe a systematic approach to performing and interpreting 4DCT and 4DMRI studies.

9.1 Introduction

Four-dimensional computed tomography (4DCT), first introduced in 2006, has since established itself as a valuable imaging modality in the setting of primary hyperparathyroidism (PHPT) [1]. By combining high-resolution anatomical detail with temporal perfusion information, 4DCT facilitates accurate localization of parathyroid adenomas. While up to 90% of PHPT cases result from a single parathyroid adenoma, the disease can also be multiglandular, e.g., in the form of double adenomas or parathyroid hyperplasia, occurring in up to 6% of cases [2]. Surgical excision remains the only definitive treatment for PHPT and can be performed through minimally invasive parathyroidectomy (MIP) should a sin-

N. Hainc (✉)
Department of Neuroradiology, Clinical Neurosciences Center, University Hospital of Zurich, Zurich, Switzerland
e-mail: Nicolin.Hainc@usz.ch

E. Yu
Medical Imaging, University Health Network, Toronto, ON, Canada
e-mail: Eugene.Yu@uhn.ca

© The Author(s), under exclusive license to Springer Nature Switzerland AG 2026

P. Petranović Ovčariček et al. (eds.), *Parathyroid Imaging*,
https://doi.org/10.1007/978-3-032-14178 1_9

gle parathyroid adenoma be identified preoperatively. MIP offers several advantages over traditional procedures and is associated with shorter operating times, shorter postoperative hospitalization, smaller surgical incisions with better cosmetic outcomes, decreased postoperative pain, and lower overall costs while maintaining similar cure rates [1, 3–5]. Should imaging be non-localizing or demonstrate multiglandular disease, the more extensive bilateral neck exploration (BNE), is warranted.

Preoperative imaging in PHPT encompasses a range of modalities including ultrasound (US), ^{99m}Tc-sestamibi SPECT/CT (hereafter referred to as sestamibi), 4DCT, and MRI. To date, no universally accepted algorithm or consensus exists regarding optimal preoperative imaging strategy, and choice of imaging usually depends on availability, local expertise, and surgeon preference. The role of preoperative imaging in PHPT is localization, not diagnosis, of a parathyroid adenoma, and all patients undergoing imaging of the parathyroid glands should have biochemically confirmed primary hyperparathyroidism. In this setting, each imaging modality offers distinct advantages and limitations.

US is widely available, cost effective, and free of ionizing radiation, making it the ideal first-line imaging modality for localization of parathyroid adenomas. However, US is limited through lower accuracies in obese patients and insensitivity for ectopic, deeper-seated adenomas located in the retropharyngeal space and lower in the mediastinum. Sestamibi offers functional tracer uptake information, but drawbacks include ionizing radiation exposure, low anatomic resolution, longer scan times, and higher costs compared to US. 4DCT addresses several of these limitations through the combination of high anatomic resolution with functional perfusion information, allowing for unrestricted assessment of ectopic and supernumerary adenomas, with the benefit of shorter scan times [6, 7]. However, like sestamibi, 4DCT is associated with exposure to ionizing radiation. In direct comparative studies, when used as a first-line imaging study, 4DCT harbors a sensitivity of up to 92% for the localization of parathyroid adenomas [8–11], exceeding first-line US [12–16] and sestamibi [14, 17]. Furthermore, when US and sestamibi were nonlocalizing or inconclusive, 4DCT boasted sensitivities of up to 89% [12, 18, 19].

MRI theoretically combines all of the advantages of the previous modalities without ionizing radiation, boasting high spatial and temporal resolution perfusion imaging. Unfortunately, its utility remains constrained due to limited availability, limited experience, and susceptibility to motion artifacts from free breathing and swallowing, as scan times are longer than 4DCT.

9.2 The 4DCT Technique: Phases, Enhancement Patterns, and Radiation Exposure Considerations

Single-phase CT provides excellent anatomical detail of the parathyroid gland and surrounding tissues to accurately detect and localize lesions. However, accurate differentiation of parathyroid adenomas from potential mimics such as lymph nodes and exophytic thyroid nodules requires additional information in the form of temporal tissue perfusion or acquisition of an "enhancement pattern." This is performed on CT through the acquisition of multiple contrast-enhanced CT phases, introducing temporal "4D" information [1, 5, 20]. A CT phase refers to a single imaging "snapshot" at a predefined timepoint after administration of intravenous iodinated contrast material, commonly including non-contrast, arterial, venous, and delayed or late phases. Phases are typically obtained at 30-second intervals, although considerable inter-institutional variability exists [21]. The optimal number of phases for parathyroid imaging remains a topic of debate, as each additional phase introduces a trade-off between information gained and increased exposure to ionizing radiation. Two-phase, three-phase, and four-phase protocols have all been described, with the three-phase protocol being the most common [15, 22].

Similar to sestamibi, 4DCT exposes the patient to ionizing radiation. Depending on the number of phases and institutional implementation, the radiation exposure from 4DCT ranges from 4 to 26 mSv; however, it can be as low as

10.4 mSv for a four-phase protocol [21]. This is comparable to sestamibi at 7–9 mSv. Model-based estimated lifetime cancer risk attributed to 4DCT in a 20-year-old woman is calculated to be 0.1% [23], while in a middle-aged female patient with PHPT, the risk is seen as negligible [24]. It is generally accepted that the benefits of 4DCT outweigh the small attributable cancer risk in this setting. [21, 24]

Using 4D information, the ideal enhancement pattern of a parathyroid adenoma includes hypoattenuation on noncontrast imaging relative to the thyroid gland, followed by arterial hyperattenuation with a rapid washout on venous and delayed phases [25]. Unfortunately, this classic pattern is only seen in 20% of cases and at least three different patterns have been described in parathyroid adenomas [8]. In contrast, lymph nodes typically exhibit slow and progressive enhancement across the CT phases, reflecting their lower vascularity relative to parathyroid adenomas.

Given the spectrum of enhancement patterns observed in parathyroid adenomas, studies have investigated reducing in the number of CT phases to minimize radiation exposure without compromising diagnostic accuracy. A single CT phase lacks temporal perfusion information and results in low confidence for differentiating lymph nodes from ectopic parathyroid tissue. Two-phase protocols (arterial and venous phases) [26] and three-phase protocols (additional noncontrast phase) have demonstrated better performance compared to single-phase imaging [21]. A recent study assessed the feasibility of eliminating the noncontrast phase scan and replacing it with dual energy CT (DECT) virtual noncontrast (VNC) images derived from contrast-enhanced phases. While radiation exposure to the patient was reduced, the virtual noncontrast images did not accurately replicate a true noncontrast scan, with limitations attributed to the natural iodine content of the thyroid gland [27, 28]. VNC algorithms implement iodine suppression to eliminate attenuation of iodinated CT contrast, creating a virtual image that appears unenhanced. However, this algorithm also affects thyroid tissue, rendering the virtual noncontrast reconstructions of little utility in 4DCT, as enhancement patterns generally require attenuation comparison with the thyroid. Further studies assessing phase reduction from four to two or three to two [26] phases found equivalent diagnostic performance in localizing parathyroid adenomas using the respective reduced-phase protocol. A meta-analysis in 2017 reported pooled sensitivities of 71% for two-phase studies, 76% for three-phase studies, and 80% for four-phase studies [21] for parathyroid adenomas. The variability in enhancement patterns of parathyroid adenomas likely explains the moderate differences in diagnostic yield using reduced-phase protocols, allowing omission of phases that offer limited additional value.

The variability of parathyroid adenoma and hyperplasia enhancement patterns was characterized by Bahl et al. in 2015 [8]. In this study, pathologically proven parathyroid adenomas or hyperplasia were correlated to preoperative imaging and three distinct enhancement patterns on 4DCT were found. Common to all patterns was the requirement that the parathyroid attenuation had to be lower than the thyroid on noncontrast images, thus making this phase irreplaceable. In addition to this requirement, "type A" lesions demonstrated hyperattenuation in the arterial phase compared to the thyroid (Fig. 9.1). Only 20% of all lesions demonstrated this "classic" pattern. "Type B" lesions did not demonstrate arterial hyperattenuation but demonstrated washout (i.e., lower attenuation than the thyroid) on the delayed phase (Fig. 9.2). This was the most common enhancement pattern at 57%. The remaining "type C" pattern (22%) showed neither arterial hyperattenuation nor washout.

The study by Bahl et al. suggests that a three-phase protocol is generally sufficient to capture the spectrum of parathyroid behaviors, and omission of one phase could compromise lesion characterization. The arbitrary timing of CT phases likely contributes to the low prevalence of the classic hypervascular enhancement pattern, as single imaging snapshots do not correct for unique inter-individual parathyroid perfusion differences. Additionally, chronic disease such as Hashimoto's thyroiditis reduces thyroidal iodine content, thereby affecting 4DCT performance.

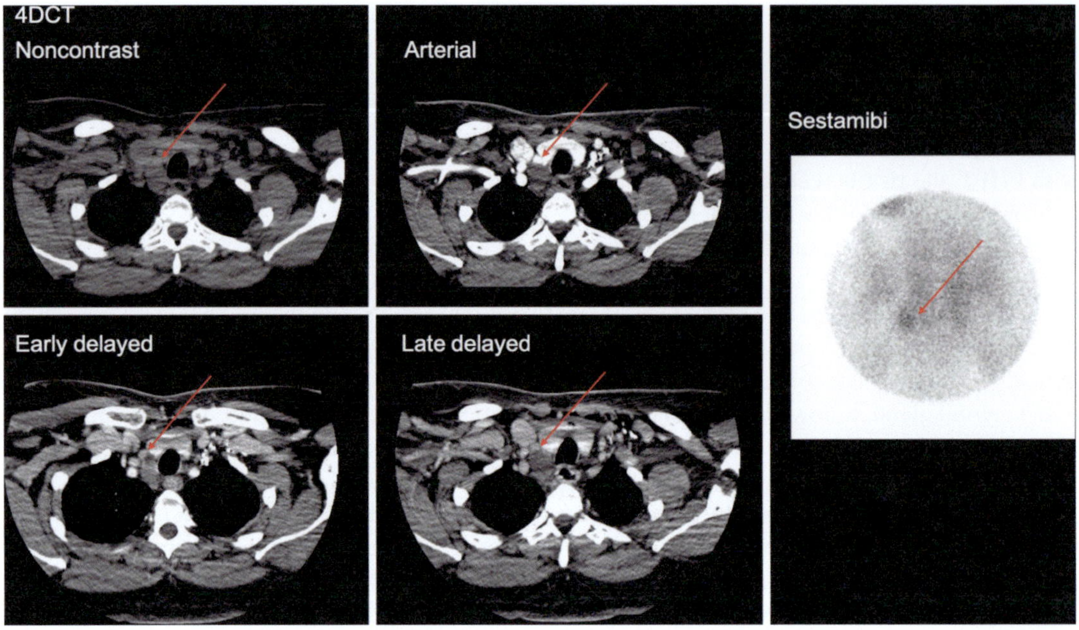

Fig. 9.1 A 59-year-old female with hyperparathyroidism. 4DCT demonstrates a parathyroid adenoma posterior to the right thyroid lobe with the following enhancement pattern relative to the thyroid gland: noncontrast phase hypoattenuating; arterial phase hyperattenuating; early delayed and late delayed phase washout. Sestamibi scan demonstrates increased uptake of the parathyroid adenoma

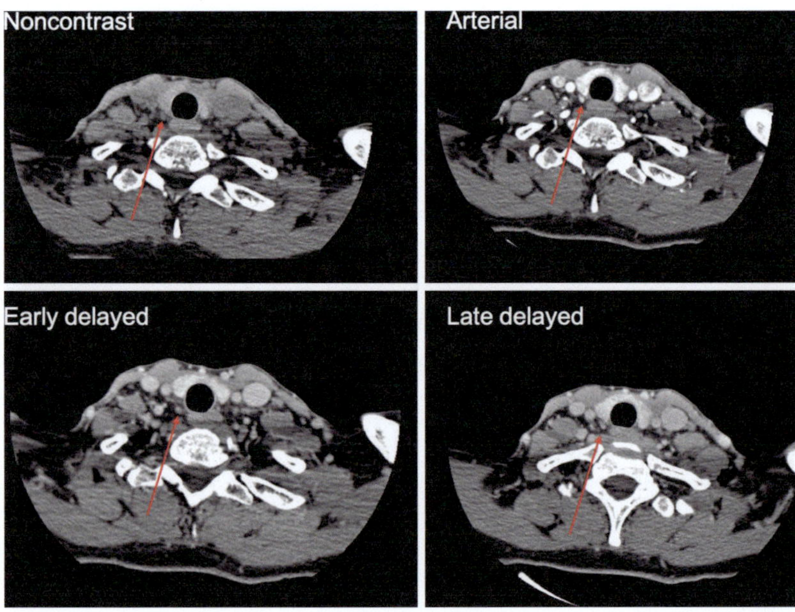

Fig. 9.2 A 54-year old female with hyperparathyroidism. 4DCT demonstrates a parathyroid adenoma posterior to the right thyroid lobe with the following enhancement pattern relative to the thyroid gland: noncontrast phase hypoattenuating; arterial phase isoattenuating; early delayed and late delayed phase washout

9.3 Anatomy, Embryology, and Imaging Features

In addition to the expected locations within the posterior aspect of the superior and inferior thyroid poles, scrutinization of the entire embryological migrational pathway is required to definitively assess for parathyroid adenomas. Embryologically, the superior parathyroid glands originate from the fourth branchial pouch, while the inferior parathyroid glands derive from the third branchial pouch. As a result, ectopic superior parathyroid tissue can be encountered in retropharyngeal, retroesophageal, and mediastinal locations. Additional ectopic sites of the superior parathyroid gland include locations within the thyroid parenchyma or scalene fat pads. In contrast, ectopic inferior parathyroid tissue is commonly found near the thymus, thyrothymic ligament, or in the carotid sheath. The relatively long migrational pathway of the inferior parathyroid glands results in a much larger variability, as ectopic locations have been reported from the angle of the mandible to the pericardium [29]. The inferior parathyroid glands are more commonly found in ectopic locations compared to the superior glands [30].

Beyond anatomical location, distinct imaging features can aid in the identification of parathyroid adenomas. One such feature is the polar vessel, which increases confidence in the identification of parathyroid adenomas when present. The polar vessel is classically described as an enlarged feeding artery based on prior sonography studies [31, 32], but it can also represent an enlarged draining vein seen on the arterial 4DCT phase [33]. This vessel is typically larger than vessels seen in similar contralateral neck locations and can be seen in up to 63% of parathyroid adenomas [33]. Parathyroid adenomas can also harbor cystic foci, fat deposition, and calcification [29].

When reporting 4D CT studies, it is recommended that radiologists describe lesions relative to the cricoid cartilage and tracheoesophageal groove, locations which represent classical surgical landmarks. The tracheooesopahgeal groove is particularly important as it represents the expected course of the recurrent laryngeal nerve (RLN) and differentiates superior from inferior parathyroid gland origin. Furthermore, it is critical to alert the surgeon of anatomical vascular anomalies such as an aberrant right subclavian artery or a right aortic arch with an aberrant left subclavian artery. In these cases, the RLN follows a nonrecurrent course and may not be found at its expected location [7].

Ultimately, the radiologist must systematically evaluate all embryologically possible ectopic parathyroid locations and be aware of the entire spectrum of enhancement patterns on 4DCT. Any lesion that cannot be confidently classified as thyroid tissue, a lymph node, or a blood vessel should be described in the radiological report. Nonetheless, even with thorough evaluation, the possibility of unidentified parathyroid tissue persists. Figures 9.3a, 9.3b, 9.4, 9.5 and 9.6 demonstrate further examples of parathyroid adenomas on 4DCT in various locations and with various enhancement patterns.

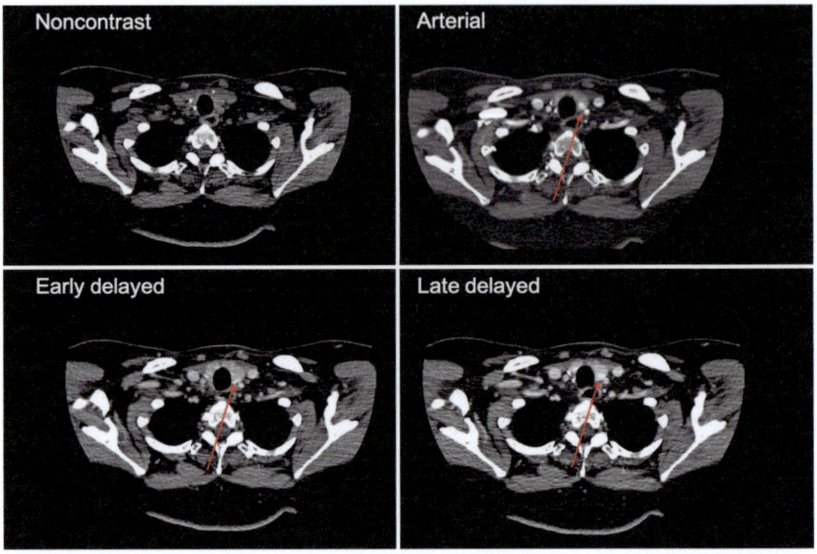

Fig. 9.3a A 51-year-old female patient with hyperparathyroidism. (**a**) 4DCT demonstrates a parathyroid adenoma within the posterior aspect of the left thyroid lobe with the following enhancement pattern relative to the thyroid gland: Noncontrast phase isoattenuating; arterial phase hyperattenuating; early delayed and late delayed phase iso- to hyperattenuating

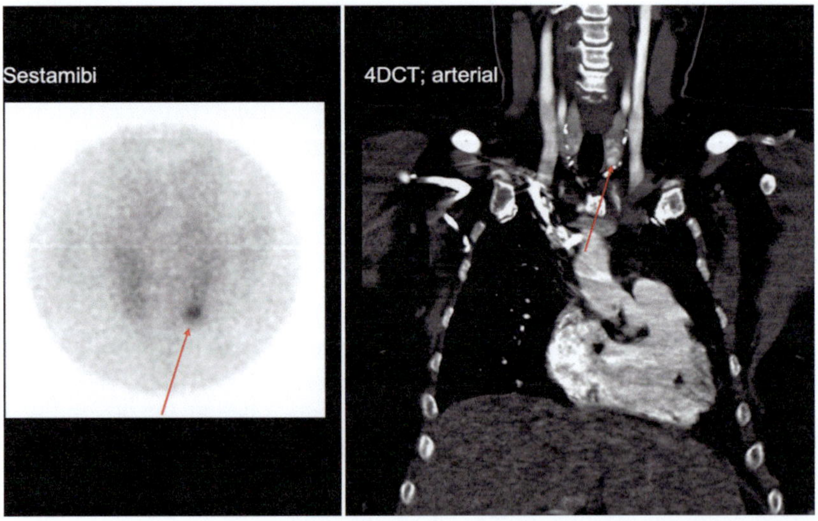

Fig. 9.3b Sestamibi demonstrates increased uptake, with localization correlated to 4DCT arterial phase, coronal reformat

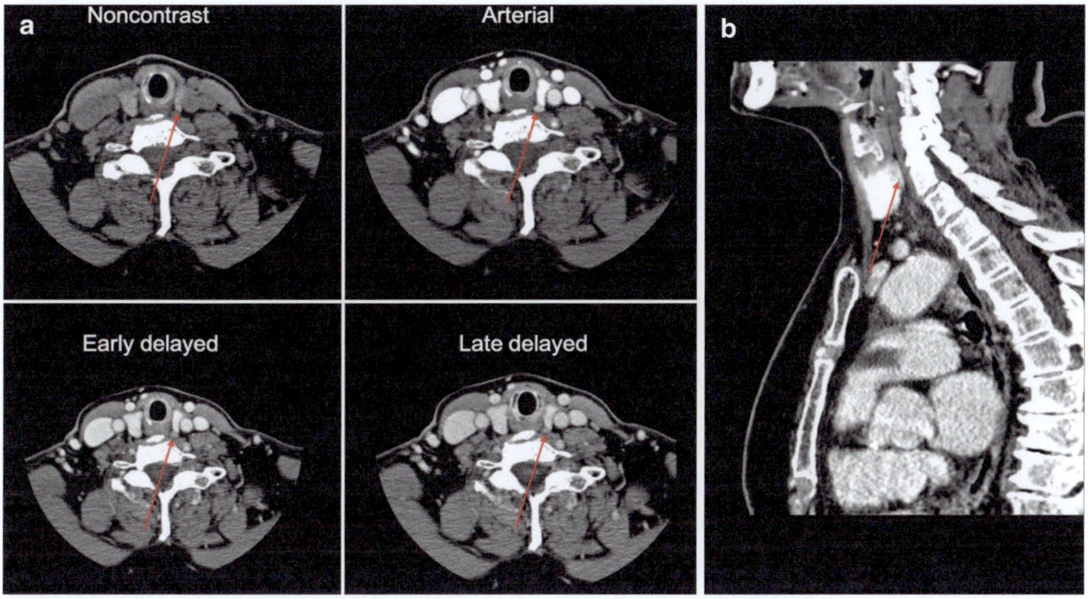

Fig. 9.4 (**a**) A 74-year-old female with hyperparathyroidism. 4DCT demonstrates a parathyroid adenoma posterior to the left thyroid lobe with the following enhancement pattern relative to the thyroid gland: noncontrast phase isoattenuating; arterial phase hypoattenuating; early delayed and late delayed phase washout. (**b**) Sagittal reformat of the arterial phase demonstrates an elongated parathyroid adenoma posterior to the thyroid gland

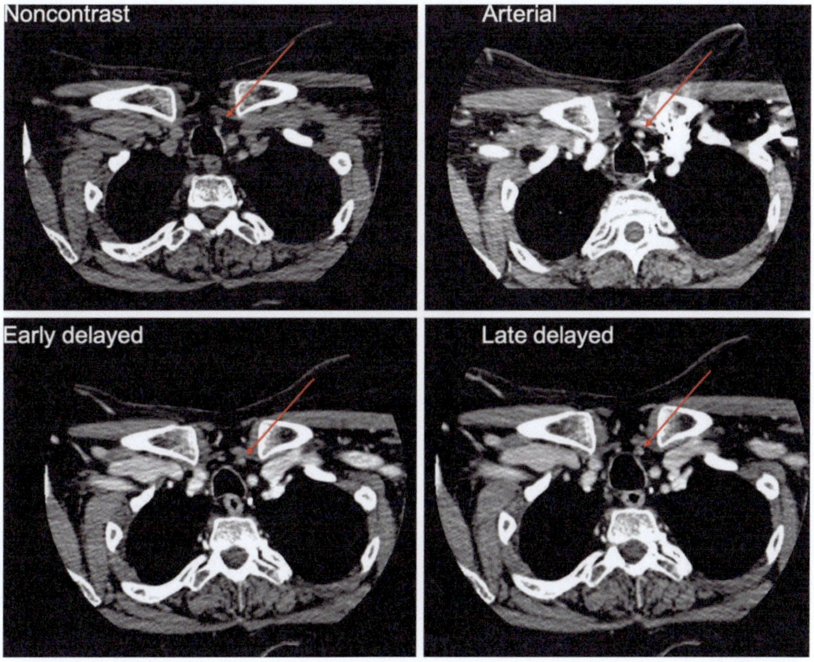

Fig. 9.5 A 58-year-old female with hyperparathyroidism. A pretracheal parathyroid adenoma inferior to the left thyroid lobe is found on 4DCT with arterial hyperattenuation and washout in the early delayed and late delayed phases

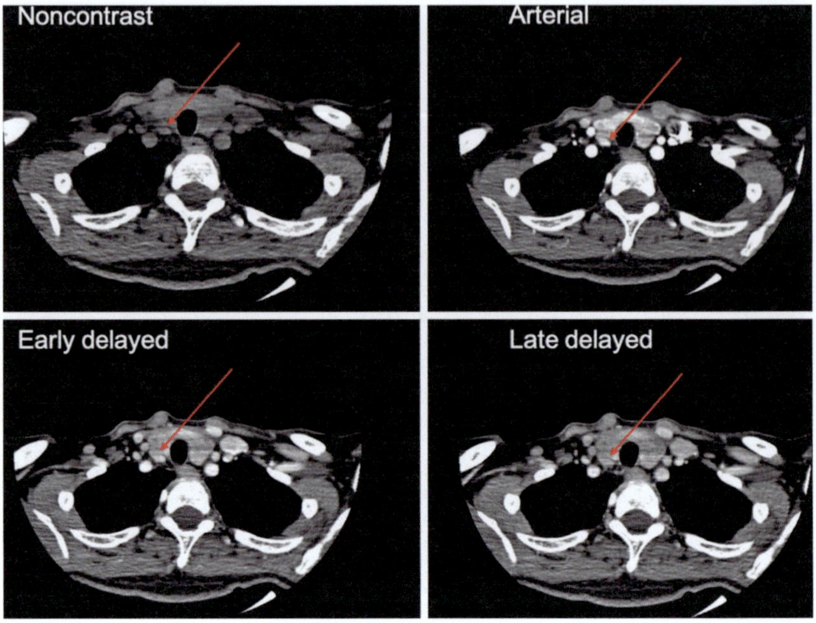

Fig. 9.6 A 54-year-old female with hyperparathyroidism. 4DCT demonstrates a parathyroid adenoma posterior to the right thyroid lobe with the following enhancement pattern relative to the thyroid gland: noncontrast phase hypoattenuating; arterial phase hyperattenuating; early delayed and late delayed phase isoattenuating

9.4 The Repeat-Surgical Candidate

Persistent or recurrent hyperparathyroidism occurs in up to 5% of patients following failed parathyroidectomy [19, 37, 38], with reoperative cervical exploration carrying an increased risk of injury to the RLN [39]. In this setting, 4DCT is preferred to US and sestamibi as post-surgical scars have been introduced and anatomical planes have been distorted, complicating the procedure. 4DCT provides accurate tumor localization and allows for improved surgical planning in reoperative candidates, boasting sensitivities of up to 88% [10, 18, 21, 40] overall and up to 42% when US and sestamibi were negative [41].

9.5 4D MRI

Theoretically, 4DMRI should outperform 4DCT by enabling near-continuous acquisition of contrast perfusion information, with temporal resolutions as high as one image every six seconds [34]. This allows for generation of high temporal resolution perfusion curves for suspected parathyroid adenomas, which can be directly compared to thyroid tissue perfusion (Fig. 9.7). 4DMRI eliminates the arbitrary snapshot-like timing of 4DCT enabling a more accurate tissue perfusion characterization. The high temporal perfusion resolution is combined with high soft-tissue contrast and high spatial resolution with voxels of under 2 mm, all without ionizing radiation. Unfortunately, MRI of the lower neck and mediastinum is limited by artifacts resulting from free breathing, swallowing, insufficient fat suppression, and pulsation of the carotid arteries [35, 36].

Although clinical experience with 4DMRI in PHPT remains limited, advances in MRI have shown promising results, most recently in a study demonstrating an area under the receiver operating characteristic curve of 0.96 for differentiating parathyroid adenomas from lymph nodes and thyroid tissue [34]. This result highlights the high potential of MRI to better characterize parathyroid adenoma hypervascularity. However, ancillary findings such as the polar vessel sign have not been described on MRI, likely due to its lower spatial resolution when compared to 4DCT or US. Thus, while 4DMRI demonstrates promise as a radiation-free alternative in parathyroid imaging, its clinical adoption suffers from low accessibility and limited clinical experience.

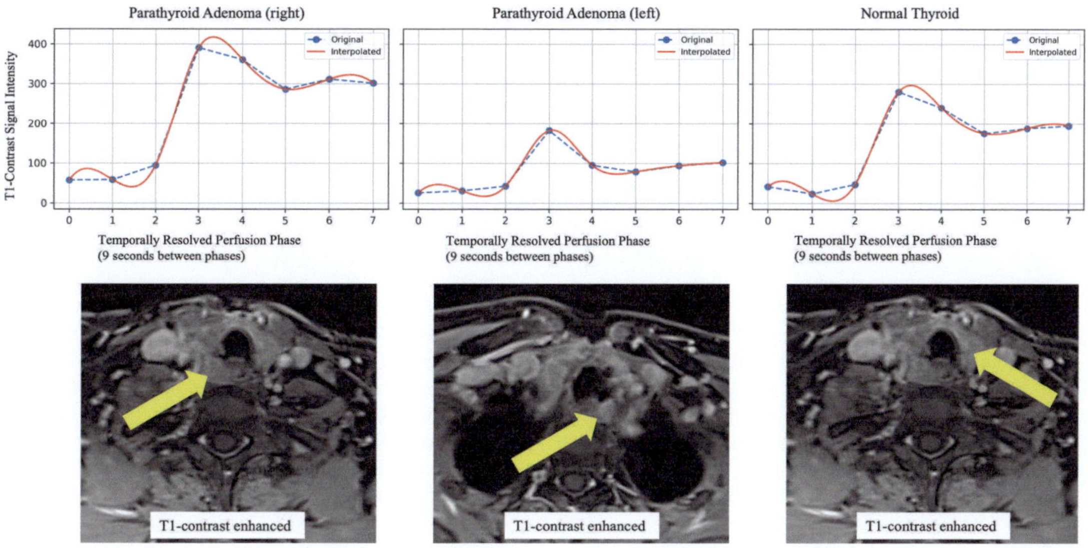

Fig. 9.7 A 72-year-old female with hyperparathyroidism harboring two parathyroid adenomas, one on each side of the trachea posterolaterally. Dynamic contrast-enhanced T1-weighted perfusion signal-intensity (SI) curves obtained using 4DMRI were acquired with a temporal resolution of 9 s between images. The right-sided parathyroid adenoma exhibited higher SI than the normal thyroid gland during the arterial phase, followed by washout. In contrast, the left-sided adenoma showed lower arterial-phase SI relative to the thyroid, also followed by washout. Peak SI for both parathyroid adenomas and the normal thyroid gland occurred at phase 3, corresponding to 27 s after injection of intravenous contrast

References

1. Rodgers SE, Hunter GJ, Hamberg LM, et al. Improved preoperative planning for directed parathyroidectomy with 4-dimensional computed tomography. Surgery. 2006;140:932–40. discussion 940–941
2. Ruda JM, Hollenbeak CS, Stack BC. A systematic review of the diagnosis and treatment of primary hyperparathyroidism from 1995 to 2003. Otolaryngol Head Neck Surg. 2005;132:359–72.
3. Abbott DE, Cantor SB, Grubbs EG, et al. Outcomes and economic analysis of routine preoperative 4-dimensional CT for surgical intervention in de novo primary hyperparathyroidism: does clinical benefit justify the cost? J Am Coll Surg. 2012;214:629–37. discussion 637–639
4. Minisola S, Cipriani C, Diacinti D, et al. Imaging of the parathyroid glands in primary hyperparathyroidism. Eur J Endocrinol. 2016;174:D1–8.
5. Hoang JK, Sung W, Bahl M, et al. How to perform parathyroid 4D CT: tips and traps for technique and interpretation. Radiology. 2014;270:15–24.
6. Lappas D, Noussios G, Anagnostis P, et al. Location, number and morphology of parathyroid glands: results from a large anatomical series. Anat Sci Int. 2012;87:160–4.
7. Phitayakorn R, McHenry CR. Incidence and location of ectopic abnormal parathyroid glands. Am J Surg. 2006;191:418–23.
8. Bahl M, Sepahdari AR, Sosa JA, et al. Parathyroid adenomas and hyperplasia on four-dimensional CT scans: three patterns of enhancement relative to the thyroid gland justify a three-phase protocol. Radiology. 2015;277:454–62.
9. Chazen JL, Gupta A, Dunning A, et al. Diagnostic accuracy of 4D-CT for parathyroid adenomas and hyperplasia. AJNR Am J Neuroradiol. 2012;33:429–33.
10. Kelly HR, Hamberg LM, Hunter GJ. 4D-CT for preoperative localization of abnormal parathyroid glands in patients with hyperparathyroidism: accuracy and ability to stratify patients by unilateral versus bilateral disease in surgery-naïve and re-exploration patients. Am J Neuroradiol. 2014;35:176–81.
11. Brown SJ, Lee JC, Christie J, et al. Four-dimensional computed tomography for parathyroid localization: a new imaging modality. ANZ J Surg. 2015;85:483–7.
12. Day KM, Elsayed M, Beland MD, et al. The utility of 4-dimensional computed tomography for preoperative localization of primary hyperparathyroidism in patients not localized by sestamibi or ultrasonography. Surgery. 2015;157:534–9.
13. Eichhorn-Wharry LI, Carlin AM, Talpos GB. Mild hypercalcemia: an indication to select 4-dimensional computed tomography scan for preoperative localization of parathyroid adenomas. Am J Surg. 2011;201:334–8. discussion 338
14. Kukar M, Platz TA, Schaffner TJ, et al. The use of modified four-dimensional computed tomography in

patients with primary hyperparathyroidism: an argument for the abandonment of routine sestamibi single-positron emission computed tomography (SPECT). Ann Surg Oncol. 2015;22:139–45.
15. Starker LF, Mahajan A, Björklund P, et al. 4D parathyroid CT as the initial localization study for patients with de novo primary hyperparathyroidism. Ann Surg Oncol. 2011;18:1723–8.
16. Suh YJ, Choi JY, Kim S, et al. Comparison of 4D CT, ultrasonography, and 99mTc sestamibi SPECT/CT in localizing single-gland primary hyperparathyroidism. Otolaryngol Head Neck Surg. 2015;152:438–43.
17. Yeh R, Tay Y-KD, Tabacco G, et al. Diagnostic performance of 4D CT and sestamibi SPECT/CT in localizing parathyroid adenomas in primary hyperparathyroidism. Radiology. 2019;291:469–76.
18. Tian Y, Tanny ST, Einsiedel P, et al. Four-dimensional computed tomography: clinical impact for patients with primary hyperparathyroidism. Ann Surg Oncol. 2018;25:117–21.
19. Lubitz CC, Hunter GJ, Hamberg LM, et al. Accuracy of 4-dimensional computed tomography in poorly localized patients with primary hyperparathyroidism. Surgery. 2010;148:1129–38.
20. Hunter GJ, Schellingerhout D, Vu TH, et al. Accuracy of four-dimensional CT for the localization of abnormal parathyroid glands in patients with primary hyperparathyroidism. Radiology. 2012;264:789–95.
21. Kluijfhout WP, Pasternak JD, Beninato T, et al. Diagnostic performance of computed tomography for parathyroid adenoma localization; a systematic review and meta-analysis. Eur J Radiol. 2017;88:117–28.
22. Griffith B, Chaudhary H, Mahmood G, et al. Accuracy of 2-phase parathyroid CT for the preoperative localization of parathyroid adenomas in primary hyperparathyroidism. Am J Neuroradiol. 2015;36:2373–9.
23. Mahajan A, Starker LF, Ghita M, et al. Parathyroid four-dimensional computed tomography: evaluation of radiation dose exposure during preoperative localization of parathyroid tumors in primary hyperparathyroidism. World J Surg. 2012;36:1335–9.
24. Hoang JK, Reiman RE, Nguyen GB, et al. Lifetime attributable risk of cancer from radiation exposure during parathyroid imaging: comparison of 4D CT and parathyroid scintigraphy. Am J Roentgenol. 2015;204:W579–85.
25. Gafton AR, Glastonbury CM, Eastwood JD, et al. Parathyroid lesions: characterization with dual-phase arterial and venous enhanced CT of the neck. Am J Neuroradiol. 2012;33:949–52.
26. Noureldine SI, Aygun N, Walden MJ, et al. Multiphase computed tomography for localization of parathyroid disease in patients with primary hyperparathyroidism: how many phases do we really need? Surgery. 2014;156:1300–6. discussion 13006–13007
27. Forghani R, Roskies M, Liu X, et al. Dual-energy CT characteristics of parathyroid adenomas on 25-and 55-second 4D-CT acquisitions: preliminary experience. J Comput Assist Tomogr. 2016;40:806–14.
28. M R, X L, Mp H, et al. 3-phase dual-energy CT scan as a feasible salvage imaging modality for the identification of non-localizing parathyroid adenomas: a prospective study. J Otolaryngol. 2015;44
29. Bunch PM, Randolph GW, Brooks JA, et al. Parathyroid 4D CT: what the surgeon wants to know. Radiographics. 2020;40:1383–94.
30. Kuzminski SJ, Sosa JA, Hoang JK. Update in parathyroid imaging. Magn Reson Imaging Clin N Am. 2018;26:151–66.
31. Wolf RJ, Cronan JJ, Monchik JM. Color Doppler sonography: an adjunctive technique in assessment of parathyroid adenomas. J Ultrasound Med Off J Am Inst Ultrasound Med. 1994;13:303–8.
32. Lane MJ, Desser TS, Weigel RJ, et al. Use of color and power Doppler sonography to identify feeding arteries associated with parathyroid adenomas. AJR Am J Roentgenol. 1998;171:819–23.
33. Bahl M, Muzaffar M, Vij G, et al. Prevalence of the polar vessel sign in parathyroid adenomas on the arterial phase of 4D CT. AJNR Am J Neuroradiol. 2014;35:578–81.
34. Nael K, Hur J, Bauer A, et al. Dynamic 4D MRI for characterization of parathyroid adenomas: multiparametric analysis. AJNR Am J Neuroradiol. 2015;36:2147–52.
35. Gotway MB, Reddy GP, Webb WR, et al. Comparison between MR imaging and 99mTc MIBI scintigraphy in the evaluation of recurrent of persistent hyperparathyroidism. Radiology. 2001;218:783–90.
36. Grayev AM, Gentry LR, Hartman MJ, et al. Presurgical localization of parathyroid adenomas with magnetic resonance imaging at 3.0 T: an adjunct method to supplement traditional imaging. Ann Surg Oncol. 2012;19:981–9. Google Search
37. Mohebati A, Shaha AR. Imaging techniques in parathyroid surgery for primary hyperparathyroidism. Am J Otolaryngol. 2012;33:457–68.
38. Udelsman R. Approach to the patient with persistent or recurrent primary hyperparathyroidism. J Clin Endocrinol Metab. 2011;96:2950–8.
39. Karakas E, Müller H-H, Schlosshauer T, et al. Reoperations for primary hyperparathyroidism—improvement of outcome over two decades. Langenbecks Arch Surg. 2013;398:99–106.
40. Mortenson MM, Evans DB, Lee JE, et al. Parathyroid exploration in the reoperative neck: improved preoperative localization with 4D-computed tomography. J Am Coll Surg. 2008;206:888–95. discussion 895–896
41. Ginsburg M, Christoforidis GA, Zivin SP, et al. Adenoma localization for recurrent or persistent primary hyperparathyroidism using dynamic four-dimensional CT and venous sampling. J Vasc Interv Radiol. 2015;26:79–86.

[18F]Fluorocholine PET/MR Imaging

10

Martin W. Huellner

Definitions

- *Primary hyperparathyroidism (PHPT):* An endocrine disorder caused by excessive secretion of parathyroid hormone (PTH), most often due to a solitary adenoma, leading to hypercalcemia.
- *Secondary hyperparathyroidism:* Parathyroid hyperplasia secondary to chronic hypocalcemia, typically associated with chronic kidney disease, sometimes also due to chronic vitamin D deficiency.
- *Tertiary hyperparathyroidism:* Persistent PTH overproduction after correction of chronic hypocalcemia and/or as a sequelae of long-standing secondary hyperparathyroidism. Often occuring after renal transplantation.
- *Orthotopic parathyroid gland:* A parathyroid gland located in its normal anatomical position in the neck, behind the thyroid gland.
- *Ectopic parathyroid gland:* A parathyroid gland located outside the typical anatomic position (e.g., in the mediastinum, along the carotid sheath).
- *Hybrid imaging:* The combination of functional (PET) and anatomical (MR, CT) imaging into a single examination for improved localization and characterization of lesions.
- *[18F]fluorocholine (FCH):* A PET radiotracer taken up by tissues with high phospholipid turnover due to increased phospholipid-dependent choline kinase activity, including hyperfunctioning parathyroid adenomas.

M. W. Huellner (✉)
Department of Nuclear Medicine, University Hospital Zurich / University of Zurich, Zurich, Switzerland
e-mail: martin.huellner@usz.ch

Learning Objectives

After reading this chapter, the reader should be able to:

1. Describe the advantages and limitations of PET/MR compared to conventional imaging modalities and PET/CT for parathyroid adenoma localization.
2. Understand the mechanisms and clinical utility of commonly used PET tracers, especially [18F]fluorocholine, in detecting parathyroid adenomas.
3. Outline the recommended PET/MR protocol for parathyroid imaging, including patient preparation, acquisition, and image fusion.
4. Recognize the typical imaging appearances of parathyroid adenomas and differentiate them from thyroid nodules, lymph nodes, and other potential mimics.
5. Identify common pitfalls, artifacts, and false-positive findings in PET/MR parathyroid imaging.

(continued)

© The Author(s), under exclusive license to Springer Nature Switzerland AG 2026
P. Petranović Ovčariček et al. (eds.), *Parathyroid Imaging*,
https://doi.org/10.1007/978-3-032-14178-1_10

6. Apply PET/MR findings to surgical planning, particularly in challenging cases such as ectopic glands or reoperative necks.
7. Discuss future developments in PET/MR technology, radiotracer design, and artificial intelligence applications in parathyroid imaging.

10.1 Introduction

Only 40 years ago, the only "localizing study" indicated for patients with untreated primary hyperparathyroidism was to localize an experienced endocrine surgeon—a remark attributed to the late John L. Doppman, then Chief of the Department of Radiology at the NIH Clinical Center [62]. This sentiment reflected the poor success rates of the noninvasive preoperative localization techniques available at the time [18]. Since then, preoperative localization methods have come a long way. Today, experienced endocrine surgeons routinely depend on precise localization by cross-sectional imaging in patients with primary hyperparathyroidism, with [18F]fluorocholine (FCH)-PET/MR now representing the pinnacle of these modalities.

Primary hyperparathyroidism is a relatively common endocrine disorder with an incidence of approximately 21 cases per 100,000 population per year, most often caused by a solitary parathyroid adenoma, less frequently by hyperplasia, and rarely by carcinoma. Surgical removal of the hyperfunctioning gland(s) is the definitive treatment, and success rates are highest when the diseased glands can be precisely localized preoperatively.

Traditional localization techniques, such as high-resolution US and [99mTc]sestamibi scintigraphy and SPECT with or without CT, are widely available but have limitations, particularly in the context of small adenomas, ectopic glands, multiglandular disease, and post-surgical necks where anatomy is distorted. In these challenging scenarios, PET using FCH as a radiotracer has emerged as a problem-solving tool and has now become a widely adopted mainstay in first-line imaging of parathyroid lesions.

PET/MR, by combining the molecular sensitivity of PET with the exquisite soft-tissue contrast of MR, can provide superior localization, especially when using tracers such as FCH, which has shown high sensitivity for parathyroid adenomas.

For several reasons, PET/MR has increasingly emerged as a valuable alternative to PET/CT in recent years. Contributing factors include the almost exclusively benign nature of parathyroid lesions, the markedly reduced radiation dose of PET/MR compared with PET/CT [2, 38, 50–53], the frequent dispensability of intravenous contrast agents often required in PET/CT for proper visualization of surrounding anatomy (particularly vessels), and—not least—the superior soft-tissue contrast offered by MR.

This chapter focuses on the hybrid imaging technique combining FCH PET with MRI for parathyroid gland localization. The chapter elaborates on the synergistic advantages of combining these two modalities. It covers image acquisition protocols, fusion techniques, and interpretation of FCH PET/MR imaging. It also describes the hybrid technique's diagnostic performance compared to other imaging modalities and addresses current limitations, such as limited availability.

10.2 Rationale for PET/MR in Parathyroid Imaging

10.2.1 Limitations of Conventional Imaging and PET/CT

The diagnostic workup of hyperparathyroidism traditionally begins with US and [99mTc]sestamibi SPECT/CT. These modalities are widely available, relatively cost-effective, and provide good accuracy in typical single-gland disease. Ultrasound offers excellent spatial resolution for superficial lesions and can simultaneously assess thyroid pathology; however, its accuracy decreases in obese patients, in those with retrotracheal or mediastinal glands, and in reoperative necks where scar tissue distorts anatomy.

Similarly, SPECT/CT is a robust first-line functional imaging technique, but its sensitivity falls sharply in small adenomas—particularly those weighing less than 500 mg—as well as in multiglandular disease. Additionally, thyroid nodules with overlapping [99mTc]sestamibi uptake can generate false-positive findings. Although PET/MR and PET/CT show comparable diagnostic accuracy in both first-line and second-line imaging [50, 53], PET/CT unnecessarily exposes patients—affected by an almost exclusively benign disease—to additional radiation from the CT component and, in many cases, to iodinated contrast agents.

10.2.2 Advantages of PET/MR

In complex clinical scenarios, the limitations of the aforementioned conventional techniques can hinder surgical planning. Reoperative necks pose a particular challenge, as altered tissue planes and postoperative fibrosis often obscure both sonographic and CT landmarks. In this context, FCH PET/MR provides significant advantages (Fig. 10.1). The metabolic sensitivity of PET, when combined with the exceptional soft-tissue contrast of MR, allows accurate localization of diseased parathyroid tissue even in anatomically complex or post-

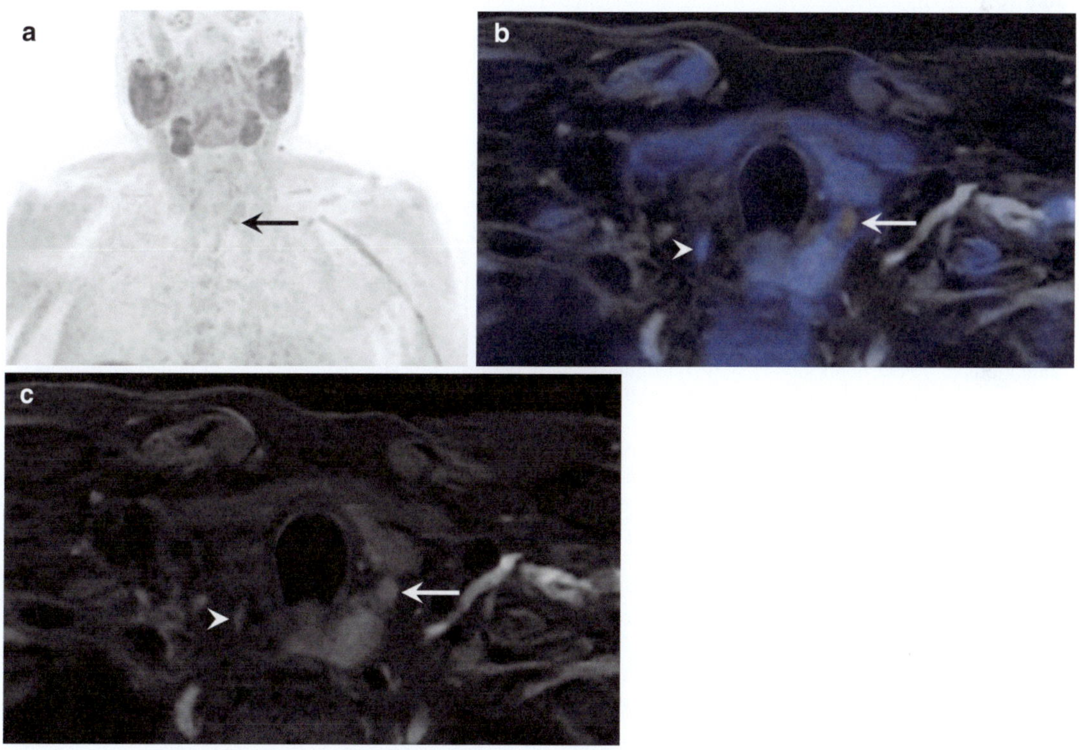

Fig. 10.1 A 71-year-old man with previous surgical resection of a right-sided upper pole parathyroid adenoma**.** (**a**) The coronal maximum intensity projection (MIP) from PET demonstrates a faintly FCH-avid focus in the neck on the left side (arrow). (**b**) Axial-fused PET/MR image and (**c**) axial T2-weighted FSE flex water image show a moderately T2w-hyperintense left-sided upper pole parathyroid adenoma (SUV_{max} 4.7; arrow) corresponding to the focus. Another spindle-shaped, T2w-hyperintense lesion with faint FCH uptake and is seen in the neck on the right side, lateral to the tracheoesophageal groove (arrowhead; SUV_{max} 3.5), corresponding to scar tissue from the previous parathyroid surgery (Fig. 10.8). The left-sided adenoma was surgically resected, and PTH and serum calcium levels remained within normal limits during follow-up

surgical environments. Furthermore, the avoidance of additional ionizing radiation from the MR component makes PET/MR an attractive alternative to PET/CT, especially in younger patients or those requiring follow-up scans. The overall radiation burden in FCH PET/MR is very low, originating solely from the PET component [21]. This hybrid approach also facilitates a comprehensive neck and mediastinal assessment, including evaluation of incidental thyroid nodules, lymphadenopathy, or other structural abnormalities that may influence the surgical strategy. Additionally, PET/MR systems feature digital PET detectors, which generally provide superior performance to analogue detectors, particularly for the detection of small lesions [23].

Table 10.1 provides an overview of key characteristics of standard first-line imaging techniques used for adenoma localization in patients with hyperparathyroidism.

Although specific cost-effectiveness studies focusing on PET/MR are currently lacking, PET/MR data have been partially incorporated into some existing analyses of FCH PET/CT cost-effectiveness, which generally demonstrate advantages over conventional localization methods [26, 40, 47, 64].

Table 10.1 Comparative overview of imaging modalities for parathyroid adenoma localization

Feature/ modality	Ultrasound (US)	SPECT/CT [99mTc] sestamibi	PET/CT [18F] fluorocholine	PET/MR [18F] fluorocholine
Principle	High-frequency sound waves; anatomy and limited functionality (e.g., tissue perfusion)	Gamma camera functional imaging + CT anatomy	PET metabolic imaging + CT anatomy	PET metabolic imaging + MR anatomy
Strengths	Widely available; inexpensive; no radiation; excellent for superficial lesions	Functional + anatomical localization; detects ectopic glands; widely available	High sensitivity for adenomas; good ectopic adenoma detection; faster acquisition than SPECT	High sensitivity + superior soft tissue contrast; reduced radiation exposure
Limitations	Poor in obesity, retrotracheal/ mediastinal glands; operator-dependent	Limited sensitivity in small adenomas, multigland disease; thyroid nodules may mimic parathyroid lesions	CT adds radiation; lower soft-tissue contrast than MR	Limited availability; potentially higher cost
Radiation dose	None	~5–8 mSv	~3–8 mSv	~2.5 mSv
Best use case	First-line, typical anatomy	First line in centers without PET/CT or PET/MR	First line in centers without PET/MR	First line
Sensitivity (single adenoma)	70–85%	>85%	>95%	>95%
Multigland disease sensitivity	40–60%	30–50%	~90%	~90%
Ectopic adenoma detection	Poor–moderate	Good	Excellent	Excellent
Anatomical thyroid evaluation	Excellent	Poor	Moderate	Excellent
Availability	Very high	High	Moderate	Low

Reported radiation dose estimates for SPECT/CT and PET/CT can vary substantially, influenced not only by the injected radiotracer dose but also by the specific acquisition protocol used for the CT component

10.3 PET Tracers for Parathyroid Imaging

The success of PET/MR in parathyroid imaging relies heavily on the choice of the radiotracer. Among available agents, FCH has emerged as the most widely used and best validated. FCH uptake reflects increased cell membrane synthesis, a characteristic of hyperfunctioning parathyroid tissue due to elevated phospholipid-dependent choline kinase activity. Multiple prospective and retrospective studies have demonstrated FCH PET to have a sensitivity exceeding 90% for solitary adenomas, with particularly strong performance in small adenomas and in patients who have had inconclusive or discordant findings from ultrasound and [99mTc]sestamibi scans. Despite its high accuracy, FCH PET is not immune to false-positive radiotracer uptake. Such uptake can occur in autonomously functioning or hyperplastic thyroid nodules and thyroid cancers, reactive cervical lymph nodes, or head and neck malignancies, making careful correlation with MR anatomy essential—an approach that typically resolves these ambiguities with ease [25, 26, 29, 50, 53].

[11C]choline was historically used in PET and PET/CT while there is no documented use in PET/MR imaging for parathyroid disease. Its short 20-minute half-life requires an on-site cyclotron, limiting its practical application and distribution to remote sites. Also, the higher positron energy compared to 18F-based tracers such as FCH negatively impacts image quality and may challenge detection of small parathyroid adenomas. [11C]methionine is another tracer with historically established use in parathyroid imaging. It targets increased amino acid transport and protein synthesis in adenomas and can be valuable in cases where FCH is unavailable. There is no documented use of this tracer in hybrid PET/MR imaging for parathyroid disease.

The amino acid PET radiotracers [18F]DOPA, used for imaging neuroendocrine tumors, and [18]fluoroethyltyrosine, used for imaging primary and secondary brain tumors, have been explored in limited PET(/CT) case series without success in parathyroid adenomas; their role in this context remains investigational at best, and no evidence is available on their utility in PET/MR [34, 36]. Incidental detection of parathyroid adenomas has been reported with nearly all available PET radiotracers, including [68Ga]PSMA and [68Ga] DOTATATE—originally developed for prostate cancer and neuroendocrine tumor imaging, respectively—sparking interest in their potential use as alternative radiotracers. While promising, these agents require further investigation before they can be adopted into routine practice, and no evidence currently suggests that they could match or exceed the remarkably high sensitivity of FCH. More recently, encouraging results have been reported for [18F]flurpiridaz, a PET radiotracer primarily developed for myocardial perfusion imaging, although no direct comparison with FCH has yet been conducted [16]. Another agent yielding positive findings in an FCH-negative case was [68Ga]trivehexin; however, this compound remains purely investigational at present [35]. The limited available data preclude a deeper understanding of these imaging phenotypes.

Taken together, incidental detection of parathyroid adenomas is possible with virtually any PET radiotracer [6, 12, 41, 54, 61]. However, only a few—apart from FCH—have demonstrated diagnostic value for prospective detection, and these generally perform inferiorly to FCH. Of note, there are reports of FCH-negative adenomas, which are positive with other clinically available radiotracers such as [68Ga] PSMA [14].

10.4 PET/MR Imaging Protocol (Including Some Tweaks)

10.4.1 Patient Preparation

Optimal results from PET/MR depend on standardized acquisition protocols that maximize lesion conspicuity [30]. For FCH PET/MR, patient preparation is straightforward and does not require fasting. Metallic objects such as jewelry and hearing aids should be removed to minimize MR artifacts. Standard MR safety precautions apply, including contraindications such as implanted electronic devices and ferromagnetic metallic foreign bodies. For further details on patient preparation, please refer to the chapter on PET/CT imaging.

10.4.2 Acquisition Workflow

In patients with benign parathyroid disorders such as primary hyperparathyroidism, imaging from the skull base to the diaphragm is typically sufficient. However, in cases of parathyroid carcinoma—particularly in patients with rising PTH levels following resection of the primary tumor—whole-body imaging is recommended to identify potential sites of recurrent or metastatic PTH secretion.

10.4.2.1 PET

Given the high sensitivity of currently available PET/MR scanners, a relatively low dose of FCH is generally sufficient (approximately 2 MBq/kg; 120–240 MBq for most adults; or alternatively a standardized dose of approximately 150 MBq). Following intravenous administration, some protocols incorporate an early dynamic neck acquisition during the first 10 min post-injection. This phase can capture rapid tracer uptake in adenomas before thyroid activity increases, thereby improving lesion-to-background contrast. Alternatively, an early static acquisition at about 5 min post-injection is used in some centers. The standard static acquisition is typically performed at 45–60 min (most commonly at 50 min) post-injection, representing the optimal imaging window, with sufficient lesion-to-background contrast against thyroid gland tissue [37]. The acquisition frame time is usually 3–6 min, usually 2 frames per patient suffice in patients with benign parathyroid disorders.

PET images are corrected in a standardized way for random, dead time, scatter, and attenuation. Since parathyroid adenomas are typically small lesions, PET datasets should be reconstructed using parameters optimized for small lesion detectability, such as block sequential regularized expectation maximization (BSREM) with appropriately adjusted β-values [3, 27, 38, 39, 50, 53]. Additionally, extending the acquisition time for the neck region—where most parathyroid adenomas are located—relative to the mediastinal frame may further improve the overall lesion detection. When a fully diagnostic, naïve MR neck protocol is used—as recommended—there is sufficient time to keep the PET acquisition running for some time during the MR scan. This approach improves count statistics, potentially resulting in optimized image quality and potentially higher lesion detectability (Figs. 10.2 and 10.3). It offers a clear advantage over PET/CT, where the anatomical component is acquired much more rapidly and not truly simultaneously, and where a prolonged PET acquisition is not possible without increasing the overall examination time.

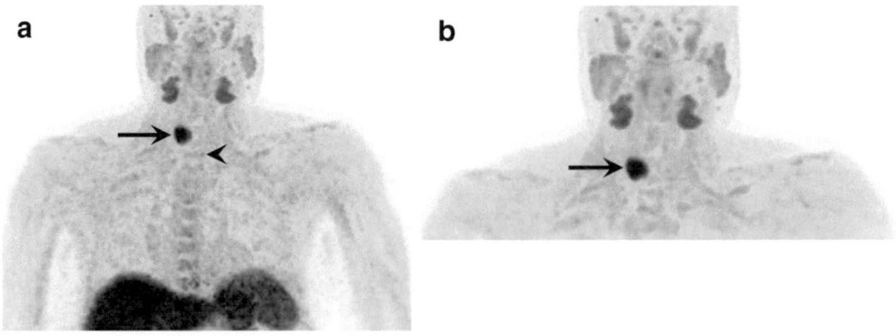

Fig. 10.2 Patient with a right-sided upper pole parathyroid adenoma. (**a**) The coronal maximum intensity projection (MIP) image from standard PET acquisition (3 min per frame) demonstrates a round, FCH-avid upper pole adenoma in the right neck (arrow; SUV_{max} 11.6) and a faintly FCH-avid focus in the left neck at the typical location of a lower pole adenoma (arrowhead). (**b**) Coronal MIP image from prolonged PET acquisition (9 min per frame) shows only the right-sided adenoma (arrow) with markedly reduced image noise. The right-sided adenoma was surgically resected, while the left neck was untouched; PTH and serum calcium levels remained within normal limits during 12 months of follow-up

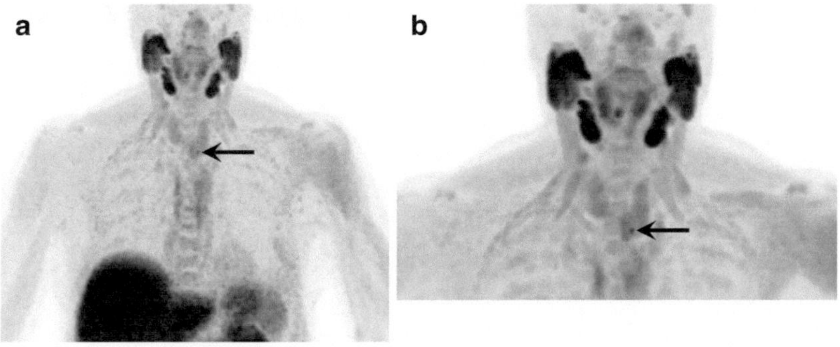

Fig. 10.3 Patient with a left-sided lower pole parathyroid adenoma. (**a**) Coronal maximum-intensity projection (MIP) from the standard PET acquisition (3 min per frame) showing a faintly FCH-avid lower pole adenoma in the left neck (arrow; SUV_{max} 6.23). (**b**) Coronal MIP from the prolonged PET acquisition (9 min per frame) demonstrating markedly improved lesion conspicuity and reduced image noise; the measured SUV_{max} (6.55) did not differ significantly from the standard acquisition. The adenoma was successfully resected

Table 10.2 Exemplary acquisition parameters of the regionalized MR protocol used in FCH-PET/MR [30]

Parameter	Axial T2w flex water	Axial T1w FSE	Coronal STIR PROPELLER	Sagittal T2w PROPELLER	Axial T1w LAVA flex
TR/TE (ms)	5120/80	640/7.4	7020/60	6400/124	659/(min/full)
Flip angle (degree)	111	111	100	142	111
TI	N/A	N/A	200	N/A	N/A
Parallel imaging acceleration factor	2.5	2.5	3	2	2
Slice thickness (mm)	2.5	3.5	3.5	2.5	3
FOV (cm)	20	20	26	22	22
Acquisition matrix (pixels)	356 × 224	300 × 236	280 × 280	340 × 340	280 × 240
Receiver bandwidth (kHz)	83.33	62.5	83.33	62.5	83.33
Fat saturation	IDEAL	N/A	STIR	N/A	IDEAL
Total acquisition time (min)	3:05	2:15	4:54	2:46	2:02

For all sequences using IDEAL methods, images with and without fat suppression are acquired simultaneously. *FOV* field of view, *IDEAL* iterative decomposition of water and fat with echo asymmetry and least-square estimation, *LAVA* liver acquisition with volume acquisition, *N/A* not applicable, *PROPELLER* periodically rotated overlapping parallel lines with enhanced reconstruction, *STIR* short tau inversion recovery, *T1w* T1-weighted, *T2w* T2-weighted, *TI* inversion time

10.4.2.2 MR

Besides the MR sequences used for attenuation correction and coarse anatomical orientation, such as a T1-weighted liver acquisition with volume acceleration–flexible (LAVA-flex) sequence and a coronal T2-weighted sequence, covering the area from the tip of the head to the upper abdomen, a regionalized, fully diagnostic MR protocol of the neck without contrast medium is recommended (Table 10.2).

This regional MR protocol covering the neck should include high-resolution axial T2w-weighted fat-suppressed and axial T1-weighted images [30]. Additional T2-weighted, STIR-weighted, or T1-weighted coronal and/or sagittal images may improve anatomical detail but are generally not considered to provide additional benefit for localizing diseased parathyroid glands. Diffusion-weighted imaging is likewise not expected to enhance lesion contrast or detectabil-

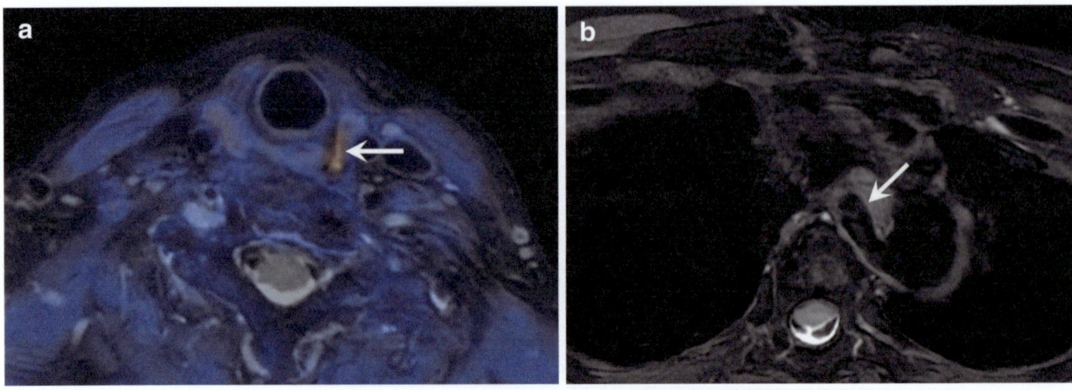

Fig. 10.4 A 67-year-old woman with a parathyroid adenoma and an aberrant right-sided subclavian artery (arteria lusoria). (**a**) Axial fused PET/MR shows a left-sided upper pole parathyroid adenoma with moderate FCH uptake (SUV_{max} 5.7). (**b**) In the same patient, an aberrant right-sided subclavian artery is present (arrow), as demonstrated on the axial T2-weighted FSE flex water image. This vascular anomaly is almost invariably associated with a non-recurrent inferior laryngeal nerve on the *right* side, which is at increased risk during parathyroid surgery due to its atypical course [57, 59]. Even when surgery is limited to the contralateral side, as in this case, potential variations in nerve anatomy should be anticipated

ity, as parathyroid adenomas typically do not exhibit distinct imaging characteristics on DWI compared with physiologic lymph nodes. There is currently no evidence that gadolinium-enhanced MR imaging improves detection of parathyroid adenomas in PET/MR. While contrast-enhanced images may aid in identifying vascular anomalies relevant for surgical planning—such as an aberrant right-sided subclavian artery, which is typically associated with a *right-sided* non-recurrent laryngeal nerve—these anomalies are usually also detectable on non-contrast images (Fig. 10.4) when carefully evaluated.

10.4.3 Image Fusion

PET and MR datasets are fused, at a minimum, in the axial plane. Additional fusion of appropriate MR and PET datasets in the sagittal and coronal planes can further assist in surgical planning by improving anatomical orientation. Maximum intensity projection (MIP) images of the PET data should be included to provide an overview and enhance sensitivity for detecting ectopic parathyroid glands. A meticulous, slice-by-slice review remains essential for identifying diseased glands.

10.5 Interpretation and Diagnostic Clues

10.5.1 Typical Findings

Interpreting PET/MR in parathyroid imaging requires integration of functional and anatomical findings. A typical adenoma appears as a well-defined, oval focus of low to intense FCH uptake, usually located posterior or inferior to the thyroid (Fig. 10.5). On MR, adenomas are characteristically hypointense on T1-weighted images and hyperintense on T2-weighted images and would demonstrate variable enhancement after contrast administration [30, 38]. Ectopic inferior parathyroid glands may be found within the thyroid, within the thymus or between the thymus and thyroid, most often in the thymic tongue or along the thyrothymic ligament [45, 46, 66]. Other inferior ectopic sites include the retroesophageal space and the mediastinum inferior to the thymus (e.g., in aorto-pulmonary position, associated with the vagus nerve), where PET plays the primary role in localization and MR provides precise anatomical detail. Superior gland ectopic locations are less common and include also intrathyroidal adenomas—most often subcapsular, less frequently completely intrathyroidal—as

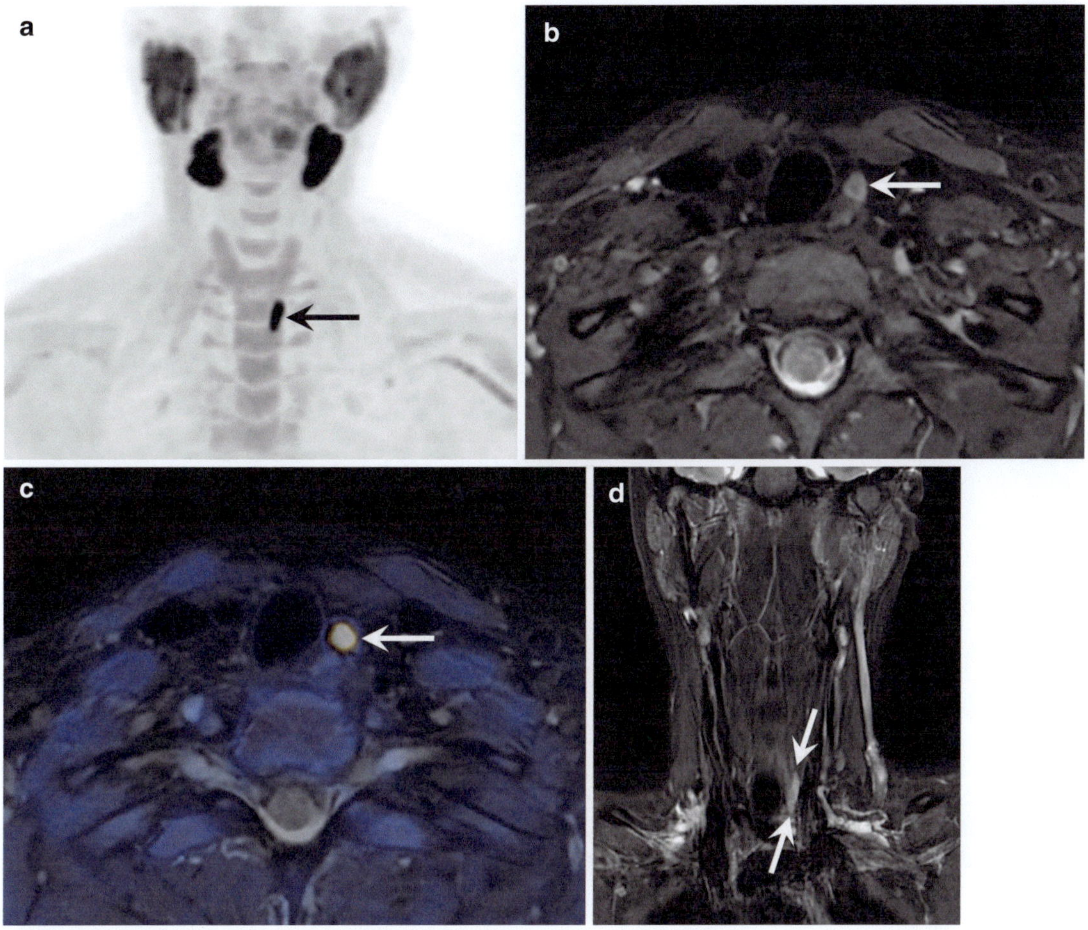

Fig. 10.5 Typical appearance of a parathyroid adenoma on FCH-PET/MR in a 28-year-old woman with primary hyperparathyroidism (PTH 120 ng/mL, albumin-corrected serum calcium 2.70 mmol/L), presenting with recurrent nephrourolithiasis. (**a**) Coronal PET MIP image demonstrates a longitudinal, FCH-avid parathyroid adenoma in the left neck adjacent to the thyroid lobe (arrow). (**b**) The lesion is hyperintense on the axial T2-weighted FSE flex water image. (**c**) Axial fused PET/MR image shows high FCH uptake (SUV_{max} 8.9) corresponding to the lesion. (**d**) The coronal STIR PROPELLER image highlights the typical longitudinal configuration of the adenoma (arrows)

well as adenomas situated along the carotid sheath up to the level of the submandibular gland. As is well known, superior gland adenomas are often "overly descended" and may be located behind, or even inferior to the lower pole of the thyroid gland, deep to the trachea [19]. PET/MR enables a dedicated assessment not only of the location of ectopic adenomas but also of the polarity of orthotopic adenomas. The trachea serves as a key landmark: superior pole adenomas lie deep to the tracheal bisecting line, whereas inferior pole adenomas are located superficial to it [31]. Remarkably, this rule of thumb also applies to the polarity of overly descended and ectopic adenomas [31] (Fig. 10.6).

Pure MR data on adenoma characteristics is relatively limited, as MR alone is seldom used for their identification due to its restricted sensitivity for small lesions and the lack of reliable criteria to distinguish them from physiologic structures such as lymph nodes. With fully diagnostic neck sequences, anatomical detail is typically excellent in the upper neck, but diminishes in the inferior neck at the level of the lung apices, and is further reduced in the mediastinum, where cardiac and vascular pulsation additionally impair image quality.

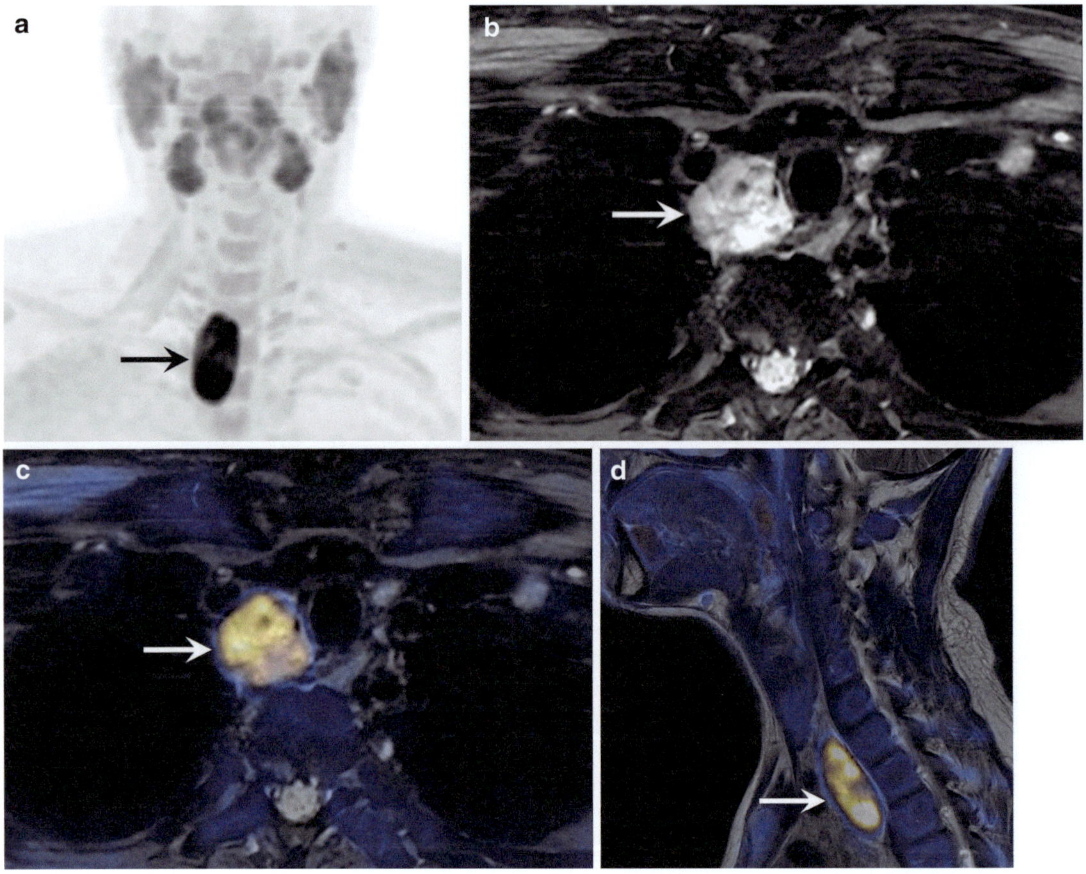

Fig. 10.6 A 45-year-old man with an overly descended giant parathyroid adenoma. (**a**) Coronal PET MIP shows a large oval FCH-avid parathyroid adenoma in the right neck (arrow). (**b**) On the axial T2-weighted FSE flex water image, the adenoma (arrow) appears hyperintense and is located predominantly inferior to the thyroid gland, positioned between the trachea, innominate artery, and prevertebral muscles. The main portion of the adenoma is located deep to the tracheal bisecting line, indicating an upper pole origin. (**c**) Axial fused PET/MR image demonstrates intense FCH uptake (arrow; SUV_{max} 15.2) of the adenoma. (**d**) Sagittal fused PET/MR T2w-weighted PROPELLER image reveals the typical longitudinal configuration of the adenoma (arrows) and its extension into the mediastinum. The lesion was successfully resected via a minimally invasive *transthoracic* approach, confirming an overly descended upper pole parathyroid adenoma; specimen weight was 10.8 g

Dynamic or time-resolved contrast-enhanced MR (4D-MR) has been described, but a head-to-head comparison with nuclear medicine techniques—particularly FCH PET—is lacking [4, 8, 43, 48]. 4D-MR is based on the reported rapid arterial contrast enhancement and subsequent washout of parathyroid adenomas, assessed by near-continuous acquisition of contrast perfusion information, unlike as in 4D-CT. In practice, however, parathyroid adenomas do not necessarily exhibit the typical pattern of hypoattenuation on naïve images, followed by arterial hyperattenuation and rapid washout on venous and delayed phases often referred to in the literature—but which is in fact present in only 20%, as shown on CT [7]. Also, the available data on their enhancement behavior on MR remain ambiguous [4, 8, 43, 48]. Moreover, analyzing such enhancement patterns essentially presupposes prior knowledge of the adenoma's location, creating a diagnostic vicious cycle. An additional limitation of 4D-MR is its increased susceptibility to motion artifacts caused by breathing, swallowing, and vascular pulsation. These artifacts can significantly degrade image quality, particularly in the lower neck and mediastinal regions, where many ectopic parathyroid glands are found. In our institutional experience, the diagnostic performance of 4D-MR for parathyroid adenoma detection is, at best, mediocre.

10.5.2 Key Differentiators

Distinguishing parathyroid adenomas from other hypermetabolic lesions in the neck is one of the most critical—and sometimes challenging—interpretive tasks in PET/MR. Intrathyroidal uptake typically points toward a thyroid nodule, such as a colloid nodule, an adenoma or carcinoma, rather than an ectopic parathyroid adenoma [25, 61]. While ectopically located intrathyroidal parathyroid adenomas do exist—predominantly in a subcapsular location—they are distinctly uncommon compared to genuine thyroidal lesions [11, 61]. This distinction is often aided by high-resolution MR sequences, which can delineate the lesion's position relative to the thyroid capsule more precisely than even contrast-enhanced CT. Particularly, opposed-phase imaging can be helpful: the presence of a complete "India ink" (chemical shift) artifact at the interface between the lesion and thyroid tissue is a strong indicator of an extrathyroidal location, favoring a parathyroid origin. On the other hand, if an FCH-positive intrathyroidal nodule is detected in a patient who also has a separate extrathyroidal lesion compatible with a parathyroid adenoma, especially if both are on the same side, this constellation strongly favors the thyroidal origin of the intrathyroidal lesion. In such cases, the PET/MR findings should be interpreted in the broader anatomical and clinical context to avoid misclassification.

Cervical lymph nodes, another common source of focal uptake, frequently display a visible fatty hilum on MR, a feature that is absent in parathyroid adenomas. Another useful clue is the "polar vessel" sign: a discrete feeding artery or draining vein seen entering one pole of the lesion, which can occasionally be identified in parathyroid adenomas—especially larger ones—on high-resolution MR angiographic sequences. In contrast, lymph nodes characteristically demonstrate vascular entry at the hilum rather than at a pole, providing a useful distinction in differential diagnosis. Additionally, lymph nodes tend to exhibit more rapid washout or different tracer uptake kinetics compared with the persistent or gradually increasing tracer uptake often seen in parathyroid tissue. Awareness of these morphological and functional patterns—especially when evaluated side-by-side in fused PET/MR datasets—helps avoid false positives and ensures accurate localization before surgical intervention.

10.5.3 Pitfalls

Several pitfalls can reduce the accuracy of PET/MR in parathyroid imaging and must be actively considered during interpretation. Very small adenomas—particularly those under 3–4 mm—may produce insufficient tracer accumulation to be distinguished from background activity, falling below the effective spatial resolution of PET. Such lesions can be especially elusive in multiglandular disease, where hyperplasia or microadenomas predominate.

Cystic adenomas do not necessarily represent a pitfall for PET/MR imaging. Although they are known for their oftentimes faint FCH uptake, they are easily identified on T2-weighted fat-suppressed MR images due to their high signal intensity (Fig. 10.7).

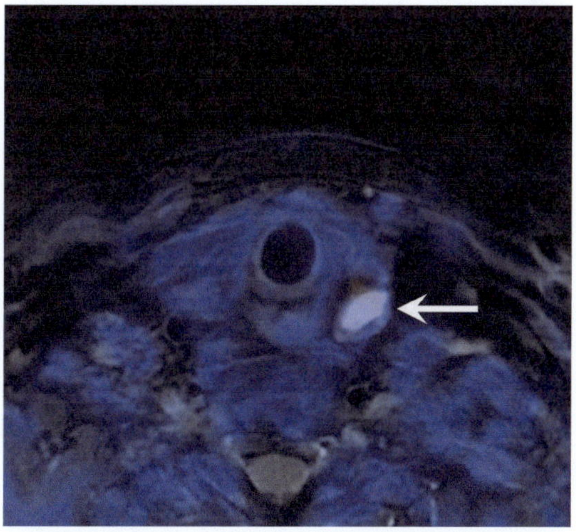

Fig. 10.7 A 64-year-old woman with primary hyperparathyroidism. The axial PET/T2-weighted FSE flex water MR image shows a comparably large and mainly cystic, left-sided upper pole parathyroid adenoma with faint to moderate FCH uptake (arrow; SUV_{max} 5.7). The central portions of the lesion represent fluid and appear hyperintense

Non-specific tracer uptake is another challenge, most commonly seen in inflammatory or reactive lymph nodes. These can mimic adenomas both in size and in metabolic activity, particularly in patients with recent upper respiratory tract infections or autoimmune thyroid disease [25]. Morphological clues on MR, such as the presence of a fatty hilum, can help, but these features are not always conspicuous.

Motion artifacts also degrade image quality [27]. Swallowing, breathing, or subtle patient movement during acquisition can blur lesion boundaries, obscure small adenomas, and complicate PET/MR co-registration. The long acquisition time of MR compared to CT makes it more susceptible to such motion-related artifacts.

Tracer-related pitfalls include focal uptake in thyroid nodules—benign or malignant—which can be mistaken for intrathyroidal adenomas (Fig. 10.8). Physiologic uptake in muscles or tracer retention in veins, particularly when early-phase imaging is performed, may also occur in the neck and upper mediastinum, potentially mimicking adenomas [12, 25, 55]. Knowledge of these patterns, combined with careful correlation to MR anatomy and, when available, prior imaging, is essential. In equivocal cases, reviewing dynamic tracer uptake curves or adding targeted

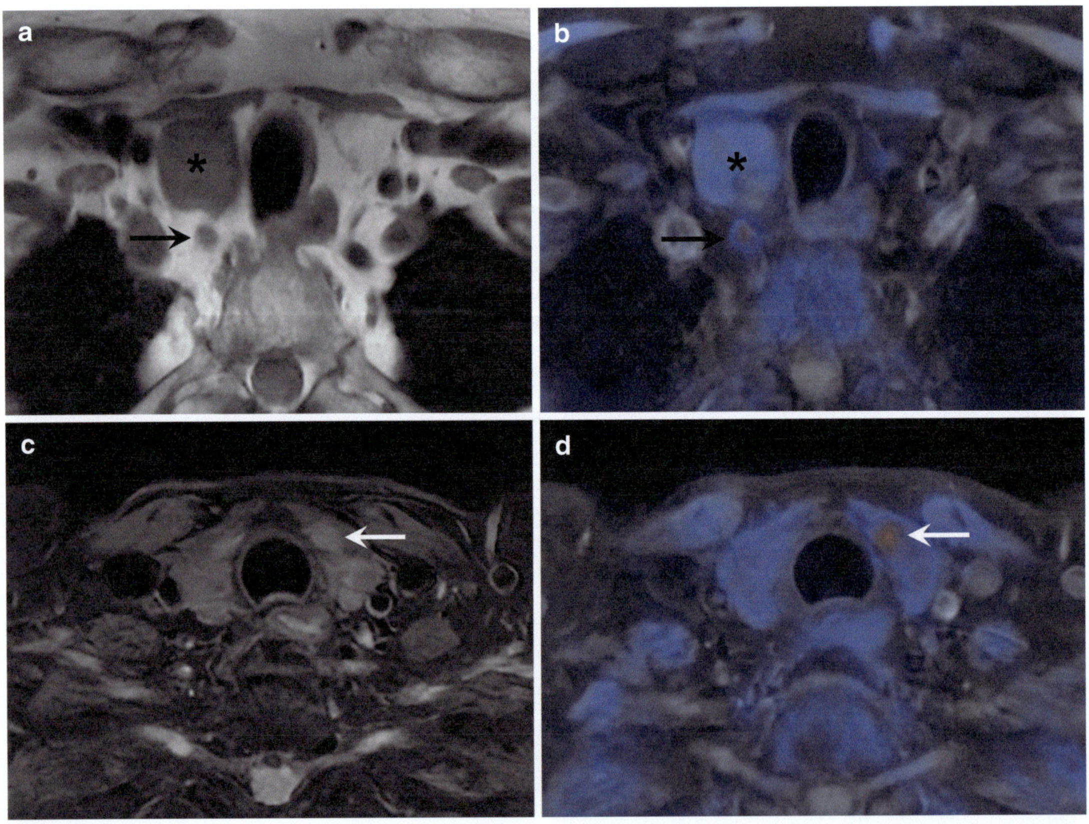

Fig. 10.8 A 69-year-old man with primary hyperparathyroidism. (**a**) The axial T1-weighted FSE image and (**b**) the axial fused PET/MR image show a T1w-isointense nodule with faint to moderate FCH uptake (arrow; SUV_{max} 5.3), lateral to the tracheoesophageal groove on the right side, corresponding to an upper pole parathyroid adenoma. An FCH-negative goiter nodule (asterisk) is seen as well. (**c**) Axial T2-weighted FSE flex water image and (**d**) axial fused PET/MR image at the level of the thyroid gland show a moderately FCH-avid, T2w-hyperintense nodule within the left lobe of the thyroid (arrow; SUV_{max} 7.0), corresponding to an incidental T1a papillary microcarcinoma of the thyroid gland. All three lesions were surgically removed and their histology confirmed

MR sequences can increase confidence and reduce the risk of misclassification.

In the unlikely event that standard FCH PET/MR is negative for a parathyroid adenoma in a patient with (overt) hyperparathyroidism, performing earlier FCH imaging (approximately 5 min after injection) may be considered the initial step in repeat PET/MR, rather than immediately switching to a different nuclear medicine technique. A subset of patients may demonstrate improved adenoma visualization on these early-phase images [2, 13]. Alternatively, the use of a different PET radiotracer may be explored [14, 35].

10.6 Clinical Applications

PET/MR has evolved from a predominantly research-based modality into a valuable clinical tool for selected patient populations [65]. The particular strength of FCH PET/MR in patients with hyperparathyroidism that need to undergo imaging lies in combining the high sensitivity of FCH PET for metabolically active parathyroid tissue with the superior soft-tissue resolution and multiparametric capabilities of MR. While adoption varies between institutions, several clinical scenarios have emerged in which PET/MR can meaningfully influence management.

10.6.1 First-Line Localization

Although PET/MR is not yet a universal first-line study, certain high-volume endocrine surgery centers have adopted it as the initial imaging modality not only in complex or high-stakes patients but also routinely in all patients with hyperparathyroidism that need to undergo imaging [2, 38, 50, 53]. Petranović Ovčariček et al. reported remarkably high performance metrics for PET/MR as first-line imaging modality in a cohort of 109 patients, with a sensitivity of 0.948, a positive predictive value of 0.978, and an accuracy of 0.936 [50, 53]. However, these results were not statistically different from those achieved with PET/CT [50, 53]. Notably, particularly complex cases may benefit from PET/MR over conventional localization techniques. This includes those with prior extensive neck dissection for thyroid cancer or other head and neck malignancy, suspected mediastinal or retroesophageal ectopic glands, or unequivocal biochemical hyperparathyroidism with a negative or equivocal ultrasound. In these situations, PET/MR offers a "one-stop" approach, replacing the need for multiple sequential imaging studies and enabling surgical planning with high confidence.

10.6.2 Problem-Solving After Inconclusive or Discordant First-Line Imaging

This remains the most common indication for PET/MR referral. Discordant results, such as a suspicious ultrasound lesion without [99mTc] sestamibi uptake or [99mTc]sestamibi uptake without a corresponding sonographic correlate, can create diagnostic uncertainty and delay surgery. FCH PET/MR can often resolve these discrepancies by clarifying whether the lesion represents a parathyroid adenoma or an unrelated thyroid nodule, lymph node, or other structure. The combination of PET's metabolic specificity and MR's anatomical detail frequently allows for definitive classification and precise localization. In the second-line setting as well, an excellent diagnostic performance was reported in a cohort of 155 patients, with a sensitivity of 0.979, a positive predictive value of 0.986, and an accuracy of 0.968, with no statistically significant difference compared to PET/CT [50, 53]. Interestingly, Araz et al. reported respectable diagnostic performance for FCH PET/MR even in cases where FCH PET/CT had yielded negative results [5].

10.6.3 Reoperative Neck Surgery

Reoperation for persistent or recurrent primary hyperparathyroidism poses technical and safety challenges due to postoperative fibrosis, altered anatomy, and a heightened risk of recurrent laryngeal nerve injury. FCH PET/MR has demonstrated high sensitivity for detecting residual or ectopic parathyroid tissue even in scarred or anatomically distorted regions, including the mediastinum [5, 50, 53]. The ability to provide precise 3D localization can reduce operative time, guide incision placement, and lower complication rates.

10.6.4 Detection of Ectopic and Supernumerary Glands

Ectopic parathyroid glands may be located anywhere between the submandibular space and the aortopulmonary region, but are usually found between the submandibular gland and the pericardium [1, 15, 24, 58]. PET/MR's extended field of view compared to conventional localization techniques, coupled with its ability to image deep and mediastinal locations without additional radiation exposure, makes it particularly effective in detecting carotid sheath, retrotracheal, paraesophageal, and intrathymic glands. In patients with persistent disease after partial parathyroidectomy, FCH PET/MR can also reveal overlooked supernumerary glands—present in up to 15% of individuals and typically small in size—which may not be detected on planar or ultrasound-based techniques [17, 20, 63].

10.6.5 Multigland Disease and Secondary and Tertiary Hyperparathyroidism

Multigland involvement is a diagnostic hurdle for all localization techniques. It is often encountered in patients with normocalcemic hyperparathyroidism (see below). FCH PET/MR can detect asymmetric hyperplasia, differentiate dominant hyperfunctioning glands from smaller hyperplastic ones, and guide selective rather than blanket resection strategies. In secondary hyperparathyroidism—common in chronic kidney disease—FCH uptake can vary to some extent between glands, reflecting differences in cellular activity and hyperplasia stage [28, 44, 63]. PET/MR may assist in identifying the most active glands, potentially enabling subtotal rather than total parathyroidectomy.

In tertiary hyperparathyroidism, typically occurring after renal transplantation, PET/MR is valuable for identifying persistent hyperfunctioning glands responsible for ongoing PTH excess despite normalization of calcium-phosphate metabolism. It is expected that PET imaging with choline-based radiotracers outperforms ultrasound and traditional scintigraphic techniques in such cases, especially when glands are deeply located or surrounded by scar tissue from prior surgery [44, 56, 63]. However, specific studies of FCH PET/MR today are missing.

In this context, a recent multicenter study provides valuable evidence supporting the use of FCH PET/CT imaging as a primary diagnostic tool for MEN1-related primary hyperparathyroidism, both prior to initial surgery and in cases of persistent or recurrent disease [10, 63]. Although specific data on PET/MR in this setting are currently lacking, its performance is expected to be at least equivalent.

For many of these indications, dedicated studies on FCH PET/MR are either absent or limited to small patient cohorts or even single reported cases. However, based on our extensive experience conducting FCH PET/MR as a first-line imaging modality in these scenarios over several years, the outcomes have been consistently favorable and superior to those achieved with any other parathyroid imaging technique.

10.6.6 Normocalcemic Primary Hyperparathyroidism

The two main causes of negative FCH PET results are small adenomas and multigland involvement, both of which are often encountered in normocalcemic pHPT. Normocalcemic primary HPT is a growing subgroup of the disease, typically associated with more subtle clinical manifestations and smaller, oftentimes multiple adenomas. It is increasingly recognized due to more widespread biochemical screening, presenting an imaging challenge because lesions may be both smaller and also less metabolically active. Despite this, reports indicate that FCH PET can detect adenomas missed on conventional imaging in such patients [9, 22, 26, 33]. Also, in the FCH PET/MR cohort reported by Petranović Ovčariček et al. several patients had normocalcemic primary HPT [50, 53]. PET/MR's sensitivity in this subgroup may derive from its ability to detect subtle tracer accumulation and precisely localize small adenomas relative to surrounding soft tissue, potentially allowing for earlier surgical intervention before overt hypercalcemia develops.

As a note of caution, imaging outcomes in patients with normocalcemic hyperparathyroidism are generally less reliable than in those with overt hyperparathyroidism. Indications for surgery in this subgroup remain debated and are not universally accepted; therefore, localization imaging should be undertaken with careful consideration.

10.6.7 Surgical Planning and Intraoperative Guidance

Beyond lesion detection, PET/MR assists in preoperative mapping of the lesion's spatial relationships to the hyroid lobes, the recurrent laryngeal nerve, and major cervical vessels. MR can provide clear vascular roadmaps and delineate the thyroid capsule with millimetric precision, while PET defines the hyperfunctioning target. This integrated anatomical-metabolic dataset can be shared directly with the surgical team, aiding decisions on minimally invasive parathyroidectomy, focused neck exploration, or even thoracoscopic surgery for deep mediastinal lesions [22, 26, 42]. In the future, PET/MR findings could guide the intraoperative use of fluorescence imaging to confirm complete excision [32, 49, 60].

10.7 Future Directions

The future of PET/MR in parathyroid imaging will likely be shaped by expanding the indications of FCH PET/MR to non-primary hyperparathyroidism, as well as by advances in radiotracer development [16, 35], particularly in the rather uncommon FCH-negative cases. Further standardization, education, and harmonization are needed in image analysis and workflow optimization. The development of novel tracers with higher adenoma-to-thyroid uptake ratios may help reduce false-positive findings and improve specificity [16, 35]. In addition, artificial intelligence–based segmentation and automated detection algorithms hold promise for standardizing image interpretation and may ultimately integrate with intraoperative navigation systems. Ongoing efforts aim to streamline PET/MR protocols to increase time efficiency in high-volume clinical settings. Finally, large-scale outcome studies are essential to determine whether PET/MR-guided surgery results in higher cure rates, shorter operative times, and fewer complications compared with conventional localization strategies and PET/CT.

10.8 Conclusion

[18F]fluorocholine PET/MR represents the pinnacle of cross-sectional imaging techniques for the noninvasive preoperative localization of parathyroid adenomas, not only in patients with challenging anatomy or inconclusive findings on conventional imaging, but particularly in standard cases in daily routine. By combining the metabolic insights of PET with the high-resolution soft-tissue imaging of MR, PET/MR facilitates accurate localization and characterization of hyperfunctioning parathyroid tissue, enhancing preoperative planning and potentially improving surgical outcomes in patients with parathyroid disease. The performance metrics of FCH PET/MR are outstanding, and the radiation dose to the patient is significantly lower than that associated with any other technique employing ionizing radiation for this indication. Further advancements in clinical indications, tracer development, and imaging protocols are likely to expand the clinical utility of PET/MR, making it a cornerstone in the management of all parathyroid cases.

References

1. Akerstrom G, Malmaeus J, Bergstrom R. Surgical anatomy of human parathyroid glands. Surgery. 1984;95(1):14–21. https://www.ncbi.nlm.nih.gov/pubmed/6691181
2. Alharbi AA, Alshehri FM, Albatly AA, Sah BR, Schmid C, Huber GF, Huellner MW. [(18)F]fluorocholine uptake of parathyroid adenoma is correlated with parathyroid hormone level. Mol Imaging Biol. 2018;20(5):857–67. https://doi.org/10.1007/s11307-018-1179-x.
3. Aljared A, Alharbi AA, Huellner MW. BSREM reconstruction for improved detection of in-transit metastases with digital FDG-PET/CT in patients with malignant melanoma. Clin Nucl Med. 2018;43(5):370–1. https://doi.org/10.1097/RLU.0000000000002024.
4. Altintop SE, Cerit MN, Cindil E, Sendur HN, Barlas T, Yalcin MM, Altinova AE, Akturk M, Toruner FB, Karakoc MA, Cerit ET. Dynamic 4 dimensional contrast enhanced MRI for localization in primary hyperparathyroidism. Endocrine. 2025;89(1):267–75. https://doi.org/10.1007/s12020-025-04239-2.
5. Araz M, Nak D, Soydal C, Peker E, Erden I, Kucuk NO. Detectability of 18F-choline PET/MR in primary hyperparathyroidism. Eur Arch Otorrinolaringol. 2022;279(5):2583–9. https://doi.org/10.1007/s00405-021-07046-3.
6. Arora S, Damle NA, Passah A, Yadav MP, Ballal S, Aggarwal V, Gupta Y, Kumar P, Tripathi M, Bal C. Incidental detection of parathyroid adenoma on somatostatin receptor PET/CT and incremental role of (18)F-fluorocholine PET/CT in MEN1 syndrome. Nucl Med Mol Imaging. 2018;52(3):238–42. https://doi.org/10.1007/s13139-018-0520-2.
7. Bahl M, Sepahdari AR, Sosa JA, Hoang JK. Parathyroid adenomas and hyperplasia on four-dimensional CT scans: three patterns of enhancement relative to the thyroid gland justify a three-phase protocol. Radiology. 2015;277(2):454–62. https://doi.org/10.1148/radiol.2015142393.
8. Becker JL, Patel V, Johnson KJ, Guerrero M, Klein RR, Ranvier GF, Owen RP, Pawha P, Nael K. 4D-dynamic contrast-enhanced MRI for preoperative localization in patients with primary hyperparathyroidism. AJNR Am J Neuroradiol. 2020;41(3):522–8. https://doi.org/10.3174/ajnr.A6482.
9. Bossert I, Chytiris S, Hodolic M, Croce L, Mansi L, Chiovato L, Mariani G, Trifiro G. PETC/CT with (18) F-choline localizes hyperfunctioning parathyroid adenomas equally well in normocalcemic hyperparathyroidism as in overt hyperparathyroidism. J Endocrinol Investig. 2019;42(4):419–26. https://doi.org/10.1007/s40618-018-0931-z.
10. Boucher A, Delabie J, Lussey-Lepoutre C, Haissaguerre M, Ouvrard E, Lavinia V, Le Bras M, Batisse-Lignier M, Cuny T, Jacquet-Francillon N, Gaujoux S, Molina O, Imperiale A, Latge A, Ansquer C, Kelly A, Borson-Chazot F, Tlili G, Sebag F, et al. Performance of [(18)F]fluorocholine PET/CT in MEN1-related primary hyperparathyroidism before initial surgery or for persistent/recurrent disease. Eur J Nucl Med Mol Imaging. 2024;51(5):1349–60. https://doi.org/10.1007/s00259-023-06537-1.
11. Bradley KM, McGowan DR, Bartley L, Scott-Coombes D, Rees JI. Ectopic, intra-thyroid parathyroid adenoma better visualised by deep learning enhanced choline PET/CT. QJM. 2025; https://doi.org/10.1093/qjmed/hcaf057.
12. Broos WAM, van der Zant FM, Knol RJJ. Incidental detection of parathyroid adenoma on 18F-PSMA PET/CT. Clin Nucl Med. 2023;48(12):1082–3. https://doi.org/10.1097/RLU.0000000000004896.
13. Broos WAM, Wondergem M, van der Zant FM, Knol RJJ. Dual-time-point (18)F-fluorocholine PET/CT in parathyroid imaging. J Nucl Med. 2019;60(11):1605–10. https://doi.org/10.2967/jnumed.118.225599.
14. Cieslewicz M, Andryszak N, Pelka K, Szczepanek-Parulska E, Ruchala M, Kunikowska J, Czepczynski R. Parathyroid adenoma detected in (68)Ga-PSMA PET/CT but not in the dedicated imaging modalities. Diagnostics (Basel). 2024;14(15) https://doi.org/10.3390/diagnostics14151690.
15. Cook MI, Qureshi YA, Todd CE, Cummins RS. An unusual ectopic location of a parathyroid carcinoma arising within the thyroid gland. J Clin Endocrinol Metab. 2012;97(6):1829–33. https://doi.org/10.1210/jc.2011-3115.
16. Derlin T, Kleine-Dopke D, Neubert L, Ross TL, Ringe BP, Schmelzle M, Bengel FM. Initial experience with dual-time-point [(18)F]flurpiridaz PET/CT for localization of parathyroid adenomas in primary hyperparathyroidism. J Nucl Med. 2025;66(6):922–5. https://doi.org/10.2967/jnumed.124.269387.
17. Dharmashaktu Y, Damle NA, Seenu V, Agarwal S, Radhakrishnan L, Wakankar R. Integrated 18F-FCH PET/4D-CT in a case of supernumerary parathyroid glandular hyperplasia with incidentally detected thymic NET. Clin Nucl Med. 2025; https://doi.org/10.1097/RLU.0000000000006067.
18. Doppman, J. L., & Miller, D. L. (1991). Localization of parathyroid tumors in patients with asymptomatic hyperparathyroidism and no previous surgery. J Bone Miner Res, 6 Suppl 2, S153-S158; discussion S159. doi:https://doi.org/10.1002/jbmr.5650061431.
19. Duke WS, Vernon HM, Terris DJ. Reoperative parathyroidectomy: overly descended superior adenoma. Otolaryngol Head Neck Surg. 2016;154(2):268–71. https://doi.org/10.1177/0194599815619625.
20. Expert Panel on Neurological I, Zander D, Bunch PM, Policeni B, Juliano AF, Carneiro-Pla D, Dubey P, Gule-Monroe MK, Hagiwara M, Hoang JK, Jain V, Kim LT, Moonis G, Parsons MS, Rath TJ, Solorzano CC, Subramaniam RM, Taheri MR, DuChene Thoma K, et al. ACR appropriateness criteria(R) parathyroid

adenoma. J Am Coll Radiol. 2021;18(11S):S406–22. https://doi.org/10.1016/j.jacr.2021.08.013.
21. Fabbri C, Galassi R, Moretti A, Sintuzzi E, Mautone V, Sarti G, Strigari L, Benassi M, Matteucci F. Radiation dosimetry of 18F-fluorocholine PET/CT studies in prostate cancer patients. Phys Med. 2014;30(3):346–51. https://doi.org/10.1016/j.ejmp.2013.10.007.
22. Ferrari SB, Morand GB, Rupp NJ, Krutzfeldt J, Vetter D, Hullner MW, Broglie MA. Clinical predictors of negative/equivocal SPECT imaging outcomes in primary hyperparathyroidism: factors calling for (18)F-choline-PET. Am J Otolaryngol. 2024;45(4):104315. https://doi.org/10.1016/j.amjoto.2024.104315.
23. Filippi L, Bianconi F, Ferrari C, Linguanti F, Battisti C, Urbano N, Minestrini M, Messina SG, Buci L, Baldoncini A, Rubini G, Schillaci O, Palumbo B. Digital versus analogue PET in parathyroid imaging: comparison of PET metrics and machine learning-based characterisation of hyperfunctioning lesions (the DIGI-PET study). Eur J Nucl Med Mol Imaging. 2025. https://doi.org/10.1007/s00259-025-07508-4. Epub ahead of print. PMID: 40844547.
24. Georgakopoulos B, Al Khalili Y. Anatomy, head and neck, parathyroid, ectopic glands. In StatPearls; 2025. https://www.ncbi.nlm.nih.gov/pubmed/31082016
25. Grunig H, Strobel K, Zander A, Perez Lago MDS, Lima T, Wicke C, Fischli S, Bhure U. Significance of incidental thyroid 18 F-fluorocholine uptake in patients with hyperparathyroidism imaged for localizing hyperfunctioning parathyroid glands. Nucl Med Commun. 2024;45(11):938–46. https://doi.org/10.1097/MNM.0000000000001887.
26. Huber GF, Hullner M, Schmid C, Brunner A, Sah B, Vetter D, Kaufmann PA, von Schulthess GK. Benefit of (18)F-fluorocholine PET imaging in parathyroid surgery. Eur Radiol. 2018;28(6):2700–7. https://doi.org/10.1007/s00330-017-5190-4.
27. Huellner MW. PET/MR in head and neck cancer—an update. Semin Nucl Med. 2021;51(1):26–38. https://doi.org/10.1053/j.semnuclmed.2020.07.006.
28. Huellner MW, Aberle S, Sah BR, Veit-Haibach P, Bonani M, Schmid C, Steinert H. Visualization of parathyroid hyperplasia using 18F-fluorocholine PET/MR in a patient with secondary hyperparathyroidism. Clin Nucl Med. 2016;41(3):e159–61. https://doi.org/10.1097/RLU.0000000000001053.
29. Imperiale A, Bani J, Bottoni G, Latge A, Heimburger C, Catrambone U, Vix M, Treglia G, Piccardo A. Does (18)F-Fluorocholine PET/CT add value to positive parathyroid scintigraphy in the presurgical assessment of primary hyperparathyroidism? Front Med (Lausanne). 2023;10:1148287. https://doi.org/10.3389/fmed.2023.1148287.
30. Isenschmid SK, Schaab JA, Gennari AG et al. MR Pulse sequences for parathyroid adenoma imaging using [18F]fluorocholine PET/MR in primary hyperparathyroidism. Nucl Med Mol Imaging 2025. https://doi.org/10.1007/s13139-025-00961-x.
31. Inukai JI, Sah BR, Beintner-Skawran S, Maurer A, Mueller SA, Morand GB, Nogami M, Murakami T, Rupp NJ, Ovčariček PP, Giovanella L, Huellner MW. Use of the tracheal bisecting line to differentiate upper pole from lower pole parathyroid adenomas: a PET/MR study using [18F]Fluorocholine. Ann Nucl Med. 2025 Oct 9. doi: 10.1007/s12149-025-02105-9. Epub ahead of print. PMID: 41066026.
32. Kose E, Rudin AV, Kahramangil B, Moore E, Aydin H, Donmez M, Krishnamurthy V, Siperstein A, Berber E. Autofluorescence imaging of parathyroid glands: an assessment of potential indications. Surgery. 2020;167(1):173–9. https://doi.org/10.1016/j.surg.2019.04.072.
33. Koumakis E, Gauthe M, Martinino A, Sindayigaya R, Delbot T, Wartski M, Clerc J, Roux C, Borderie D, Cochand-Priollet B, Cormier C, Gaujoux S. FCH-PET/CT in primary hyperparathyroidism with discordant/negative MIBI scintigraphy and ultrasonography. J Clin Endocrinol Metab. 2023;108(8):1958–67. https://doi.org/10.1210/clinem/dgad073.
34. Krakauer M, Kjaer A, Bennedbaek FN. (18)F-FET-PET in primary hyperparathyroidism: a pilot study. Diagnostics (Basel). 2016;6(3) https://doi.org/10.3390/diagnostics6030030.
35. Kuyumcu S, Denizmen D, Has-Simsek D, Poyanli A, Uzum AK, Buyukkaya F, Isik EG, Onder S, Aksakal N, Ozkan ZG, Sanli Y. (68)Ga-Trivehexin PET/CT uptake in malignant and fibrotic lung tissue: refining diagnostic applications. Eur J Nucl Med Mol Imaging. 2025;52(10):3513–14. https://doi.org/10.1007/s00259025-07193-3. PMID: 40082263; PMCID: PMC12316737.
36. Lange-Nolde A, Zajic T, Slawik M, Brink I, Reincke M, Moser E, Hoegerle S. PET with 18F-DOPA in the imaging of parathyroid adenoma in patients with primary hyperparathyroidism. A pilot study. Nuklearmedizin. 2006;45(5):193–6. https://www.ncbi.nlm.nih.gov/pubmed/17043728
37. Lezaic L, Rep S, Sever MJ, Kocjan T, Hocevar M, Fettich J. (1)(8)F-Fluorocholine PET/CT for localization of hyperfunctioning parathyroid tissue in primary hyperparathyroidism: a pilot study. Eur J Nucl Med Mol Imaging. 2014;41(11):2083–9. https://doi.org/10.1007/s00259-014-2837-0.
38. Liberini V, Morand GB, Rupp NJ, Orita E, Deandreis D, Broglie Dappen M, Hofbauer M, Maurer A, Husmann L, Mader CE, Grunig H, Alharbi AA, Messerli M, Huellner MW. Histopathological features of parathyroid adenoma and 18F-choline uptake in PET/MR of primary hyperparathyroidism. Clin Nucl Med. 2022;47(2):101–7. https://doi.org/10.1097/RLU.0000000000003987.
39. Lohaus N, Enderlin F, Skawran S, Maurer A, Abukwaik AMA, Franzen D, Huellner MW, Messerli M. Impact of Bayesian penalized likelihood reconstruction on quantitative and qualitative aspects for pulmonary nodule detection in digital 2-[(18)F]FDG-PET/CT. Sci Rep. 2022;12(1):8308. https://doi.org/10.1038/s41598-022-09904-4.

40. Mamou A, Chkair S, Gilly O, Maimoun L, Mamou Y, Sheppard SC, Kotzki PO, Lallemant B, Boudousq V. Economic evaluation of [(18)F]fluorocholine PET/CT in pre operative assessment of hyperfunctional parathyroids in primary hyperparathyroidism: a cost effectiveness analysis. EJNMMI Rep. 2025;9(1):11. https://doi.org/10.1186/s41824-025-00244-w.
41. Mendoza PL, Ongkeko EE, Santiago JF. Silent parathyroid adenoma mistakenly interpreted on FDG-PET as thyroid cancer metastasis in a patient with elevated thyroglobulin and negative I-131 whole body scan and removed by radioguided minimally invasive surgery. Clin Nucl Med. 2008;33(1):23–5. https://doi.org/10.1097/RLU.0b013e31815c50c0.
42. Morand GB, Rupp NJ, Huellner MW, Gerber PA, Soyka MB, Broglie MA, Holzmann D. Transnasal-transpterygoid endoscopic removal of an 18F-choline-avid parathyroid carcinoma metastasis in the Skull Base. JAMA Otolaryngol Head Neck Surg. 2019;145(10):978–80. https://doi.org/10.1001/jamaoto.2019.2352.
43. Nael K, Hur J, Bauer A, Khan R, Sepahdari A, Inampudi R, Guerrero M. Dynamic 4D MRI for characterization of parathyroid adenomas: multiparametric analysis. AJNR Am J Neuroradiol. 2015;36(11):2147–52. https://doi.org/10.3174/ajnr.A4425.
44. Noskovicova L, Balogova S, Aveline C, Tassart M, Zhang-Yin J, Kerrou K, Jaksic I, Montravers F, Talbot JN. (18)F-fluorocholine-positron emission tomography/computerized tomography (FCH PET/CT) imaging for detecting abnormal parathyroid glands: indication, practice, interpretation and diagnostic performance. Semin Nucl Med. 2024;54(6):875–95. https://doi.org/10.1053/j.semnuclmed.2024.08.002.
45. Noussios G, Anagnostis P, Natsis K. Ectopic parathyroid glands and their anatomical, clinical and surgical implications. Exp Clin Endocrinol Diabetes. 2012;120(10):604–10. https://doi.org/10.1055/s-0032-1327628.
46. Okada M, Tominaga Y, Yamamoto T, Hiramitsu T, Narumi S, Watarai Y. Location frequency of missed parathyroid glands after parathyroidectomy in patients with persistent or recurrent secondary hyperparathyroidism. World J Surg. 2016;40(3):595–9. https://doi.org/10.1007/s00268-015-3312-1.
47. Ortega-Serrano J, Serrano-Lopez S, Alfonso-Ballester R, Marti-Fernandez R, Lapena-Rodriguez M, Exposito RD, Cassinello-Fernandez N. Is the (18)F-choline PET-CT more cost-effective than standard protocol for locating a parathyroid adenoma? Langenbeck's Arch Surg. 2025;410(1):235. https://doi.org/10.1007/s00423-025-03824-3.
48. Ozturk M, Polat AV, Celenk C, Elmali M, Kir S, Polat C. The diagnostic value of 4D MRI at 3T for the localization of parathyroid adenomas. Eur J Radiol. 2019;112:207–13. https://doi.org/10.1016/j.ejrad.2019.01.022.
49. Pace-Asciak P, Russell J, Solorzano C, Berber E, Singer M, Shaha AR, Khafif A, Angelos P, Nixon I, Tufano RP. The utility of parathyroid autofluorescence as an adjunct in thyroid and parathyroid surgery 2023. Head Neck. 2023;45(12):3157–67. https://doi.org/10.1002/hed.27538.
50. Petranovic Ovcaricek P, Campenni A, Giovanella L, Huellner MW. Parathyroid carcinoma: a comprehensive analysis with focus on molecular imaging. Eur J Nucl Med Mol Imaging. 2025a;52(8):2754–8. https://doi.org/10.1007/s00259-025-07162-w.
51. Petranovic Ovcaricek P, Giovanella L, Carrio Gasset I, Hindie E, Huellner MW, Luster M, Piccardo A, Weber T, Talbot JN, Verburg FA. The EANM practice guidelines for parathyroid imaging. Eur J Nucl Med Mol Imaging. 2021;48(9):2801–22. https://doi.org/10.1007/s00259-021-05334-y.
52. Petranovic Ovcaricek P, Giovanella L, Hindie E, Huellner MW, Talbot JN, Verburg FA. An essential practice summary of the new EANM guidelines for parathyroid imaging. Q J Nucl Med Mol Imaging. 2022;66(2):93–103. https://doi.org/10.23736/S1824-4785.22.03427-6.
53. Petranovic Ovcaricek P, Schaab J, Beintner-Skawran S, Maurer A, Rupp NJ, Ikenberg K, Morand GB, Mueller SA, Vetter D, Liberini V, Giovanella L, Huellner MW. [(18)F]Fluorocholine PET/MRI and [(18)F]Fluorocholine PET/CT as first- and second-line imaging in primary hyperparathyroidism—who takes the lead? Eur J Nucl Med Mol Imaging. 2025b; https://doi.org/10.1007/s00259-025-07373-1.
54. Pfob CH, Karimov I, Jesinghaus M, Novotny A, Weber WA, Eiber M, Feuerecker B. Pitfalls in Ga-68-PSMA-PET/CT: incidental finding of parathyroid adenoma. Eur J Nucl Med Mol Imaging. 2019;46(4):1041. https://doi.org/10.1007/s00259-018-4239-1.
55. Prabhu M, Damle NA. Fluorocholine PET imaging of parathyroid disease. Indian J Endocrinol Metab. 2018;22(4):535–41. https://doi.org/10.4103/ijem.IJEM_707_17.
56. Raitza M, Alshalali AAN, Glaudemans A, Gans ROB, Slart R. Use of [(11)C]choline PET/CT for visualization of four hyperactive parathyroid glands in a patient with renal hyperparathyroidism. Eur J Nucl Med Mol Imaging. 2022;49(13):4750–1. https://doi.org/10.1007/s00259-022-05885-8.
57. Saxe A, Idris M, Gemechu J. Does the use of intraoperative neuromonitoring during thyroid and parathyroid surgery reduce the incidence of recurrent laryngeal nerve injuries? A systematic review and meta-analysis. Diagnostics (Basel). 2024;14(9) https://doi.org/10.3390/diagnostics14090860.
58. Shan H, Jiang Z, Xu J, Li J, Zhu X. Ectopic parathyroid adenoma on sternocleidomastoid muscle: a case report. Front Oncol. 2024;14:1410057. https://doi.org/10.3389/fonc.2024.1410057.
59. So JT, Thompson CSG. Non-recurrent laryngeal nerve: surgical risk of injury in comparison with the normal recurrent laryngeal nerve—a systematic review and

meta-analysis. Clin Otolaryngol. 2025;50(4):654–63. https://doi.org/10.1111/coa.14312.

60. St Amour TC, Demarchi MS, Thomas G, Triponez F, Kiernan CM, Solomicronrzano CC. Educational review: intraoperative parathyroid fluorescence detection technology in thyroid and parathyroid surgery. Ann Surg Oncol. 2023;30(2):973–93. https://doi.org/10.1245/s10434-022-12807-3.
61. Thanseer NTK, Bhadada SK, Sood A, Parihar AS, Dahiya D, Singh P, Basher RK, Das A, Mittal BR. Dual pathologies of parathyroid adenoma and papillary thyroid cancer on fluorocholine and fluorodeoxyglucose PET/CT. Nucl Med Mol Imaging. 2018;52(2):154–8. https://doi.org/10.1007/s13139-017-0488-3.
62. Thompson NW. Localization studies in patients with primary hyperparathyroidism. Br J Surg. 1988;75(2):97–8. https://doi.org/10.1002/bjs.1800750202.
63. Treglia G, Rizzo A, Piccardo A. Expanding the clinical indications of [(18)F]fluorocholine PET/CT in primary hyperparathyroidism: the evidence cannot be evaded. Eur J Nucl Med Mol Imaging. 2024;51(5):1345–8. https://doi.org/10.1007/s00259-023-06573-x.
64. van Mossel S, Saing S, Appelman-Dijkstra N, Quak E, Schepers A, Smit F, de Geus-Oei LF, Vriens D. Cost-effectiveness of one-stop-shop [(18)F]Fluorocholine PET/CT to localise parathyroid adenomas in patients suffering from primary hyperparathyroidism. Eur J Nucl Med Mol Imaging. 2024;51(12):3585–95. https://doi.org/10.1007/s00259-024-06771-1.
65. Veit-Haibach P, Ahlstrom H, Boellaard R, Delgado Bolton RC, Hesse S, Hope T, Huellner MW, Iagaru A, Johnson GB, Kjaer A, Law I, Metser U, Quick HH, Sattler B, Umutlu L, Zaharchuk G, Herrmann K. International EANM-SNMMI-ISMRM consensus recommendation for PET/MRI in oncology. Eur J Nucl Med Mol Imaging. 2023;50(12):3513–37. https://doi.org/10.1007/s00259-023-06406-x.
66. Wang X, Si Y, Cai J, Lu H, Tong H, Zhang H, Wen J, Shen M. Proactive exploration of inferior parathyroid gland using a novel meticulous thyrothymic ligament dissection technique. Eur J Surg Oncol. 2022;48(6):1258–63. https://doi.org/10.1016/j.ejso.2022.03.011.

Parathyroid Cancer Imaging

11

Virginia Liberini and Martin W. Huellner

▶ **Definitions**

Parathyroid Carcinoma (PC)
- Rare and aggressive endocrine malignancy
- Represents <1% of PHPT cases and <0.005% of all cancers
- Often functional, with excessive PTH secretion and severe hypercalcemia
- High risk of local invasion, recurrence, and distant metastases

Epidemiology
- Most common in the 5th–6th decade of life
- Slight male predominance
- Frequently under-recognized, with diagnostic delays

This chapter focuses on imaging techniques used to detect and stage parathyroid cancer, a rare but aggressive malignancy. It discusses the imaging features of parathyroid carcinoma and the challenges in differentiating parathyroid cancer from atypical adenomas by imaging. The role of each imaging modality in initial diagnosis, preoperative planning, and post-treatment surveillance is addressed, with a focus on whole-body imaging.

V. Liberini
Nuclear Medicine Unit, ASO S. Croce e Carle Cuneo, Cuneo, Italy
e-mail: liberini_v@ospedale.cuneo.it

M. W. Huellner (✉)
Department of Nuclear Medicine, University Hospital Zurich / University of Zurich, Zurich, Switzerland
e-mail: martin.huellner@usz.ch

Sites of Metastasis and Recurrence
- Regional lymph nodes (15–20%), lungs, bones, liver
- Local recurrence is common (up to 80%)

Genetic Associations
- Frequent inactivating mutations in *CDC73* (parafibromin)
- Germline testing and immunohistochemistry (IHC) are recommended in all confirmed cases

Atypical Parathyroid Tumor (APT)
- Intermediate entity between benign adenoma and carcinoma
- May share molecular features with PC, especially *CDC73* mutations
- Lacks definitive features of malignancy (e.g., angioinvasion, metastasis)

© The Author(s), under exclusive license to Springer Nature Switzerland AG 2026
P. Petranović Ovčariček et al. (eds.), *Parathyroid Imaging*,
https://doi.org/10.1007/978-3-032-14178-1_11

Learning Objectives

Recognize high-risk clinical and biochemical features of PC

- Markedly elevated serum calcium and PTH
- Palpable neck mass >3 cm
- Signs of local invasion or severe systemic hypercalcemia

Understand implications for surgical management

- Early suspicion supports immediate *en bloc* resection
- Minimally invasive approaches may be inadequate or detrimental in malignant cases

Describe typical imaging findings across modalities

- *Ultrasound*: hypoechoic, lobulated, inhomogeneous mass, often >3 cm
- *CT/MRI*: irregular margins, capsular invasion, soft tissue infiltration, calcifications
- *[^{99m}Tc]Tc-MIBI scintigraphy*: persistent tracer uptake
- *[^{18}F]fluorocholine PET/CT*: high sensitivity for locoregional and distant disease
- *[^{18}F]FDG PET/CT*: valuable for poorly differentiated or aggressive tumors

Define the role of imaging in staging and surgical planning

- CT and MRI are essential for restaging and local extension assessment
- [^{18}F]fluorocholine PET/CT enables accurate whole-body evaluation

Recognize imaging limitations and pitfalls

- Possible false positives (e.g., thyroid nodules, reactive lymph nodes) on [^{99m}Tc]Tc-MIBI and [^{18}F]fluorocholine PET
- Importance of histological confirmation in equivocal findings
- FDG-avid bone lesions may mimic metastases but represent brown tumors (osteolytic lesions secondary to severe hyperparathyroidism)
- Dual-tracer PET imaging ([^{18}F]FDG + [^{18}F]fluorocholine or [^{99m}Tc]Tc-MIBI) may improve specificity

Integrate multimodal data

- Combine imaging, clinical, laboratory, and histopathological findings
- Optimize diagnosis, staging, and treatment planning for personalized care

11.1 Introduction

Parathyroid carcinoma (PC) is a rare endocrine malignancy of the parathyroid glands. It may arise in any of the parathyroid glands, with no known preference for the superior, inferior, or ectopic glands. Nevertheless, the rarity of the disease results in a limited understanding of its incidence, distribution, and risk factors [53, 89, 93, 160, 169].

PC accounts for approximately 0.005% of all malignant neoplasms in Western populations and reportedly for approximately 1% of primary hyperparathyroidism (PHPT) cases. Although its incidence is low, parathyroid cancer presents considerable clinical challenges due to its diverse manifestations, diagnostic uncertainties, and the risk of local recurrence and distant metastases [53, 156].

Most PCs are functionally active, with excessive and dysregulated parathyroid hormone (PTH) secretion. A highly increased serum PTH level, not uncommonly in the thousands, is a biochemical hallmark rarely seen in benign hyperparathyroid disorders. The clinical burden of the disease is significantly increased by resulting severe hypercalcemia, which is a primary cause of morbidity [17, 73, 161].

According to the literature, organ metastases are rather uncommon, occurring in approximately 5% of cases. By contrast, lymph node involvement has been documented in the literature at an overall rate of 6.5%, and in approximately 30% of cases where this was specifically evaluated. However, local recurrence is more prevalent, with rates ranging from 25% to 80% [134]. Mortality is mainly due to complications arising from hypercalcemia rather than from local aggressive behavior of the tumor. Survival rates at 5 and 10 years have been reported with 76–85% and 49–77%, respectively. Adverse prognostic factors encompass age older than 40 years, tumor size exceeding 4 cm, male sex, presence of distant metastasis, and poor histological differentiation [13, 102, 141, 156].

Parathyroid carcinoma remains poorly defined in the literature, with limited consensus regarding its clinical presentation, diagnostic criteria, optimal imaging techniques, and recommended treatment approaches. Nevertheless, in 2024, the European Society for Medical Oncology (ESMO) released guidelines for the diagnosis, management, and monitoring of PC [62]. Diagnostic challenges emerge due to considerable overlap with parathyroid adenoma and hyperplasia, both in their clinical presentation and radiological findings. Confirmation of diagnosis generally relies on clear evidence of local tissue invasion on histopathology or proven metastatic spread [23, 169].

The management of parathyroid carcinoma necessitates a multidisciplinary approach that includes endocrinologists, endocrine surgeons, radiologists, nuclear medicine physicians, and pathologists. Imaging is integral to each phase of the diagnostic and therapeutic process, encompassing the initial localization and characterization of lesions, surgical planning, intraoperative guidance, and postoperative monitoring. Radiological techniques, including ultrasound, CT, and MRI, alongside functional imaging modalities such as scintigraphy, SPECT/CT, and PET/CT or PET/MR, offer complementary information essential for precise diagnosis and informed clinical decision-making. This chapter examines the critical role of imaging, highlighting how the combination of anatomic and functional imaging improves diagnostic precision, informs surgical decisions, and aids in long-term patient care. The strengths, limitations, and appropriate indications of each imaging modality in the context of this rare but clinically significant malignancy will be examined with particular attention.

11.2 Epidemiology

Despite its rarity, the Surveillance, Epidemiology, and End Results (SEER) program has documented a notable increase in the incidence of parathyroid carcinoma in the United States in recent years. The incidence rose from 3.5 cases per 10 million people per year in 1988 to 5.7 cases per 10 million people per year in 2003. There is an absence of the significant gender disparity that is observed in benign parathyroid adenomas, which are more prevalent in females. The prevalence of aggressive forms of primary HPT, such as parathyroid carcinoma, peaks in the fifth decade of life [94].

According to a more recent retrospective SEER analysis, which included 609 PC cases identified between 1975 and 2016, the incidence was slightly greater in males (52.2%) and more common in Caucasian individuals (75.4%). At the time of diagnosis, the average age was 62 years, with only 14 percent of individuals younger than 40. Histological analysis revealed that 99.7% of tumors were adenocarcinomas, with 36.8% of cases identified as organ-confined at diagnosis [156].

The National Cancer Database (NCDB) provides additional insights by functioning as a comprehensive registry that documents over 60% of all newly diagnosed cancer cases in the United States (286 cases of PC diagnosed between 1985 and 1995), accounting PC for 0.005% of all cancers recorded in the database. The overall relative survival rates at 5 and 10 years were reported as 85.5% and 49.1%, respectively [71].

11.3 Etiology

PC generally manifests sporadically. Although its precise etiology remains largely elusive, stage V chronic renal disease and prior cervical irradiation have been associated with an

Table 11.1 Hereditary syndromes associated with parathyroid carcinoma

Syndrome	Inheritance, mutations	Main features	Parathyroid involvement
HPT-JT (hyperparathyroidism-jaw tumor syndrome)	Autosomal dominant; germline mutation in CDC73	Primary hyperparathyroidism, ossifying jaw fibromas, renal/uterine lesions	High risk of PC (15–37.5%); requires genetic counseling
MEN1 (multiple endocrine neoplasia type 1)	Autosomal dominant; mutation in MEN1 (chromosome 11q13)	Parathyroid hyperplasia/adenomas, pancreatic NETs, pituitary tumors	Parathyroid pathology in ~95%; PC is rare
MEN2A (multiple endocrine neoplasia type 2A/Sipple syndrome)	Autosomal dominant; activating mutation in RET (chromosome 10q11.21)	Medullary thyroid carcinoma (>99%), pheochromocytoma (~40%), parathyroid tumors (~30%)	Parathyroid pathology in ~30%; PC is rare
FIHP (familial isolated hyperparathyroidism)	Autosomal dominant; genetic basis heterogeneous (sometimes MEN1, CDC73, or unknown)	Hyperparathyroidism without other MEN tumors	Rarely associated with PC; accounts for ~1% of pHPT cases

Note: *CDC73* cell division cycle 73 gene, *FIHP* familial isolated hyperparathyroidism, *HPT-JT* hyperparathyroidism-jaw tumor syndrome, *MEN1/MEN2A* multiple endocrine neoplasia type 1/type 2A, *NETs* neuroendocrine tumors, *PC* parathyroid carcinoma, *pHPT* primary hyperparathyroidism, *RET* rearranged during transfection proto-oncogene

increased prevalence, suggesting the possible involvement of systemic and environmental risk factors [75, 77].

The development of PC has been linked to several genetic alterations [24, 107]. A mutation in the cell division cycle 73 gene (CDC73), also referred to as HRPT2, is most frequently linked to PC and is essential to its molecular etiology. The parafibromin protein is encoded by the tumor suppressor gene CDC73, which is located on chromosome 1q31.2. Immunohistochemistry is a technique that can be used to identify parafibromin deficiency caused by loss-of-function mutations in this gene. Decreased parafibromin expression has been associated with enhanced cellular proliferation, disrupted apoptosis, and chromosomal instability, all of which facilitate carcinogenesis [29].

In addition to CDC73, molecular investigations have identified further alterations in gene expression associated with the development of PC. As of now, a total of 144 genes have been linked to the progression from non-metastatic to metastatic PC. This encompasses the expression of MMP9, ANGPTL4, BMP7, FGFR1, and SOX2, alongside the downregulation of ERBB3, TBX1, FBP1, and RAB25, indicating that these genes may play a role in the metastatic phenotype of PC [107].

Inherited syndromic diseases have been observed to be associated with PC. As indicated in Table 11.1, the most significant inherited diseases include familial isolated hyperparathyroidism (FIHP), multiple endocrine neoplasia types 1 and 2A (MEN1 and MEN2A), and hyperparathyroidism-jaw tumor syndrome (HPT-JT) [5, 25, 108, 112, 150].

11.4 Anatomy and Pathology

11.4.1 Histology

Differentiating benign from malignant parathyroid disease remains a significant diagnostic challenge, particularly preoperatively, as no specific clinical or cytological features reliably distinguish PC [45, 148]. Fine-needle aspiration is generally discouraged due to limited diagnostic utility and the risk of tumor seeding [1, 9, 86, 119]. Histologically, a definitive diagnosis of malignancy often requires evidence of invasive growth or metastasis or angioinvasion, which may be absent at initial presentation [156].

Advances in molecular pathology and genetics have expanded the understanding of parathyroid neoplasia, leading to the 2022 WHO classification, which offers a more refined perspective on parathyroid tumors by incorporating emerging clinicopathological and genetic association [48].

The WHO 2022 classification defines seven distinct entities, emphasizing both morphological and molecular characteristics [43, 48, 62, 79, 93, 160]:

1. *Parathyroid Adenoma (PA):* a benign, typically solitary lesion without evidence of genetic syndromes or multiglandular involvement. Histology reveals a cellular nodule often surrounded by a rim of normal parathyroid tissue. Distinction from hyperplasia is hardly possible by histopathology alone but typically requires clinical and cross-sectional imaging correlation.
2. *Atypical Parathyroid Tumor (APT)*: previously termed atypical parathyroid adenoma, APT is a noninvasive neoplasm of uncertain malignant potential. It exhibits features that are intermediate between adenoma and carcinoma, including fibrous bands, high mitotic activity (> 5 mitoses/10 mm^2), trabecular or monotonous sheet-like growth, coagulative necrosis, presence of tumor cells in the tumor capsule or adherence to adjacent tissues. Immunohistochemistry (IHC) may reveal loss of parafibromin and elevated Ki-67 (>5%), indicating increased recurrence risk, particularly in CDC73-mutated cases.
3. *Parathyroid Carcinoma (PC)*: a diagnosis requires histologic evidence of malignancy, such as angioinvasion, lymphatic or perineural invasion, local tissue infiltration, or confirmed metastases. Diagnosis is further supported by IHC, including loss of parafibromin, APC, RB, E-cadherin, and p27, and positivity for galectin-3, PGP9.5, and p53 overexpression. However, no single marker is considered definitive.
4. *Parafibromin-Deficient Tumors*: often corresponding to APT or PC, these are defined by loss of parafibromin on IHC and may exhibit eosinophilic cytoplasm, sheet-like growth architecture, and prominent vascularization. Their identification is important due to associated genetic predisposition and recurrence risk, but diagnostic accuracy remains limited by IHC variability.
5. *Multiglandular Parathyroid Disease*: previously called "hyperplasia," this entity is now recognized as a clonal, often germline-driven neoplasm involving multiple glands. The WHO endorses classifying such cases—especially in primary hyperparathyroidism—as multiglandular adenomatous disease.
6. *Parathyroid Hyperplasia*: this entity refers to reactive, non-clonal enlargement secondary to chronic stimuli.
7. *Parathyromatosis*: Refers to small, often iatrogenic, parathyroid tissue foci that may mimic malignancy and have a high recurrence rate.

11.4.2 Immunohistochemistry

The 2022 WHO classification highlights immunohistochemistry (IHC) as a pivotal tool in distinguishing parathyroid carcinoma (PC) from benign lesions. Among the most informative markers are parafibromin, Ki-67, and galectin-3 [43, 48, 62, 79, 93, 160].

Parafibromin, encoded by the *CDC73* gene, is of central importance in PC diagnosis. A complete loss of nuclear staining is a strong indicator of malignancy and correlates with underlying *CDC73* mutations. As a result, the WHO recommends routine parafibromin IHC and *CDC73* germline testing in all cases of PC, regardless of familial history [29, 53, 57, 68, 153]. Galectin-3 is frequently overexpressed in PC and may contribute to immune evasion, while Ki-67 levels above 5% indicate increased proliferative activity, though specificity is limited [47, 153].

Additional markers show variable utility: overexpression of PGP9.5 and p53, and loss of APC, p27, and CaSR expression, have been observed in subsets of PC. Increased cytoplasmic expression of filamin A has also been suggested as a potential discriminator from adenoma. While benign lesions typically retain parafibromin, APC, and p27, PCs often exhibit reduced or absent expression of these markers [69, 153]. Given the overlap in individual marker expression, a panel-based approach—integrating IHC with clinical, biochemical, and histopathological data—is essential for accurate diagnosis [29, 53, 57, 68, 69, 153].

11.4.3 Cancer Stem Cells (CSCs)

The integration of cancer stem cells (CSCs) markers into the investigation of PC is an emerging area of translational research with potential implications for diagnosis, prognosis, and therapy. CSCs constitute a subpopulation of tumor cells characterized by self-renewal, multilineage differentiation, and resistance to chemotherapy and radiotherapy. In PC, prominent CSCs markers of tumor aggressiveness, recurrence, or treatment-refractory phenotypes include CD44, CD133, ALDH1, and pluripotency-associated transcription factors such as SOX2, OCT4, and NANOG. While clinical validation remains limited, these findings suggest that CSCs may contribute to tumor persistence and progression, warranting further investigation as both biomarkers and potential therapeutic targets [53].

11.5 The WHO Classification

Currently, no standardized TNM staging system for PC exists. Unlike other endocrine malignancies, a formal TNM classification has not been established, primarily due to the rarity of the disease and the limited availability of robust prognostic data. The American Joint Committee on Cancer (AJCC), in its 2017 edition of the TNM classification manual, explicitly states that it is premature to implement a staging system for PC ([4, 45, 62, 175]; [CSL STYLE ERROR: reference with no printed form]).

Despite the absence of an official system, several efforts have been made to propose TNM-like classifications, based on observed patterns of tumor spread and anatomical involvement (Table 11.2) [62, 130, 133, 148].

Table 11.2 Staging systems for parathyroid carcinoma adapted from AJCC eighth edition (2017) [45] and Schulte studies [133, 148], as proposed by Roser et al. in *Diagnosis and management of parathyroid carcinoma* [130]

	Adapted from and based on the AJCC Version 8, 2017	Schulte classification
T		*Low risk* capsular invasion, invasion of surrounding soft tissue
Tx	No information available	
T1	Localized to the parathyroid gland with limited extension to soft tissue	
T2	Direct invasion into the thyroid gland	
T3	Direct invasion into recurrent laryngeal nerve, esophagus, trachea, skeletal muscle, adjacent lymph nodes, or thymus	
T4	Direct invasion into major blood vessel or spine	*High risk* vascular invasion and/or lymph node metastases and/or invasion of vital organs and/or distant metastases
N		
Nx	Lymph node not assessed	
N0	No regional lymph node metastases	
N1	Regional lymph node metastases	
N1a	… including metastasis to level VI or VII	
N1b	… including levels I, II, III, IV, V, or retropharyngeal nodes	
M		
Mx	Distant metastases not assessed	
M0	No evidence of distant metastasis	
M1	Evidence of distant metastasis	
Stage		
I	T1 or T2 N0 M0	
II	T3 N0 M0	
III	Any T, N1 M0, or T4	
IV	Any N, M1	

11.6 Clinical Presentation

In contrast to parathyroid adenomas, PC is typically characterized by markedly elevated PTH levels, often 5–10 times the upper limit of normal, resulting in severe hypercalcemia with serum calcium concentrations frequently exceeding 14 mg/dL (3.5 mmol/L). This biochemical profile is often accompanied by a more aggressive clinical presentation, including hypercalcemic crisis, oligoanuria, as well as neurological and psychiatric symptoms [21, 53, 156, 160, 169].

Clinical manifestations of PHPT in PC primarily include skeletal complications (e.g., osteoporosis, fractures, and bone and muscle pain in ~46%) and renal involvement (e.g., nephrolithiasis and kidney failure in ~37%). Fatigue and psychiatric problems are not uncommon (~11–12%). Gastrointestinal symptoms, such as nausea, vomiting, polyuria, and pancreatitis, are rather uncommon and correlate with the severity of hypercalcemia [130].

On clinical examination, a palpable neck mass is present in up to 70% of cases, occasionally associated with compressive symptoms or vocal cord paralysis due to recurrent laryngeal nerve involvement [21, 23, 53, 93, 156, 160, 169].

Although most PCs are functional, 5–10% are non-functioning and present later, often due to local invasion. In these cases, tumors are usually solid and adherent, measuring approximately 3 cm at diagnosis, sometimes infiltrating the thyroid, trachea, or strap muscles [54, 163, 166].

Metastases are most commonly involve cervical lymph nodes (15–20%), while distant spread to the lungs, liver, or bone is rare (1%) [21, 23, 53, 93, 156, 160, 169].

Given the overlapping features with benign parathyroid disease, maintaining a high degree of clinical alertness is essential to ensure timely recognition and diagnosis of PC.

11.7 Serum Biomarkers

Multiple lines of evidence highlight the diagnostic relevance of various serum biomarkers in PC.

A recent systematic review by Davies et al. identified five serum biomarkers with potential diagnostic value. Among these, serum calcium and parathyroid hormone (PTH) levels demonstrated the most consistent associations, with diagnostic thresholds defined as serum calcium levels exceeding 14 mg/dL (3.5 mmol/L) and PTH concentrations greater than three times the upper limit of normal (ULN). Additionally, elevated levels of alkaline phosphatase (ALP) and creatinine, along with decreased concentrations of 25-hydroxyvitamin D, were frequently observed. While these markers may reflect disease severity, they are not specific to PC [40, 130, 170].

The role of ALP as a supportive biochemical indicator in the clinical assessment of suspected PC has been validated in a cohort study by Bae et al., which demonstrated that ALP levels exceeding 285 IU/L yield a sensitivity of 83% and a specificity of 97% for PC [14].

In addition, several studies have investigated the diagnostic utility of the third- to second-generation PTH assay ratio. This ratio reflects the overproduction of amino-terminal PTH (amino-PTH), a pattern more commonly observed in PC and rarely seen in benign parathyroid adenomas (BPA). Cavalier et al. proposed a more nuanced approach to PTH assessment, showing that an assay ratio greater than 1.0 offers 82% sensitivity and 97% specificity in distinguishing PC from other forms of PHPT. This biomarker strategy may be particularly valuable in diagnostically challenging cases where absolute PTH levels are inconclusive [27, 130, 142].

In summary, markedly elevated serum calcium and PTH levels, supported by increased ALP and an elevated third–/second-generation PTH ratio, remain key biochemical indicators suggestive of parathyroid carcinoma [130].

11.8 Imaging

In general, imaging for patients with parathyroid carcinoma (PC) should encompass whole-body evaluation (unlike in patients with benign parathyroid adenomas), with particular emphasis on assessing the bones and lungs. As a result, the utility of regional imaging modalities—such as ultrasound, 4D-CT, or MRI—is limited, given their inability to visualize areas beyond the neck or evaluate lung and skeletal involvement.

11.8.1 Ultrasound (US)

Ultrasound (US) is the first-line imaging modality for preoperative examination in PC. Despite being heavily operator-dependent, it is widely used for surgery planning due to its availability, lack of ionizing radiation, and non-invasiveness [34]. According to a meta-analysis by Cheung et al. [33], neck US showed a sensitivity of 76.1% and a positive predictive value (PPV) of 93.2% for localizing hyperfunctioning parathyroid glands in PHPT.

Hyperfunctioning glands typically appear as hypoechoic, lentiform lesions deep to the thyroid, sometimes with cystic changes, echogenic areas, or calcifications [131]. While US is effective in detecting single-gland disease, it cannot reliably distinguish between benign and malignant lesions without evidence of invasion. Important features to assess include shape, calcifications, vascularity, infiltration, and internal texture. Neck US should also check for suspicious lymph nodes in both central and lateral compartments [64, 99, 118, 140]. Elastography may highlight increased stiffness in suspicious lesions, but remains of limited diagnostic utility [157].

To date, the 2017 retrospective study by Christakis et al. remains the only work specifically evaluating the diagnostic accuracy of preoperative imaging modalities in parathyroid carcinoma. In this series, neck ultrasound—performed in 18 of 20 patients—achieved a sensitivity of 80% and an accuracy of 73%, highlighting its usefulness as an accessible first-line tool, though limited by operator dependence and reduced reliability in complex cases [37].

11.8.2 Computed Tomography (CT)

Computed tomography (CT) has traditionally been employed to detect parathyroid adenomas, albeit with limited sensitivity. A late arterial phase, approximately 25 seconds after contrast injection, is considered optimal for lesion detection, whereas non-contrast CT and other contrast phases generally provide little to no additional diagnostic benefit. Parathyroid carcinomas may resemble adenomas but may also appear ill-defined and demonstrate macroscopic infiltration of adjacent structures, such as the thyroid gland and subcutaneous adipose tissue, and are often considerably larger than adenomas. They may also exhibit calcifications inconsistently and can contain necrotic or cystic components, which typically demonstrate reduced contrast enhancement [34, 84, 92, 159]. Whole-body staging in patients with PC is feasible using CT; however, its sensitivity remains limited, especially in the context of suspected disease recurrence indicated by rising PTH levels [51].

Four-dimensional computed tomography (4D-CT) integrates three-dimensional anatomical imaging with dynamic contrast enhancement, enabling detailed multiphase evaluation of parathyroid lesions. The most widely adopted protocol involves three phases: non-contrast, arterial (25–30 seconds post-contrast injection), and venous (60–90 seconds post-injection) acquisitions. Among these, arterial phase imaging is generally the most informative, particularly for the localization of hyperfunctioning parathyroid glands. To adequately assess ectopic locations, at least one imaging series—ideally the arterial phase—should extend from the skull base to the carina [34, 84, 92, 159].

Parathyroid adenomas are reported as hypoattenuating relative to thyroid tissue on non-contrast scans, with strong arterial enhancement and venous washout. However, this classical pattern is seen in only ~20% of cases, and diagnostic performance may be affected by hypothyroidism, cystic changes, or motion artifacts [34, 84, 92, 159]. Moreover, accurate assessment of a lesion and generation of time-enhancement curves following volume of interest (VOI) placement require prior lesion identification—an often circular challenge in clinical practice. Meta-analyses report a per-lesion sensitivity of 75–85% and specificity of 85–93%. 4D-CT is reported to be particularly valuable in reoperative cases, ectopic locations, and multiglandular disease. Limitations of 4D-CT include radiation exposure, variability in protocols, and reduced diagnostic accuracy in patients with thyroid dysfunction, a history of prior neck surgery, contraindication to contrast media, or chronic kidney disease [33, 83, 146].

In clinical practice, however, 4D-CT has limited impact, as it rarely influences decision-making compared to other modalities such as ultrasound or PET imaging, and specific data on its performance in PC are currently lacking. In the previously mentioned retrospective study by Christakis et al. involving 20 patients with PC, 4D-CT was performed in 18 cases and demonstrated a sensitivity of 79% and an accuracy of 82% for preoperative tumor localization; when combined with other modalities, diagnostic accuracy improved significantly, reaching up to 100% [37].

11.8.3 Magnetic Resonance Imaging (MRI)

Magnetic resonance imaging (MRI) is generally regarded as a second- or third-line modality for localizing parathyroid lesions, particularly in persistent or recurrent disease. Its superior soft-tissue contrast can improve diagnostic accuracy, and the absence of ionizing radiation makes it a safer option for patients with impaired renal function. While accessibility and scan duration may limit its use in some countries, MRI remains a valuable tool, especially for complex cases and surgical planning [61, 115, 173].

On conventional MRI, parathyroid adenomas typically appear as well-defined, ovoid, hyperintense lesions on T2-weighted images and enhance during the arterial phase following gadolinium administration. Diffusion-weighted imaging (DWI) aids lesion characterization but cannot reliably differentiate adenomas from lymph nodes. Parathyroid carcinomas, as on CT, may appear similar as adenomas, may show macroscopic infiltration of adjacent tissues such as the thyroid gland and the subcutaneous adipose tissue, and/or may be considerably larger than adenomas [34, 115, 132].

Four-dimensional MRI (4D-MRI), with dynamic contrast-enhanced imaging, has shown diagnostic performance comparable to 4D-CT. Unlike 4D-CT, 4D-MRI can provide continuous dynamic enhancement data. Small studies report sensitivities up to >90% and PPV of 95% for detecting adenomas, particularly with 3T MRI systems and optimized protocols [121], while specific data on PC is missing to date. However, similar to 4D-CT, 4D-MRI depends on prior lesion identification and may not detect atypical enhancement patterns.

4D-MRI has shown particular utility in multiglandular disease (MGD) and ectopic glands, especially in younger patients [111, 117]. MR spectroscopy has demonstrated potential in differentiating metabolic profiles of parathyroid lesions: though data on PC remain unavailable, elevated phosphorylcholine, choline, glycerophosphocholine, fumarate, succinate, lactate, glucose, glutamine, and ascorbate may help distinguish single-gland disease from multigland disease [16].

Despite promising findings, MRI-based techniques are not yet widely adopted in routine practice for parathyroid imaging. A notable exception is MRI with positron emission tomography (PET), particularly using [^{18}F]fluorocholine as radiotracer: although still limited in availability, [^{18}F]fluorocholine PET/MRI has shown high diagnostic accuracy in detecting parathyroid lesions and significantly enhances the clinical utility of MRI in this imaging setting [8, 70, 97, 125, 126, 128].

11.8.4 [^{99m}Tc]Tc-MIBI Scintigraphy

The most widely used imaging technique globally, except ultrasound, for the detection of parathyroid lesions in PHPT is scintigraphy and/or single photon emission computed tomography/computed tomography (SPECT/CT) with [^{99}mTc]Tc-Methoxy-IsoButyl-Isonitrol ([^{99m}Tc]Tc-MIBI) or less commonly with [^{99m}Tc]Tc-1,2-bis[bis(2-ethoxyethyl)phophino]ethane) ([^{99m}Tc]Tc-tetrofosmin) [126].

As lipophilic cations, [^{99m}Tc]Tc-MIBI accumulate in mitochondria-rich oxyphilic cells and chief cells, reflecting perfusion and metabolic activity. Hyperfunctioning parathyroid tissue demonstrates higher uptake and slower wash-out than thyroid tissue. Consequently, areas of increased radiotracer uptake observed on delayed images (60–180 minutes post-injection) indicate parathyroid tissue [3, 18, 52, 88, 110]. Notably, the retention patterns of [^{99m}Tc]Tc-MIBI can serve as an indicator of malignant transformation within parathyroid tissue. Usually, this pattern is evident in delayed imaging; however, in some cases, lesions are visible only in early images due to rapid washout, particularly in parathyroid adenomas or hyperplasia with high mitochondrial activity and fast clearance [122].

Hybrid SPECT/CT improves lesion localization, particularly for ectopic glands and reoperative cases, with a pooled lesion-based detection rate (DR) for parathyroid adenoma of 88% when compared to stand-alone SPECT [152]. However, its sensitivity decreases in small lesions (<1.4 ml), multiglandular hyperplasia (~44%), and double adenomas (30%), and false positives can occur due to thyroid pathology or reactive lymph nodes [10, 66, 90].

In the retrospective study by Christakis et al., [^{99m}Tc]Tc-MIBI SPECT/CT, performed in 9 cases, demonstrated a sensitivity of 81% and an accuracy of 78% for preoperative tumor localization; when combined with CT and/or ultrasound, sensitivity and accuracy increased to 94–100%, highlighting the value of multimodal imaging in these patients [37].

Additionally, intraoperative radioguidance using [^{99m}Tc]Tc-MIBI and a gamma probe, typically 2–3 hours post-injection, enhances surgical precision and complements intraoperative PTH monitoring [26, 31].

11.8.5 [^{18}F]Fluorocholine PET/CT or PET/MRI

While [^{99m}Tc]Tc-MIBI remains the traditional standard in nuclear imaging for primary hyperparathyroidism, emerging evidence supports the superior sensitivity of PET imaging with fluorine-18-fluorocholine ([^{18}F]fluorocholine–[^{18}F]F-FCH) or, in some centers, with carbon-11-choline ([^{11}C]choline–[^{11}C]C-CH) in detecting hyperfunctioning parathyroid glands, especially in cases with small, ectopic, or multiple lesions. The high lesion-to-thyroid contrast improves the detection of smaller lesions. A meta-analysis reported per-patient pooled sensitivity, pooled PPV, and DR of 95%, 97% and 91%, respectively, and per-lesion pooled sensitivity and PPV of 92% [151]. [^{18}F]fluorocholine PET is expected to become a "one-stop-shop" technique in the detection of hyperfunctioning parathyroid glands in the coming years, gradually replacing [^{99m}Tc]Tc-MIBI SPECT/CT in many larger centers. This transition is already underway in several European countries [58, 127].

The mechanisms underlying choline uptake are not fully understood. Choline, a positively charged lipophilic molecule essential for phospholipid synthesis, accumulates in mitochondria and is phosphorylated by choline kinase, an enzyme overexpressed in hyperparathyroidism. This enables its incorporation into cell membranes. The dual uptake mechanism, mitochondrial accumulation, and membrane biosynthesis may offer a significant advantage of choline-PET over SPECT/CT imaging [52]. The mechanisms underlying [^{99m}Tc]Tc-MIBI and [^{18}F]fluorocholine or [^{11}C]choline uptake in hyperfunctioning parathyroid glands are summarized and schematically illustrated in Fig. 11.1.

Histopathological correlations remain under investigation. While some studies link [^{18}F]fluorocholine uptake to lesion size and follicular growth patterns, others emphasize the role of cellular composition, particularly the number of chief cells [11, 97]. Discrepancies likely arise from methodological variability in histological quantification. Additionally, focal thyroidal uptake of [^{18}F]fluorocholine may indicate differentiated thyroid carcinoma (DTC), which should be considered in the differential diagnosis. Uptake in inflammatory lymph nodes has also been observed, though its clinical significance remains unclear [34, 92, 115, 162].

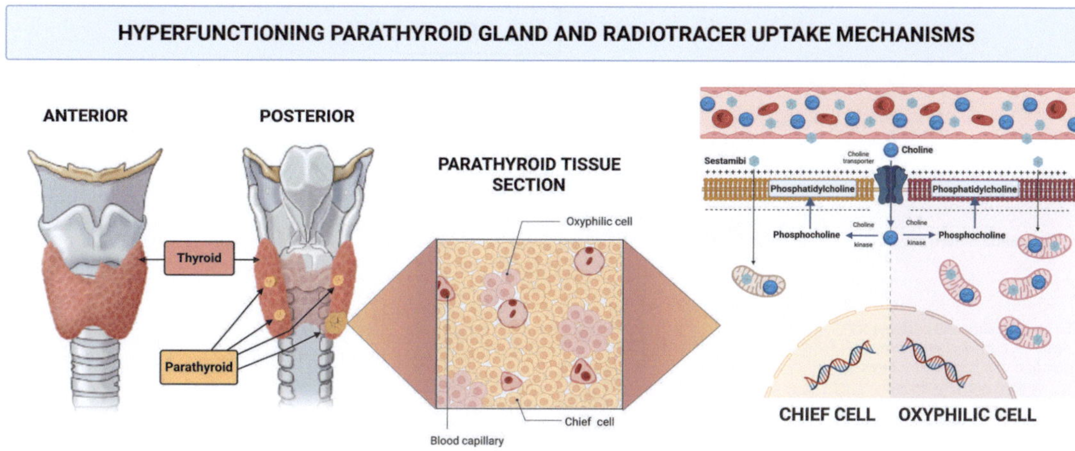

Fig. 11.1 Schematic representation of the cellular uptake mechanisms of [^{99m}Tc]Tc-MIBI and [^{18}F]fluorocholine in hyperfunctioning parathyroid tissue. Both radiotracers accumulate in metabolically active cells, with [^{99m}Tc] Tc-MIBI concentrating in mitochondria-rich cells via passive diffusion and electrochemical gradients, and [^{18}F]fluorocholine undergoing active transport and phosphorylation for incorporation into phospholipid membranes

Given the extensive data supporting [^{18}F] fluorocholine-PET in parathyroid adenomas, its application in parathyroid carcinoma appears promising; however, current evidence is limited to isolated case reports, and robust data on diagnostic accuracy in this specific context are still lacking [56, 67, 72, 114, 145].

11.8.6 [^{18}F]F-FDG PET/CT

2-deoxy-2-[^{18}F]fluoro-D-glucose (2-[^{18}F]FDG) is a radioactive glucose analogue used to image lesions with increased metabolic activity. After cellular uptake via glucose transporters (primarily GLUT-1 and GLUT-3), [^{18}F]FDG is phosphorylated but not further metabolized, leading to intracellular trapping. In cancer cells, glucose metabolism is often dominated by inefficient aerobic glycolysis rather than oxidative phosphorylation, resulting in the upregulation of glycolytic pathways—a phenomenon known as the Warburg effect [19].

Although widely available, [^{18}F]FDG PET/CT is not recommended for routine imaging in PHPT due to considerably lower sensitivity compared to other modalities. However, [^{18}F]FDG PET/TC is particularly useful for assessing regional or distant metastases in poorly differentiated parathyroid carcinomas, which show high glucose metabolism, a hallmark of malignant transformation [34, 92, 115, 125, 162].

11.9 Treatment

The treatment of parathyroid carcinoma is a complex process influenced by multiple factors and requires a multidisciplinary team, ideally within a specialized tumor board setting. Figure 11.2 summarizes this approach by using a management algorithm adapted from the 2024 ESMO Clinical Practice Guideline [62].

11.9.1 Medical Treatment of Hypercalcemia

Correcting hypercalcemia and associated metabolic disturbances is an immediate priority prior to surgery and remains a long-term goal for patients with incurable parathyroid carcinoma. First-line therapy often consists of intravenous fluids, loop diuretics, and bisphosphonates to effectively lower serum calcium levels [103, 106, 130].

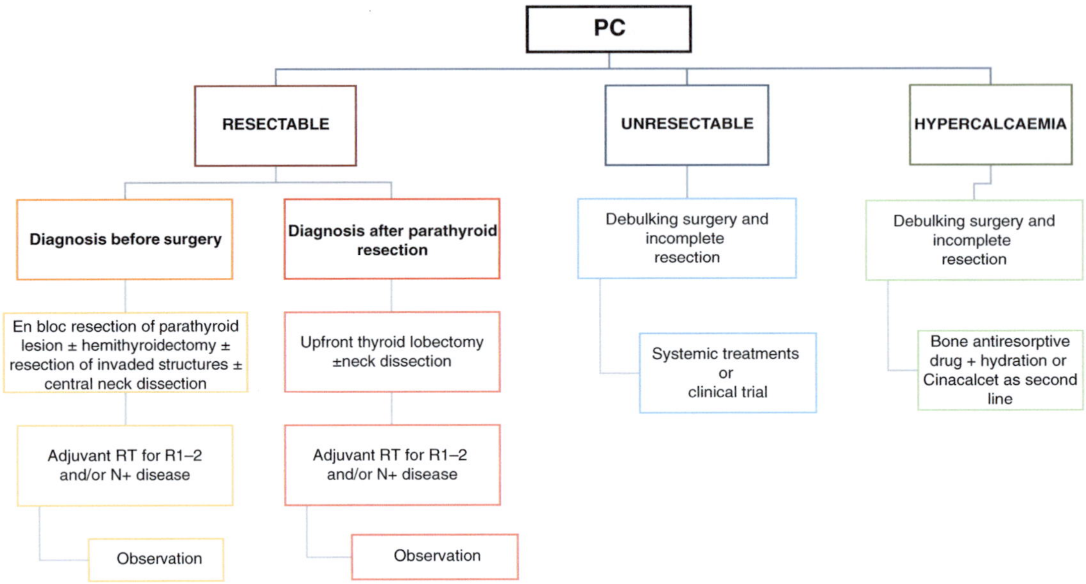

Fig. 11.2 Management algorithm of PC adapted from the 2024 ESMO Clinical Practice Guideline [62]

If first-line therapy proves ineffective, second-line treatment with calcimimetic drugs, such as cinacalcet, is recommended. Cinacalcet has demonstrated efficacy in managing PC-induced hypercalcemia by suppressing parathyroid hormone (PTH) release [103, 106, 130]. The typical starting dose is 30 mg twice daily, which may be titrated up to 90 mg four times daily based on clinical response. Notably, more advanced tumors may show reduced expression of CASR, potentially limiting the effectiveness of this treatment [147].

11.9.2 Surgery

Surgical resection remains the gold standard and the only curative treatment for PC. To achieve optimal outcomes, surgery should be performed in specialized, high-volume centers with expertise in managing this rare malignancy [103, 106, 130].

The preferred surgical approach is en bloc (radical) resection, which involves removal of the primary tumor along with the ipsilateral thyroid lobe, thyroid isthmus, central neck lymph nodes, and any involved prethyroidal musculature [124, 137]. Central neck lymph node metastases are observed in approximately 10% of patients, whereas involvement of the lateral compartment is uncommon [134]. Emerging intraoperative diagnostic tools, such as immune colloidal gold techniques (ICGT), have shown potential in improving surgical accuracy. ICGT allows real-time identification of malignant parathyroid tissue, particularly in cases with unclear tumor boundaries or large, invasive lesions. This technique may reduce the reliance on frozen section analysis and assist surgeons in making more informed intraoperative decisions [171].

Radical resection reduces the risk of capsular rupture and provides a clear margin of uninvolved tissue, thereby improving disease-free survival compared to limited excision, which has been linked to poorer oncological outcomes [103, 130]. While some authors suggest that radical surgery may not be necessary after an incidental diagnosis of PC following minimally invasive parathyroidectomy (MIP), current data are limited, and long-term outcomes remain uncertain [63, 82, 104, 120]. A large retrospective register study by Leonard-Murali et al., which included 555 patients, found no significant difference in overall survival between local excision and radical surgery. However, the study's limitations—such as the lack of progression-free and disease-specific survival data, along with inadequate detail regarding surgical techniques—limit the strength of its conclusions [95].

Reoperation may be warranted if calcium and iPTH levels remain elevated after initial surgery and there is no evidence of distant metastases. However, it requires meticulous planning due to the heightened risk of complications. Postoperative care should involve close monitoring and correction of eventual hypocalcemia, long-term surveillance of biochemical markers (PTH and calcium levels), and evaluation of quality of life (QoL), which has been shown to improve markedly following parathyroidectomy [74, 91, 160].

In PC, distant metastases occur synchronously in approximately 5% of cases and metachronously in up to 50% of cases. The lungs, bones, liver, and distant lymph nodes are the most commonly affected sites. For patients with localized or oligometastatic disease, repeated surgical resection of metastases—when technically feasible—remains the preferred strategy. Given the typically slow progression of PC, this approach can improve biochemical control and potentially extend survival, especially when treatment decisions are guided by an experienced multidisciplinary tumor board [23, 160, 171].

11.9.3 Radiotherapy

Locoregional radiotherapy (RT) has limited efficacy in PC, which is generally considered a radioresistant tumor. Its role remains controversial, primarily due to the lack of randomized controlled trials [23, 103, 106, 160]. Nonetheless, small retrospective studies have suggested that adjuvant RT may help reduce locoregional recurrence in selected high-risk patients, particularly those with positive surgical margins (R1/R2 resections), nodal metastases, or persistent hypercalcemia [20, 36, 49, 87, 116, 136]. Current evidence does not support the use of RT for metastatic PC, and large registry-based analyses have not demonstrated a survival benefit [13, 98]. Additionally, RT carries risks, such as fibrosis, which may complicate future surgical interventions. Therefore, the decision to use adjuvant RT should be individualized and made within the context of a multidisciplinary tumor board [62].

11.9.4 Chemotherapy

Chemotherapy has historically shown minimal to no efficacy in PC, whether in localized or metastatic disease. A recent literature review encompassing systemic treatments in 79 patients with metastatic PC between 1951 and 2020 reaffirmed the consistently poor response rates to chemotherapy [7]. While isolated case reports have suggested that temozolomide may lead to transient disease stabilization—particularly in patients exhibiting MGMT promoter methylation—these findings remain anecdotal and lack robust clinical validation [160]. Various cytotoxic regimens, including dacarbazine (alone or in combination with 5-FU), cyclophosphamide monotherapy, and multi-agent protocols involving methotrexate, doxorubicin, or lomustine, have been explored with uniformly disappointing outcomes [7, 62]. As such, chemotherapy should be considered only in highly selected cases within a multidisciplinary framework.

11.9.5 Targeted Therapy

Targeted therapies, including tyrosine kinase inhibitors (TKIs) directed at VEGFR and inhibitors of the mTOR pathway, such as everolimus, are emerging as promising treatment options for advanced PC, particularly in cases harboring specific molecular alterations [7, 23, 130, 160]. TKIs such as sunitinib, sorafenib, cabozantinib, lenvatinib, and surufatinib have shown variable success in controlling tumor progression and associated hypercalcemia in patients with VEGFR, FGFR, or related mutations. However, current evidence is largely limited to case reports and small series, with no prospective clinical trials available to validate these findings [49, 50]. Everolimus, an mTOR inhibitor, has shown biochemical and radiologic disease stabilization in selected patients with alterations in the PI3K/AKT/mTOR pathway—mutations seen in up to 20% of PC cases. These preliminary observations underscore the potential of precision oncology in the management of refractory PC, although further research is needed to better define indications, efficacy, and long-term outcomes [48, 50].

11.9.6 Immunotherapy

Immunotherapy remains an investigational but promising strategy for treating PC, especially in metastatic cases with high tumor mutational burden (TMB). Although data are sparse, two published case reports involving pembrolizumab, an immune checkpoint inhibitor (ICI), demonstrated biochemical improvement and disease stabilization, even in the absence of PD-L1 expression [44, 123]. However, one of these cases was complicated by treatment-related immune toxicity (severe colitis), resulting in early therapy discontinuation. Retrospective data suggest that PD-L1 expression is present in only about 22% of PC cases, while high TMB is observed in approximately 18% [42, 80]. These findings underscore the importance of biomarker-based patient selection. Further prospective studies are necessary to clarify the efficacy, safety, and ideal timing of ICIs in PC, as well as to explore potential benefits of combination regimens that might enhance antitumor immune responses.

11.10 Clinical Approach

11.10.1 Local Assessment and Differential Diagnosis

The definitive diagnosis of PC remains particularly challenging due to its extreme rarity, limited representation in the literature, and substantial clinical and morphological overlap with BPA. Both entities can present with PHPT and hypercalcemia, making differentiation difficult in routine clinical practice. Although a comprehensive, multidisciplinary assessment—including epidemiological context, clinical features, histopathological and immunohistochemical analysis, and biochemical markers—can provide valuable diagnostic clues, no single parameter is pathognomonic for PC. As illustrated in Fig. 11.3, these diagnostic features often intersect across BPA, APT, and PC, blurring the lines between benign, borderline, and malignant disease. This frequent overlap significantly complicates the diagnostic process and underscores the need for expert path-

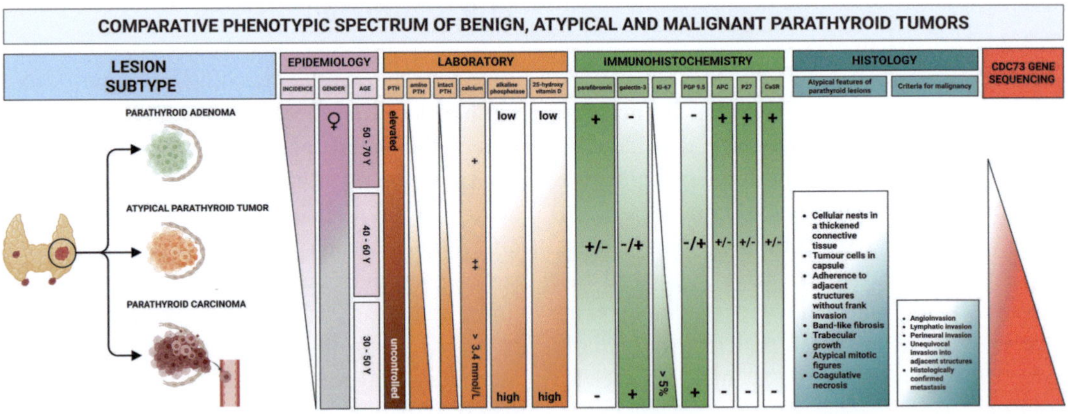

Fig. 11.3 Summary of epidemiological, clinical, histopathological, immunohistochemical, and biochemical key features used to differentiate benign parathyroid adenoma (BPA), atypical parathyroid tumor (APT), and parathyroid carcinoma (PC). Although these parameters may assist in diagnosis, none are pathognomonic, and significant overlap may occur among these three entities [43, 48, 62, 79, 93, 160]

ological review, and potentially molecular profiling to improve diagnostic confidence [43, 48, 62, 79, 93, 160].

As previously highlighted, FNA is generally contraindicated due to its limited diagnostic utility and the potential risk of tumor seeding [1, 9, 86, 119]. Accurate preoperative imaging is crucial for the optimal management of patients with suspected or confirmed PC. When combined with clinical suspicion, precise localization and characterization of parathyroid lesions facilitate appropriate surgical planning. In contrast to BPA, which typically requires limited local excision, PC requires an oncologic en-bloc resection with curative intent. This approach is currently considered the gold standard, as it is associated with improved local disease control and superior long-term outcomes.

At this stage, the principal objectives of imaging are twofold: first, to localize the parathyroid lesion with high precision; and second, to support differentiation between malignant and benign pathology. When specific clinical features are present, such as a palpable cervical mass, severe hypercalcemia (serum calcium >14 mg/dL or 3.5 mmol/L), hypercalcemic crisis, markedly elevated plasma PTH levels (>10 times the upper limit of normal), or vocal cord paralysis due to laryngeal nerve involvement, imaging assessment should prioritize the identification of radiological features suggestive of PC [130].

Ultrasound (US) is widely regarded as the first-line imaging modality for evaluating parathyroid lesions, due to its broad availability, real-time capabilities, and excellent spatial resolution [165].

Harari et al. reported 71.4% sensitivity and 100% specificity for US in localizing parathyroid carcinoma, based on data from a highly experienced national referral center (the University of California, San Francisco), which managed 37 PC cases during a 43-year period. However, the reported specificity refers to the accuracy in lesion localization, not in distinguishing between benign and malignant parathyroid lesions. In fact, none of the imaging modalities used in their series, including ultrasound, were able to suggest malignancy preoperatively [65]. In fact, differentiating benign adenomas from malignant lesions remains a diagnostic challenge with US, owing to substantial overlap in clinical and imaging features.

Several B-mode ultrasound features have been associated with malignancy: a hypoechoic, heterogeneous lesion exceeding 15 mm in size, irregular or lobulated lesion margins, capsular disruption, a depth-to-width ratio ≥ 1:1, presence of coarse calcifications, and evidence of infiltration into adjacent soft tissues [28].

Tumor size has traditionally been considered a key discriminative parameter, with a threshold of ≥30 mm demonstrating strong predictive value for malignancy (sensitivity 91%, specificity 92%), according to Bae et al. [14]. However, data from a large national US database involving 520 patients showed that approximately one-third of PCs (33.8%) were smaller than 30 mm [102], suggesting that size alone is insufficient for reliable diagnosis. Furthermore, Calapkulu et al. proposed that tumor volume may serve as a more sensitive and specific metric than maximal diameter in differentiating PC from BPA [22].

Sidhu et al. demonstrated that infiltration and calcification were highly specific indicators of PC, each showing a 100% positive predictive value (PPV). Conversely, features such as absence of suspicious vascularity (NPV 97.6%), absence of a thick capsule (NPV 96.7%), and lesion homogeneity (NPV 100%) were associated with high negative predictive values, effectively excluding malignancy [140]. Supporting these findings, Hara et al. reported that malignant lesions tend to be large, hypoechoic, and inhomogeneous with irregular margins, whereas benign adenomas usually present as small, homogeneous, hypoechoic nodules with smooth, well-defined borders [64].

The advent of advanced ultrasonography systems has further improved diagnostic accuracy. High-resolution B-mode imaging, in combination with modern vascular mapping technologies—notably detective flow imaging (DFI)—enables the visualization of low-velocity blood flow and microvascular networks, which are often undetectable using conventional Doppler techniques. These innovations allow for more detailed evaluation of capsular integrity, intralesional vascularity, and local tissue invasion. Nevertheless, ultrasonography remains an operator-dependent modality, and accurate interpretation in parathyroid disease requires specialized training and experience [2, 109].

Parathyroid carcinomas typically present with a high short-to-long axis ratio, irregular shape, peritumoral infiltration, calcifications, and limited contrast enhancement [15, 37, 78, 115, 130, 146, 159]. 4D-CT offers dynamic contrast-enhanced multiphasic imaging of a limited region of interest that captures arterial enhancement and venous washout, along with structural characteristics from plain CT. Notably, PCs were reported to demonstrate slower washout than benign adenomas, with mean reductions of approximately 9% in the early delayed phase, and 17% in the late delayed phase compared to arterial peak enhancement. Although significant contrast uptake is observed across all imaging phases, no significant difference was found between arterial, early delayed, and late delayed phases. These distinctive enhancement kinetics may aid in differentiating PC from other parathyroid and thyroid pathologies [37]. However, the available evidence is limited, based on only a few studies with small patient cohorts.

Previous research has demonstrated high diagnostic accuracy of 4D-CT in identifying parathyroid lesions, with lateralization accuracy ranging from 84% to 94% and quadrant-level accuracy from 87% to 88% in non-operated patients [78, 84, 124]. Although the overall diagnostic accuracy is slightly lower for parathyroid carcinoma (approximately 82%), it remains uncertain whether 4D-CT will establish itself as a consistently valuable component of a multimodal imaging approach in this context; therefore, it should not be used in isolation [30, 37].

While 4D-CT provides important information for lesion characterization, especially in anatomically complex cases, its role in the broader staging process of PC appears more limited. Cross-sectional imaging, particularly contrast-enhanced CT, remains a valuable tool in the assessment of suspected malignancy, surgical planning, and in cases of recurrent disease or distant metastases. For whole-body evaluation, standard contrast-enhanced CT is often sufficient (see below). However, nuclear medicine techniques may offer additional value in detecting distant metastatic spread, particularly to the bones, suggesting that CT alone is probably insufficient in the comprehensive staging strategy for parathyroid carcinoma. The primary utility of CT, therefore, lies in its capacity to define local disease extent and guide surgical management, particularly in cases involving retrosternal extension, lymphadenopathy, or suspected local invasion, where accurate anatomical localization is essential [30, 37]. For the detection and localization of tumor recurrence in cases with increasing PTH levels, CT should be combined with nuclear medicine techniques or be replaced by [^{18}F]fluorocholine PET/CT or PET/MR (see below).

Radionuclide imaging with [^{99m}Tc]Tc-MIBI scintigraphy serves as a well-established and valuable complement to anatomical studies. PCs typically show increased and prolonged tracer retention compared to benign lesions. Zhang et al. reported that both mean and peak retention indices were significantly higher in malignant parathyroid tissue [172]. However, caution is warranted, as small PC lesions may exhibit retention indices that overlap with those of benign adenomas. As a result, [^{99m}Tc]Tc-MIBI scintigraphy may be less sensitive in detecting early-stage or small-volume malignancies [6, 26, 37, 115, 125, 160]. Notably, unlike ultrasound, both 4D-CT and [^{99m}Tc]Tc-MIBI scintigraphy are not confined to the cervical region and can detect metastatic lesions, including pulmonary metastases, due to routine imaging of the mediastinum to evaluate for ectopic mediastinal parathyroid tissue [174].

As previously emphasized by Lo et al. [102], the study of Christakis et al. [37] demonstrated that combining CT and [^{99m}Tc]Tc-MIBI yields a diagnostic accuracy of 95% for PC, while the combination of US and CT offers an accuracy of 88%. Notably, when all three modalities—US, [^{99m}Tc]Tc-MIBI, and 4D-CT—are used together, localization sensitivity can reach 100%, significantly outperforming any single imaging technique.

Although atypical parathyroid neoplasms (APN) are histologically distinct from PC, they may exhibit aggressive behavior in rare instances. While APNs generally follow a benign course—with 5-year disease-free survival rates approaching 90.9% compared to 59.6% for PC—features such as soft tissue invasion on initial pathology warrant prolonged surveillance. Given the diagnostic and therapeutic challenges associated with PC, a multimodal imaging strategy remains critical for accurate lesion characterization, optimal surgical planning, and long-term oncologic monitoring [35, 143]. Key imaging features differentiating BPA from PC across these modalities are summarized in Table 11.3.

11.10.2 Staging

Patients presenting with severe clinical symptoms, a personal or family history of HPT-JT syndrome, or suspicious lesions on ultrasound should undergo a thorough diagnostic assessment. This should include screening for common systemic

Table 11.3 Comparative imaging characteristics of benign parathyroid adenoma (BPA) and parathyroid carcinoma (PC)

Modality	Features	Benign parathyroid adenoma	Parathyroid carcinoma
Ultrasound (US)	Size	Typically <30 mm	Often >30 mm (but may be <30 mm)
	Echogenicity	Hypoechoic, homogeneous, well circumscribed	Hypoechoic, heterogeneous
	Margins/capsule	Smooth margins, intact capsule	Irregular/lobulated margins, thick capsule, capsular invasion
	Calcifications	Rare	Intralesional coarse calcifications (15–100%)
	Vascular pattern (color Doppler)	Single polar vessel	Abnormal/disordered vascularity, decreased polar vessels
	CEUS (contrast-enhanced US)	Early peripheral enhancement with central wash-out in later phases	Early heterogeneous enhancement; delayed homogeneous wash-out
	Elastography (USE)	Stiffer than normal parathyroid glands and hyperplastic glands	Stiffer than normal, hyperplastic, and adenomatous glands
4D-CT	Hounsfield units (HU)	Typically high in arterial phase, decreasing in delayed phases	Contrast-enhanced phases show higher HU than non-contrast; no significant variation among post-contrast phases
	Contrast enhancement	Intense arterial enhancement, significant decrease in delayed phases	Significant enhancement vs. baseline (non-contrast), but minimal differences between phases
	Contrast wash-out	Rapid washout after arterial peak	Slow or minimal washout (slower compared to BPA and thyroid tissue)
	Structural features	Well-defined margins No invasive signs Usually homogeneous or mildly heterogeneous	Irregular shape High short-to-long axis ratio Capsular disruption Peritumoral infiltration, calcifications
[^{99m}Tc]Tc-MIBI scintigraphy	Radiotracer uptake	Variable uptake (low to high) Positively correlated with lesion volume and PTH levels Depends on cellular composition of adenomas May mimic PC	High uptake and retention Uptake range may overlap with adenomas
[^{18}F]fluorocholine PET/CT or PET/MRI	Radiotracer uptake		High uptake Uptake range may overlap with adenomas Useful for detecting local and distant metastases

complications, particularly those affecting the bones and kidneys. The prognosis of PC remains variable, with reported overall survival rates of approximately 80% at 5 years and between 40% and 80% at 10 years following surgery. Early diagnosis and complete surgical excision during initial treatment are associated with more favorable outcomes, whereas advanced patient age and lymph node metastases have been identified as adverse prognostic factors [62, 65, 71]. Although not yet externally validated, the logarithmic formula proposed by Karakas et al. may offer a useful tool for the preoperative assessment of parathyroid carcinoma. By incorporating preoperative serum calcium levels, parathyroid hormone concentrations, and patient age, the model provides an individualized risk of PC and demonstrates a sensitivity of 100% and specificity of 30% in a cohort of patients with primary hyperparathyroidism [81].

Further diagnostic evaluation should include second- or third-generation parathyroid hormone assay ratios (comparing amino-terminal and intact PTH). This work-up traditionally includes conventional imaging, such as CT of the neck, chest, and abdomen and [^{99m}Tc]Tc-MIBI scintigraphy. Since 4D-CT is limited to a small anatomical area, it is not useful for staging. Total-body [^{99m}Tc]Tc-MIBI imaging can reveal unexpected lesions outside the neck region and support the accurate staging process [167, 174]. More recently, [^{18}F]fluorocholine PET combined with CT or MRI (PET/CT, PET/MRI) has emerged as a valuable tool with high sensitivity for PC [125]. Choline-based radiotracers demonstrate intense uptake in malignant parathyroid tissue, enabling the detection of both locoregional disease and distant metastases, as shown in Figs. 11.4 and 11.5 [41, 56, 114, 145].

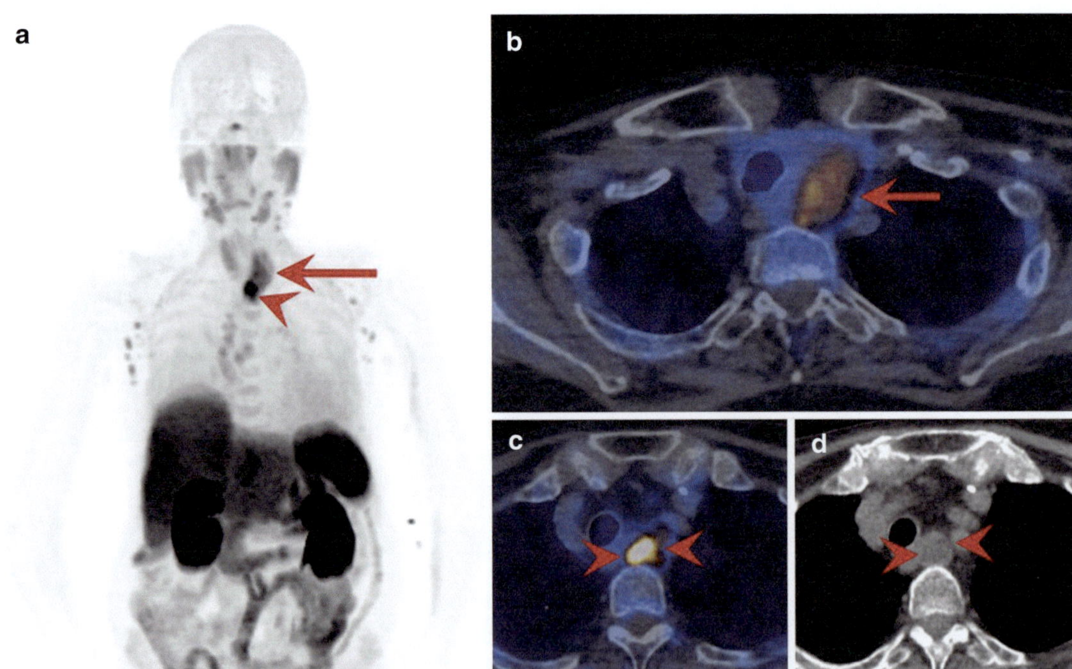

Fig. 11.4 A 91-year-old woman with parathyroid carcinoma, a serum PTH level of 665 pg/ml, and an albumin-corrected serum calcium level of 4.1 mmol/L (16.4 mg/dL). The patient presented with a hypercalcemic crisis. The coronal [^{18}F]fluorocholine PET maximum intensity projection (MIP) image (**a**) shows a moderately [^{18}F]fluorocholine-avid tumor (maximum standard uptake value (SUV_{max}) 10.1; arrow) adjacent to the left lobe of the thyroid gland. The axial PET/CT image (**b**) shows that the mass (arrow) is infiltrating the left lobe of the thyroid gland. Below the tumor, the MIP image (**a**), axial PET/CT image (**c**), and axial CT image (**d**) show intensely [^{18}F]fluorocholine-avid paratracheal lymph node metastases (arrowheads) in the upper mediastinum

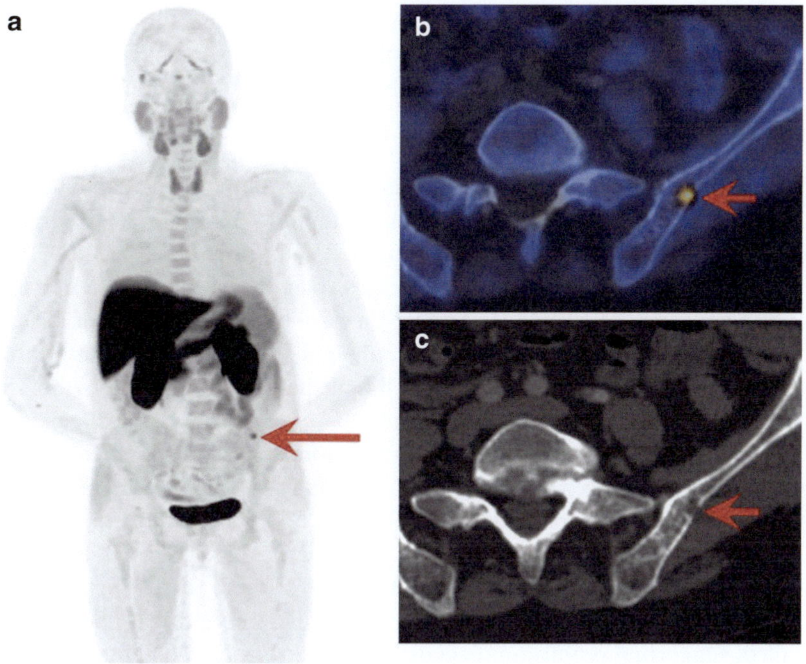

Fig. 11.5 A 61-year-old woman with parathyroid carcinoma, resected years ago, and currently increasing serum PTH level (253 pg/ml). The coronal [^{18}F] fluorocholine PET MIP image (**a**) shows a moderately [^{18}F] fluorocholine-avid focus (SUV_{max} 8.8; arrow) in the left pelvic area (SUV_{max} 8.8), which localizes to a lysis in the left-sided iliac bone on axial PET/CT (**b**; arrow) and CT image (**c**; arrow). PTH level dropped after local ablative stereotactic radiotherapy

Unlike conventional parathyroid imaging for BPA, which is typically restricted to the neck and upper mediastinum, whole-body imaging is essential in suspected PC to assess for metastatic dissemination. PET/MRI provides additional benefit by offering superior soft-tissue resolution in the neck as well as for detecting bone, while it may also be used to detect lung metastases. In PET/MRI protocols, MRI sequences should be specifically tailored to enhance sensitivity for detecting local recurrence as well as skeletal and pulmonary lesions, which are among the most common metastatic sites in PC [46, 56, 113, 125]. [^{18}F]FDG PET/CT may serve as a complementary imaging modality, particularly useful for identifying aggressive, poorly differentiated tumors with elevated glucose metabolism. It can aid conventional imaging during initial staging and in the evaluation of persistent or recurrent disease, although supporting clinical evidence remains limited [12, 51, 55, 96, 139, 158]. Importantly, [^{18}F]FDG PET/CT may also incidentally detect brown tumors—osteolytic bone lesions associated with severe hyperparathyroidism—which can mimic skeletal metastases due to their similar FDG uptake patterns as well as lesion morphology. In such cases, MRI is valuable for more accurate characterization of these lesions [85, 105, 155]. A dual-tracer PET approach, combining [^{18}F]FDG PET with [^{18}F]fluorocholine PET, may improve diagnostic sensitivity by capturing parathyroid tumors with heterogeneous metabolic profiles—those exhibiting both high glycolytic activity and increased phospholipid membrane turnover [67, 72].

If both PTH assay results and imaging findings are negative, a diagnosis of benign primary hyperparathyroidism should be considered, and active surveillance is recommended. Conversely, if either assessment yields positive findings, an oncologic en bloc resection with curative intent is recommended [62]. Following a confirmed diagnosis of PC, surgical specimens should undergo genetic and immunohistochemical analysis. Genetic testing should primarily assess for CDC73 mutations, which are key drivers in PC pathogenesis. Immunohistochemical evaluation should include assessing parafibromin expression, the Ki-67 proliferation index, and galectin-3 staining to support diagnostic confirmation and risk stratification [24, 130, 160].

Local and regional therapies, including surgical debulking in not curatively resectable tumors, should be considered to reduce tumor burden and control PTH secretion, as complete remission is rare in the setting of distant metastases. In patients with persistent hypercalcemia, cinacalcet should be continued. Evidence on systemic treatment for metastatic PC remains limited and is primarily derived from 79 reported cases spanning from 1898 to 2018 [7]. Among these, the most frequently administered systemic therapies include dacarbazine- or anthracycline-based chemotherapy and anti-angiogenic agents [62].

Notably, only a few case reports have explored alternative radiotracers for PC. One case study demonstrated the potential of [^{18}F]-FAPI (fluorodeoxyglucose-labeled Fibroblast Activation Protein Inhibitor) PET/CT to detect PC metastases when conventional radiotracers failed, suggesting promising diagnostic and therapeutic implications for fibroblast activation protein-targeted imaging [32]. Another study by Storvall et al. evaluated somatostatin receptor (SSTR) expression in PC, typical adenomas, and atypical adenomas, revealing that all of these tumor types expressed SSTRs, albeit with low membrane localization. While SSTR 1 expression was comparable across groups, SSTRs 2–5 displayed distinct patterns, with PC exhibiting the highest overall expression. Notably, cytoplasmic SSTR 5 was significantly more pronounced in carcinomas than in adenomas, indicating its potential as a malignancy marker. These findings support further investigation of SSTR-targeted imaging and therapies—such as peptide receptor radionuclide therapy (PRRT)—in the management of PC [144].

11.10.3 Restaging and Follow-Up

The risk of recurrence in PC is estimated at approximately 50% within 2 to 5 years, particularly in cases where initial surgery was non-radical. Lifelong biochemical monitoring is essential and should include serum calcium and PTH levels. Current guidelines recommend testing every 3–4 months during the first 2 years, every 6 months for the subsequent 3 years, and annually thereafter. This long-term surveillance strategy is intended to detect both early and late recurrences, the majority of which occur within the first 2–3 years post-operatively. However, late recurrences—up to 20 years after surgery—have also been documented [7, 13, 60, 95, 156].

An increase in PTH and serum calcium levels is indicative of disease recurrence and should prompt comprehensive cross-sectional imaging. At a minimum, this should include neck US and CT of the neck, chest, and abdomen. If negative, MRI of the neck might be added. Although published data remain limited—likely due to the rarity of the disease—[^{18}F]fluorocholine PET/CT or PET/MRI appears to be the most effective modality for detecting recurrent sources of abnormal PTH secretion. As whole-body imaging techniques, they are increasingly used as first-line investigations, potentially replacing other cross-sectional modalities and even ultrasound in this setting. Optimized pre-therapeutic imaging remains crucial in the context of persistent or recurrent PC following initial surgery. Precise localization of the recurrence enables a targeted and oncologically sound reoperation or radiotherapy, potentially increasing the likelihood of complete recurrence treatment while minimizing post-treatment morbidity and potentially also optimizing long-term recurrence-free survival [39, 154]. Since treatment of initial recurrences typically involves local ablative approaches—such as surgery and/or radiotherapy—targeting each recurrent or metastatic lesion individually, accurate detection of all lesions is essential. However, this is rarely achieved with CT or MRI alone, due to their relatively low sensitivity for detecting small-volume disease in this setting and their susceptibility to the well-known "red herring" effect, which may mislead clinical interpretation.

Particularly in rapidly progressive cases, scintigraphic techniques such as [^{18}F]fluorocholine PET/CT or PET/MRI as well as traditional [^{99m}Tc]Tc-MIBI scintigraphy—if [^{18}F]fluorocholine is unavailable—are useful to localize recurrent disease [62].

Liu et al. [100] evaluated the sonographic findings of locoregional recurrences of PC and identified hypoechoic solid nodules in 28 relapses (96.6%), inhomogeneous echotexture in 28 relapses (96.6%), and intralesional echogenic septa-like structures in 21 relapses (72.4%). Additional findings included irregular shape in 22 relapses (75.9%), marked vascularization on color Doppler imaging in 19 relapses (65.5%), and multiple lesions in 26 relapses (89.7%). Notably, none of the recurrent lesions exhibited calcification. The cumulative size of recurrent lesions at each relapse showed a mild correlation with serum intact parathyroid hormone levels ($r = 0.450$; $P = 0.014$) [101]. However, the diagnostic evaluation in this clinical context presents substantial challenges. Many patients with recurrent PC have a history of prior neck surgery, which often results in distorted anatomy, fibrotic changes, and altered or obliterated tissue planes. These factors can significantly impair the accuracy of all cross-sectional imaging techniques. Such limitations likely contribute to the reduced diagnostic sensitivity of these modalities for recurrent disease compared to their performance in localizing primary parathyroid tumors [46, 149, 164].

A study by Clark et al. reported a diagnostic accuracy of 67% (10/15 lesions) for [^{99m}Tc]Tc-MIBI scintigraphy in detecting recurrent PC, compared to 53% (9/17) for CT [38]. [^{99m}Tc]Tc-MIBI scintigraphy as well as CT can detect parathyroid carcinoma metastases within and beyond the neck. However, an advantage of [^{99m}Tc]Tc-MIBI scintigraphy over CT lies in its ability to highlight ectopic or atypically located lesions based on functional uptake, which can be particularly valuable in cases where anatomical imaging yields inconclusive results. However, some tumors may undergo dedifferentiation over time, leading to decreased uptake on [^{99m}Tc]Tc-MIBI scintigraphy and [^{18}F]fluorocholine PET. In such cases, [^{18}F]FDG PET can serve as a valuable adjunct, particularly for identifying metabolically active lesions that are not visible by the aforementioned imaging techniques [6, 129, 135].

11.10.4 Non-functional Parathyroid Carcinoma (NFPC)

Non-functional parathyroid carcinoma (NFPC) is an exceptionally rare endocrine malignancy (<10% of all PC), defined by the absence of hyperparathyroidism and normal serum parathyroid hormone (PTH) levels. Fewer than 40 well-documented cases have been reported in the literature [163]. In the absence of biochemical markers, NFPC is typically diagnosed at a more advanced stage, often presenting as a neck or mediastinal mass detected on imaging. Tumor size frequently ranges between 5 and 11 cm, and patients may exhibit symptoms related to local invasion, such as neck swelling, hoarseness, and dysphagia [71, 138]. The non-secretory nature of these tumors may result from impaired hormone synthesis, production of an inactive PTH variant, or defective secretion [166].

The lack of PTH-driven clinical signs delays detection and complicates postoperative monitoring. Imaging modalities including ultrasound (US), computed tomography (CT), and magnetic resonance imaging (MRI) are used for localization, but definitive diagnosis relies on histopathological evidence of capsular or vascular invasion. En bloc surgical resection remains the cornerstone of management [163, 166]. Prognosis is generally worse than for functional parathyroid carcinoma, owing to late diagnosis, high rates of recurrence—particularly in the lungs, bone, and lymph nodes—and the absence of reliable biochemical follow-up markers. In cases with dedifferentiated or non-secretory tumors, both [^{18}F]FDG and [^{18}F]fluorocholine PET/CT or PET/MRI may aid in surveillance by detecting metabolically active disease and can serve as a surrogate indicator of tumor burden and progression when PTH is not informative [51, 59, 76, 130, 160, 163, 166].

11.11 Overall Survival and Prognosis

Overall survival (OS) in PC is highly variable. Data from US cancer registries (SEER and NCDB) indicate 5-year and 10-year OS rates of approximately 83% and 57–66%, respectively. Meta-analyses report a broader 5-year OS range of 60–93%, reflecting heterogeneity in patient populations and treatment strategies [7, 13, 60, 95, 156]. Several clinical and pathological features have been associated with poor prognosis, including tumor size greater than 3–4 cm, lymph node involvement (N1), distant metastases (M1), capsular rupture, vascular invasion, markedly elevated serum calcium levels (>15 mg/dL or 3.74 mmol/L), high PTH levels (>700 pg/mL), poorly differentiated histology, and somatic CDC73 mutations or loss of parafibromin expression. Additionally, a Ki-67 proliferation index above 5% and the absence of CD8+ T-cell infiltration have been linked to increased risk of recurrence and reduced OS [62, 130, 133, 148, 160].

Recurrence is common in PC, occurring in 30–67% of patients, most frequently within 2–5 years following initial surgery, though late recurrences—up to 20 years postoperatively—have been reported. Identified risk factors for recurrence include younger or older age (<47 or >65 years), male sex, incomplete surgical resection (R1, R1), and histopathological features indicative of aggressive tumor behavior [23]. The extent and quality of surgical intervention—particularly en bloc resection versus local excision—are critical prognostic determinants. Nevertheless, even with aggressive re-intervention, however, reoperation is rarely curative, and recurrent disease continues to represent a major clinical challenge [164].

To enhance risk stratification, several prognostic staging systems have been proposed. Among these, the Schulte classification—which incorporates a dichotomous risk grouping (low vs. high risk) and a TNM-like staging system (stages I–IV)—has been validated across multiple studies as a reliable predictor of recurrence and survival. Notably, its application is associated with marked survival differences, with 5-year OS rates of 98.6% for stage I compared to 40% for stage IV. These findings support the routine use of the Schulte classification in clinical decision-making and patient counselling [133, 134, 148, 168].

11.12 Conclusion

Parathyroid carcinoma is a rare malignancy that typically presents with severe hypercalcemia and necessitates prompt recognition. Accurate preoperative assessment—integrating imaging, biochemical, and genetic data—is critical for diagnosis and surgical planning. En bloc resection remains the standard of care and should ideally be performed in specialized centers with relevant expertise. Given the limited efficacy of secondary interventions, early referral to such centers is strongly recommended. Advances in molecular profiling and the development of targeted therapies offer promising avenues for future treatment, underscoring the importance of multidisciplinary management. This includes the appropriate use of imaging techniques to ensure comprehensive disease assessment. In cases of metastatic or recurrent parathyroid carcinoma, whole-body imaging with PET/CT or PET/MRI is recommended. When serum PTH levels are elevated, [^{18}F]fluorocholine is generally the radiotracer of choice. In contrast, for anaplastic disease, in the absence of significant PTH elevation or in [^{18}F]fluorocholine-negative cases, [^{18}F]FDG PET imaging represents a suitable alternative.

Acknowledgments Figures 11.1 and 11.3 included in this chapter were created using BioRender.com.

References

1. Agarwal G, Dhingra S, Mishra SK, Krishnani N. Implantation of parathyroid carcinoma along fine needle aspiration track. Langenbeck's Arch Surg. 2006;391(6):623–6.
2. Akasu H, Jikuzono T, Matsui M, Sen M, Saitou M, Ishibashi O, et al. Ultrasonographic detective flow Imaging for evaluating Parathyroid adenoma in patients with primary hyperparathyroidism. J Nippon Med Sch. 2024;91(2):227–32. Medical Association of Nippon Medical School.
3. Akin M, Atasever T, Kurukahvecioglu O, Dogan M, Gokaslan D, Poyraz A, et al. Preoperative detection of parathyroid adenomas with Tc-99m MIBI and Tc-99m pertechnetate scintigraphy: histopathological and biochemical correlation with Tc-99m MIBI uptake. Bratislava Med J. 2009;110(3):166–9.

4. Akirov A, Asa SL, Larouche V, Mete O, Sawka AM, Jang R, et al. The clinicopathological spectrum of parathyroid carcinoma. Front Endocrinol (Lausanne) [Internet]. 2019 Oct 23 [cited 2025 May 28];10:731. Available from: https://pmc.ncbi.nlm.nih.gov/articles/PMC6819433/. Frontiers Media S.A.
5. Al-Salameh A, Cadiot G, Calender A, Goudet P, Chanson P. Clinical aspects of multiple endocrine neoplasia type 1 [Internet]. Nat Rev Endocrinol. 2021 [cited 2025 May 28];207–24. Available from: https://www.nature.com/articles/s41574-021-00468-3. Nature Publishing Group.
6. Alabed YZ, Rakheja R, Novales-Diaz JA, Lisbona R. Recurrent parathyroid carcinoma appearing as FDG negative but MIBI positive. Clin Nucl Med. 2014;39(7):e362–4. Lippincott Williams and Wilkins.
7. Alberti A, Smussi D, Zamparini M, Turla A, Laini L, Marchiselli C, et al. Treatment and outcome of metastatic parathyroid carcinoma: a systematic review and pooled analysis of published cases [Internet]. Front Oncol; 2022 [cited 2025 May 26];997009. Available from: http://www.ncbi.nlm.nih.gov/pubmed/36226055. Frontiers Media SA.
8. Alharbi AA, Alshehri FM, Albatly AA, Sah BR, Schmid C, Huber GF, et al. [18F]Fluorocholine uptake of parathyroid adenoma is correlated with parathyroid hormone level. Mol Imaging Biol [Internet]. 2018 Oct 1 [cited 2021 Apr 10];20(5):857–67. Available from: https://pubmed.ncbi.nlm.nih.gov/29508264/. Springer New York LLC.
9. Alwaheeb S, Rambaldini G, Boerner S, Coiré C, Fiser J, Asa SL. Worrisome histologic alterations following fine-needle aspiration of the parathyroid. J Clin Pathol. 2006;59(10):1094–6.
10. Anderson H, Lim KH, Simpson D, Gull S, Oprean R, Lee F, et al. Correlation between biochemical features and outcomes of preoperative imaging (SPECT-CT and ultrasound) in primary hyperparathyroidism. Acta Endocrinol (Copenh) [Internet]; 2021 Jul 1 [cited 2022 Jul 3];17(3):323–30. Available from: http://www.ncbi.nlm.nih.gov/pubmed/35342467. Acta Endocrinologica Foundation.
11. Araz M, Soydal Ç, Sütçü G, Kıvrak H, Sak SD, Kır KM, et al. The relationship between 18F-FCH uptake intensity and cell content in parathyroid lesions. Eur Arch Oto-Rhino-Laryngology [Internet]. 2023 Jun 1 [cited 2023 Jun 23];280(6). Available from: https://pubmed.ncbi.nlm.nih.gov/36790722/.
12. Arslan N, Rydzewski B. Detection of a recurrent parathyroid carcinoma with FDG positron emission tomography. Clin Nucl Med. 2002;27(3):221–2.
13. Asare EA, Sturgeon C, Winchester DJP, Liu L, Palis B, Perrier ND, et al. Parathyroid carcinoma: an update on treatment outcomes and prognostic factors from the National Cancer Data Base (NCDB). Ann Surg Oncol [Internet]. 2015 Nov 1 [cited 2025 May 26];22(12):3990–5. Available from: https://link.springer.com/article/10.1245/s10434-015-4672-3. Springer New York LLC.
14. Bae JH, Choi HJ, Lee Y, Moon MK, Park YJ, Shin CS, et al. Preoperative predictive factors for parathyroid carcinoma in patients with primary hyperparathyroidism. J Korean Med Sci [Internet]. 2012 Aug [cited 2025 May 29];27(8):890–5. Available from: https://pubmed.ncbi.nlm.nih.gov/22876055/.
15. Bahl M, Sepahdari AR, Sosa JA, Hoang JK. Parathyroid adenomas and hyperplasia on fourdimensional CT scans: three patterns of enhancement relative to the thyroid gland justify a three-phase protocol. Radiology. 2015;277(2):454–62. Radiological Society of North America Inc.
16. Battini S, Imperiale A, Taïeb D, Elbayed K, Cicek AE, Sebag F, et al. High-resolution magic angle spinning 1H nuclear magnetic resonance spectroscopy metabolomics of hyperfunctioning parathyroid glands. Surgery (United States) [Internet]. 2016 Aug 1 [cited 2025 Jun 5];160(2):384–94. Available from: https://pubmed.ncbi.nlm.nih.gov/27106795/. Mosby Inc.
17. Bilezikian JP, Bandeira L, Khan A, Cusano NE. Hyperparathyroidism [Internet]. Lancet. 2018 [cited 2025 May 26];168–78. Available from: https://pubmed.ncbi.nlm.nih.gov/28923463/. Lancet Publishing Group.
18. Bleier BS, LiVolsi VA, Chalian AA, Gimotty PA, Botbyl JD, Weber RS. Technetium Tc 99m sestamibi sensitivity in oxyphil cell-dominant parathyroid adenomas. Arch Otolaryngol - Head Neck Surg. 2006;132(7):779–82.
19. Boellaard R, Delgado-Bolton R, Oyen WJG, Giammarile F, Tatsch K, Eschner W, et al. FDG PET/CT: EANM procedure guidelines for tumour imaging: version 2.0. Eur J Nucl Med Mol Imaging. 2015:328–54.
20. Busaidy NL, Jimenez C, Habra MA, Schultz PN, El-Naggar AK, Clayman GL, et al. Parathyroid carcinoma: a 22-year experience. Head Neck [Internet]. 2004 Aug [cited 2025 May 26];26(8):716–26. Available from: https://pubmed.ncbi.nlm.nih.gov/15287039/.
21. Byrd C, Kashyap S, Kwartowitz G. Parathyroid cancer. StatPearls [Internet]. 2023 Jul 24 [cited 2025 May 21]. Available from: https://www.ncbi.nlm.nih.gov/books/NBK519038/. StatPearls Publishing.
22. Çalapkulu M, Sencar ME, Unsal IO, Sakiz D, Duger H, Özbek M, et al. Tumor volume can be used as a parameter indicating the severity of disease in parathyroid cancer. Endocr Pract. 2021;27(7):706–9. Elsevier B.V.
23. Do Cao C, Christou N, Hadoux J, Deandreis D. Chapter 8: Management of aggressive forms of primary HPT: parathyroid carcinoma and atypical parathyroid tumor. Ann Endocrinol (Paris) [Internet]. 2025 Feb 1 [cited 2025 May 14];86(1). Available from: https://pubmed.ncbi.nlm.nih.gov/39818300/. Elsevier Masson s.r.l.

24. Cardoso L, Stevenson M, Thakker RV. Molecular genetics of syndromic and non-syndromic forms of parathyroid carcinoma [Internet]. Hum Mutat. 2017 [cited 2025 May 27];1621–48. Available from: https://pubmed.ncbi.nlm.nih.gov/28881068/. John Wiley and Sons Inc.
25. Carpten JD, Robbins CM, Villablanca A, Forsberg L, Presciuttini S, Bailey-Wilsons J, et al. HRPT2, encoding parafibromin, is mutated in hyperparathyroidism-jaw tumor syndrome. Nat Genet. 2002;32(4):676–80.
26. Casara D, Rubello D, Piotto A, Pelizzo MR. (99m) Tc-MIBI radio-guided minimally invasive parathyroid surgery planned on the basis of a preoperative combined (99m)Tc-pertechnetate/(99m)Tc-MIBI and ultrasound imaging protocol. Eur J Nucl Med [Internet]. 2000 [cited 2025 Jun 5];27(9):1300–4. Available from: https://pubmed.ncbi.nlm.nih.gov/11007510/.
27. Cavalier E, Betea D, Schleck ML, Gadisseur R, Vroonen L, Delanaye P, et al. The third/second generation PTH assay ratio as a marker for parathyroid carcinoma: evaluation using an automated platform. J Clin Endocrinol Metab [Internet]. 2014 [cited 2025 May 29];99(3). Available from: https://pubmed.ncbi.nlm.nih.gov/24423313/. Endocrine Society.
28. Centello R, Sesti F, Feola T, Sada V, Pandozzi C, Di Serafino M, et al. The dark side of ultrasound imaging in parathyroid disease [Internet]. J Clin Med. 2023 [cited 2025 Jun 2];2487. Available from: https://pmc.ncbi.nlm.nih.gov/articles/PMC10095081/. Multidisciplinary Digital Publishing Institute (MDPI).
29. Cetani F, Banti C, Pardi E, Borsari S, Viacava P, Miccoli P, et al. CDC73 mutational status and loss of parafibromin in the outcome of parathyroid cancer. Endocr Connect. 2013;2(4):186–95. Bioscientifica.
30. Chakrabarty N, Mahajan A, Basu S, D'Cruz AK. Imaging recommendations for diagnosis and management of primary parathyroid pathologies: a comprehensive review. Cancers (Basel). 2024;16(14):2593. Multidisciplinary Digital Publishing Institute (MDPI).
31. Chen J, Feng J, Zhou Q, Zheng W, Meng X, Wang Y, et al. Intraoperative 99mTc-MIBI-guided parathyroidectomy improves curative effect of parathyroidectomy, bone metabolism, and bone mineral density. Am Surg [Internet]. 2021 Mar 1 [cited 2025 Jun 5];87(3):463–72. Available from: https://doi.org/10.1177/0003134820951467. SAGE Publications Inc.
32. Chen J, Zhao M, An Q, Wei L, Chen B. Detection of muscular metastasis in a case of parathyroid carcinoma using 18F-FAPI-04 PET/CT. Clin Nucl Med [Internet]; 2024 Oct 1 [cited 2025 May 18];49(10):e501–2. Available from: https://pubmed.ncbi.nlm.nih.gov/39192519/. Lippincott Williams and Wilkins.
33. Cheung K, Wang TS, Farrokhyar F, Roman SA, Sosa JA. A meta-analysis of preoperative localization techniques for patients with primary hyperparathyroidism [Internet]. Ann Surg Oncol. 2012 [cited 2025 Jun 2];577–83. Available from: https://pubmed.ncbi.nlm.nih.gov/21710322/.
34. Chevalier B, Ghander C, Ladsous M, Gaujoux S, Taieb D, Buffet C, et al. Chapter 10: What parathyroid imaging is required for hyprepratahyroidism? Ann Endocrinol (Paris) [Internet]. 2025 Feb 1 [cited 2025 Jun 2];86(1):101699. Available from: https://www.sciencedirect.com/science/article/pii/S0003426625000186. Elsevier Masson.
35. Christakis I, Bussaidy N, Clarke C, Kwatampora LJ, Warneke CL, Silva AM, et al. Differentiating atypical parathyroid neoplasm from parathyroid cancer. Ann Surg Oncol. 2016;23(9):2889–97. Springer New York LLC.
36. Christakis I, Silva AM, Williams MD, Garden A, Grubbs EG, Busaidy NL, et al. Postoperative local-regional radiation therapy in the treatment of parathyroid carcinoma: the MD Anderson experience of 35 years. Pract Radiat Oncol [Internet]; 2017a Nov 1 [cited 2025 May 31];7(6):e463–70. Available from: https://pubmed.ncbi.nlm.nih.gov/28751227/. Elsevier Inc.
37. Christakis I, Vu T, Chuang HH, Fellman B, Silva-Figueroa AM, Williams MD, et al. The diagnostic accuracy of neck ultrasound, 4D-Computed tomographyand sestamibi imaging in parathyroid carcinoma. Eur J Radiol [Internet]. 2017b Oct 1 [cited 2025 Jun 2];95:82–8. Available from: https://pubmed.ncbi.nlm.nih.gov/28987702/. Elsevier Ireland Ltd.
38. Clark P, Wooldridge T, Kleinpeter K, Perrier N, Lovato J, Morton K. Providing optimal preoperative localization for recurrent parathyroid carcinoma: a combined parathyroid scintigraphy and computed tomography approach [Internet]. Clin Nucl Med; 2004 [cited 2025 Jun 8];681–4. Available from: https://pubmed.ncbi.nlm.nih.gov/15483477/.
39. Čolović Z, Krnić M, Kljajić Z, Kontić M, Kolja Poljak N, Tafra R, et al. Surgical treatment of recurrent metastatic parathyroid gland carcinoma. Acta Clin Croat. 2020;59:96–101. Dr. Mladen Stojanovic University Hospital.
40. Davies MP, John Evans TW, Tahir F, Balasubramanian SP. Parathyroid cancer: a systematic review of diagnostic biomarkers [Internet]. Surgeon. 2021 [cited 2025 May 18];e536–48. Available from: https://pubmed.ncbi.nlm.nih.gov/33642204/. Elsevier Ltd.
41. Deandreis D, Terroir M, Al Ghuzlan A, Berdelou A, Lacroix L, Bidault F, et al. 18Fluorocholine PET/CT in parathyroid carcinoma: a new tool for disease staging? Eur J Nucl Med Mol Imaging. 2015;42(12):1941–2.
42. Du X, Wang L, Shen B, He H, Chang H, Wei B. Clinical significance of pd-l1 expression in parathyroid cancer. Acta Endocrinol (Copenh) [Internet]; 2016 Oct 1 [cited 2025 Jun 1];12(4):383–6. Available

from: https://pubmed.ncbi.nlm.nih.gov/31149119/. Acta Endocrinologica Foundation.

43. Dupeux M, Aubert S. Chapter 13: Changes in 2022 WHO classification of parathyroid tumors. Ann Endocrinol (Paris) [Internet]. 2025 Feb 1 [cited 2025 May 18];86(1):101702. Available from: https://www.sciencedirect.com/science/article/pii/S0003426625000216?fr=RR-2&ref=pdf_download&rr=946e2a42cf7bea5f. Elsevier Masson s.r.l.
44. Ebrahiminik H, Chegeni H, Mosadegh Khah A, Salouti R, Ghomashchi G, Deldar Pasikhani M, et al. Radiofrequency ablation of parathyroid adenomas causing primary hyperparathyroidism: a report of 27 patients. J Clin Ultrasound [Internet]. 2022 May 1 [cited 2025 Jun 1];50(4):540–6. Available from: https://pubmed.ncbi.nlm.nih.gov/35278235/. John Wiley and Sons Inc.
45. Egner JR. AJCC cancer staging manual. JAMA [Internet]. 2010 [cited 2025 May 28];304(15):1726. Available from: https://link.springer.com/book/9783319406176.
46. Eldaya RW, Calle S, Wong FC, Learned KO, Wintermark M. Parathyroid carcinoma: imaging features of initial presentation and recurrence. A single center experience. Neuroradiol J [Internet]; 2024 Feb 1 [cited 2025 May 21];37(1):92–106. Available from: https://pmc.ncbi.nlm.nih.gov/articles/PMC10863576/. SAGE Publications Inc.
47. Erickson LA, Mete O. Immunohistochemistry in diagnostic parathyroid pathology. Endocr Pathol. 2018:113–29. Humana Press Inc.
48. Erickson LA, Mete O, Juhlin CC, Perren A, Gill AJ. Overview of the 2022 WHO classification of parathyroid tumors. Endocr Pathol. 2022:64–89. Springer.
49. Erovic BM, Goldstein DP, Kim D, Mete O, Brierley J, Tsang R, et al. Parathyroid cancer: outcome analysis of 16 patients treated at the princess margaret hospital [Internet]. Head Neck. 2013 [cited 2025 May 31];35–9. Available from: https://pubmed.ncbi.nlm.nih.gov/22290780/.
50. Erovic BM, Harris L, Jamali M, Goldstein DP, Irish JC, Asa SL, et al. Biomarkers of parathyroid carcinoma. Endocr Pathol [Internet]. 2012 Dec [cited 2025 Jun 1];23(4):221–31. Available from: http://www.ncbi.nlm.nih.gov/pubmed/23001705. Humana Press Inc.
51. Evangelista L. FDG-PET/CT and parathyroid carcinoma: review of literature and illustrative case series. World J Clin Oncol [Internet]. 2011 Oct 10 [cited 2025 May 18];2(10):348. Available from: http://www.ncbi.nlm.nih.gov/pubmed/22022662. Baishideng Publishing Group Inc.
52. Ferrari C, Santo G, Mammucci P, Pisani AR, Sardaro A, Rubini G. Diagnostic value of choline PET in the preoperative localization of hyperfunctioning parathyroid gland(s): a comprehensive overview. Biomedicines [Internet]. 2021 Feb 25 [cited 2021 May 7];9(3):231. Available from: https://doi.org/10.3390/biomedicines9030231. MDPI AG.
53. Fuenzalida L, Indo S, Contreras HR, Rappoport D, Cabané P. Basic-clinical analysis of parathyroid cancer [Internet]. Biomedicines. 2025 [cited 2025 May 14];687. Available from: https://www.mdpi.com/2227–9059/13/3/687/htm. Multidisciplinary Digital Publishing Institute.
54. Gao WC, Ruan CP, Zhang JC, Liu HM, Xu XY, Sun YP, et al. Nonfunctional parathyroid carcinoma. J Cancer Res Clin Oncol. 2010;136(7):969–74.
55. Gardner CJ, Wieshmann H, Gosney J, Carr HM, Macfarlane IA, Cuthbertson DJ. Localization of metastatic parathyroid carcinoma by18F FDG PET scanning. J Clin Endocrinol Metab [Internet]. 2010 Nov [cited 2025 May 18];95(11):4844–5. Available from: http://www.ncbi.nlm.nih.gov/pubmed/21051579. Endocrine Society.
56. Morand GB, Helmchen BM, Steinert HC, Schmid C, Broglie MA. 18F-Choline-PET in parathyroid carcinoma. Oral Oncol. 2018a;86:314–5.
57. Gill AJ, Lim G, Cheung VKY, Andrici J, Perry-Keene JL, Paik J, et al. Parafibromin-deficient (HPT-JT Type, CDC73 Mutated) parathyroid tumors demonstrate distinctive morphologic features. Am J Surg Pathol. 2019;43(1):35–46. Lippincott Williams and Wilkins.
58. Giovanella L, Bacigalupo L, Treglia G, Piccardo A. Will 18F-fluorocholine PET/CT replace other methods of preoperative parathyroid imaging? [Internet]. Endocrine; 2021 [cited 2022 Jun 2];285–97. Available from: https://pubmed.ncbi.nlm.nih.gov/32892309/.
59. Givi B, Shah JP. Parathyroid carcinoma. Clin Oncol. 2010;22(6):498–507.
60. Goldner E, Fingeret A. Parathyroid carcinoma: a national cancer database analysis. J Surg Res [Internet]. 2023 Jan 1 [cited 2025 Jun 1];281:57–62. Available from: https://pubmed.ncbi.nlm.nih.gov/36116208/. Academic Press Inc.
61. Gulati S, Chumber S, Puri G, Spalkit S, Damle NA, Das C. Multi-modality parathyroid imaging: a shifting paradigm. World J Radiol [Internet]. 2023 Mar 28 [cited 2025 Jun 4];15(3):69–82. Available from: https://pmc.ncbi.nlm.nih.gov/articles/PMC10080580/. Baishideng Publishing Group Inc.
62. Hadoux J, Lamarca A, Grande E, Deandreis D, Kaltsas G, Janson ET, et al. Neuroendocrine neoplasms of head and neck, genitourinary and gynaecological systems, unknown primaries, parathyroid carcinomas and intrathyroid thymic neoplasms: ESMO Clinical Practice Guideline for diagnosis, treatment and follow-up. ESMO open [Internet]. 2024 Oct 1 [cited 2025 May 26];9(10):103664. Available from: http://www.ncbi.nlm.nih.gov/pubmed/39461777. Elsevier.
63. Haq ZJ, Ahmed A, Abdelsalam A, Chegini S, Kurzawinski TR, Morley S, et al. The development of patient-specific 3D anatomical models in minimally invasive parathyroidectomy. Front Endocrinol (Lausanne) [Internet]. 2024 [cited 2025 May 18];15:1514451. Available from: http://www.ncbi.

nlm.nih.gov/pubmed/39722808. Frontiers Media SA.
64. Hara H, Igarashi A, Yano Y, Yashiro T, Ueno E, Aiyoshi Y, et al. Ultrasonographic features of parathyroid carcinoma. Endocr J Japan. 2001;48(2):213–7. Endocrine Society.
65. Harari A, Waring A, Fernandez-Ranvier G, Hwang J, Suh I, Mitmaker E, et al. Parathyroid carcinoma: a 43-year outcome and survival analysis. J Clin Endocrinol Metab. 2011;96(12):3679–86.
66. Hargitai L, Schefner M, Traub-Weidinger T, Haug A, Arikan M, Scheuba C, et al. Accessing the influence of 99mTc-Sesta-MIBI-positive thyroid nodules on preoperative localisation studies in patients with primary hyperparathyroidism. Langenbeck's Arch Surg. 2022;407(3):1183–91. Springer Science and Business Media Deutschland GmbH.
67. Hatzl M, Röper-Kelmayr JC, Fellner FA, Gabriel M. 18F-fluorocholine, 18F-FDG, and 18F-fluoroethyl tyrosine PET/CT in parathyroid cancer. Clin Nucl Med. 2017;42(6):448–50. Lippincott Williams and Wilkins.
68. Hosny Mohammed K, Siddiqui MT, Willis BC, Zaharieva Tsvetkova D, Mohamed A, Patel S, et al. Parafibromin, APC, and MIB-1 are useful markers for distinguishing parathyroid carcinomas from adenomas. Appl Immunohistochem Mol Morphol [Internet]; 2017 [cited 2025 May 28];25(10):731–735. Available from: https://pubmed.ncbi.nlm.nih.gov/27490759/. Lippincott Williams and Wilkins.
69. Hu Y, Mo S, Xiao J, Cui M, Zheng Q, Chen T, et al. The significance of an immunohistochemical marker-based panel in assisting the diagnosis of parathyroid carcinoma. Endocrine [Internet]; 2024 Jun 1 [cited 2025 May 28];84(3):1146–53. Available from: https://pubmed.ncbi.nlm.nih.gov/38340242/. Springer.
70. Huellner MW, Aberle S, Sah BR, Veit-Haibach P, Bonani M, Schmid C, et al. Visualization of parathyroid hyperplasia using 18F-fluorocholine PET/MR in a patient with secondary hyperparathyroidism. Clin Nucl Med [Internet]. Lippincott Williams and Wilkins; 2016 [cited 2021 Apr 29];41(3):e159–61. Available from: https://pubmed.ncbi.nlm.nih.gov/26462047/.
71. Hundahl SA, Fleming ID, Fremgen AM, Menck HR. Two hundred eighty-six cases of parathyroid carcinoma treated in the U.S. between 1985-1995: a National Cancer Data Base report. Cancer [Internet]. Cancer; 1999 Aug 1 [cited 2025 May 26];86(3):538–44. Available from: https://pubmed.ncbi.nlm.nih.gov/10430265/.
72. Iacovitti CM, Cuzzocrea M, Gianola L, Paone G, Treglia G. Dual-tracer positron emission tomography/computed tomography with [18F]FDG and [18F]fluorocholine in a patient with metastatic parathyroid carcinoma. Diagnostics [Internet]. 2024 Jul 1 [cited 2025 May 21];14(14). Available from: https://pubmed.ncbi.nlm.nih.gov/39061685/. Multidisciplinary Digital Publishing Institute (MDPI).
73. Insogna KL. Primary hyperparathyroidism. Solomon CG, editor. N Engl J Med [Internet]. 2018 Sep 13 [cited 2025 May 26];379(11):1050–9. Available from: https://pubmed.ncbi.nlm.nih.gov/30207907/.
74. Ionova TI, Buzanakov DM, Chernikov RA, Efremov SM, Gladkova IN, Nikitina TP, et al. Quality of life in patients with primary hyperparathyroidism before and after parathyroidectomy: long term single center experience. BMC Endocr Disord [Internet]; 2023 Dec 1 [cited 2025 May 31];23(1). Available from: https://pubmed.ncbi.nlm.nih.gov/37085858/. BioMed Central Ltd.
75. Ireland JP, Fleming SJ, Levison DA, Cattell WR, Baker L. Parathyroid carcinoma associated with chronic renal failure and previous radiotherapy to the neck. J Clin Pathol [Internet]. 1985 Oct 1 [cited 2025 May 27];38(10):1114–8. Available from: https://jcp.bmj.com/content/38/10/1114. BMJ Publishing Group.
76. Ivaniš S, Jovanović M, Dunđerović D, Zorić G, Odalović B, Slijepčević N, et al. Case presentation of the smallest non-functional parathyroid carcinoma and review of the literature. Eur Arch Oto-Rhino-Laryngology. 2023;280(12):5637–47.
77. Iványi G, Christofi A, Sipka G, Zombori T, Kuthi L, Simon A, et al. Radiation-induced synchronous parathyroid carcinoma and papillary thyroid carcinoma: clinical, morphological, and genetic insights. Int J Mol Sci [Internet]. 2025 May 1 [cited 2025 May 28];26(9). Available from: https://pubmed.ncbi.nlm.nih.gov/40362680/. Multidisciplinary Digital Publishing Institute (MDPI).
78. Jategaonkar AA, Lerner DK, Cooke P, Kirke D, Genden EM, Trosman SJ. Implementation of a 4-dimensional computed tomography protocol for parathyroid adenoma localization. Am J Otolaryngol. 2021;42(3). Head Neck Med Surg WB Saunders.
79. Jo SY, Hong N, Lee S, Jeong JJ, Won J, Park J, et al. Genomic and transcriptomic profiling reveal molecular characteristics of parathyroid carcinoma. Exp Mol Med [Internet]; 2023 May 1 [cited 2025 May 28];55(5):886–97. Available from: https://www.nature.com/articles/s12276-023-00968-4. Nature Publishing Group.
80. Kang H, Pettinga D, Schubert AD, Ladenson PW, Ball DW, Chung JH, et al. Genomic profiling of parathyroid carcinoma reveals genomic alterations suggesting benefit from therapy. Oncologist [Internet]. 2019 Jun 1 [cited 2025 Jun 1];24(6):791–7. Available from: https://pubmed.ncbi.nlm.nih.gov/30373905/. Oxford University Press (OUP).
81. Karakas E, Müller HH, Lyadov VK, Luz S, Schneider R, Rothmund M, et al. Development of a formula to predict parathyroid carcinoma in patients with primary hyperparathyroidism. World J Surg [Internet]. 2012 Nov [cited 2025 Jun 8];36(11):2605–11. Available from: https://pubmed.ncbi.nlm.nih.gov/22777415/.

82. Kartini D, Kurnia A, Yulian ED, Panigoro SS, Wibisana IGNG, Wardana J. Case series of diagnosis and surgery challenges in parathyroid carcinoma [Internet]. Int J Surg Case Rep. 2022 [cited 2025 May 18];107390. Available from: http://www.ncbi.nlm.nih.gov/pubmed/35863283. Elsevier Ltd.
83. Kattar N, Migneron M, Debakey MS, Haidari M, Pou AM, McCoul ED. Advanced computed tomographic localization techniques for primary hyperparathyroidism: a systematic review and meta-analysis. JAMA Otolaryngol. 2022:448–56. Head Neck Surg American Medical Association.
84. Kelly HR, Bunch PM. Parathyroid computed tomography: pearls, pitfalls, and our approach. Neuroimaging Clin N Am. 2022:413–31. WB Saunders.
85. Kemps B, Quarles Van Ufford H, Creyghton W, De Haas M, Baarslag HJ, Borel Rinkes I, et al. Brown tumors simulating metastases on FDG PET in a patient with parathyroid carcinoma. Eur J Nucl Med Mol Imaging [Internet]; 2008 Apr [cited 2025 May 18];35(4):850. Available from: https://pubmed.ncbi.nlm.nih.gov/18265978/.
86. Kim J, Horowitz G, Hong M, Orsini M, Asa SL, Higgins K. The dangers of parathyroid biopsy. J Otolaryngol - Head Neck Surg [Internet]. 2017 Jan 7 [cited 2025 May 28];46(1):4. Available from: https://pmc.ncbi.nlm.nih.gov/articles/PMC5219743/. BioMed Central Ltd.
87. Kirkby-Bott J, Lewis P, Harmer CL, Smellie WJB. One stage treatment of parathyroid cancer. Eur J Surg Oncol [Internet]. 2005 Feb [cited 2025 May 31];31(1):78–83. Available from: https://pubmed.ncbi.nlm.nih.gov/15642430/.
88. Kobylecka M, Koperski Ł, Chudziński W, Pihowicz P, Mączewska J, Płazińska MT, et al. Relationship between parathyroid gland scintigraphy and its histopathology, oxyphil cell content and volume: a retrospective study. Nucl Med Rev Via Medica. 2019;22(1):29–33.
89. Kubal M, Lech M, Lajeunesse-Trempe F, Drakou EE, Grossman AB, Dimitriadis GK. Advances in the management of parathyroid carcinoma. Mol Cell Endocrinol. 2024. Elsevier Ireland Ltd.
90. Kunstman JW, Kirsch JD, Mahajan A, Udelsman R. Parathyroid localization and implications for clinical management. J Clin Endocrinol Metab [Internet]; 2013 Mar [cited 2022 Jul 3];98(3):902–12. Available from: https://pubmed.ncbi.nlm.nih.gov/23345096/.
91. Laforgia R, Tomasicchio G, Cavalera F, Sblendorio M, Spadone A, Anelli FM, et al. Management and surgical treatment of parathyroid carcinoma: a 6-year experience of a single centre of endocrine surgery unit. Front Endocrinol (Lausanne) [Internet]. 2023 [cited 2025 May 31];14. Available from: https://pubmed.ncbi.nlm.nih.gov/38027123/. Frontiers Media SA.
92. Lalonde MN, Correia RD, Syktiotis GP, Schaefer N, Matter M, Prior JO. Parathyroid imaging. Semin Nucl Med. 2023:490–502. WB Saunders.
93. Lazzaro A, Zhao G, Kulke M. Diagnosis and management of parathyroid carcinoma [Internet]. Clin Pharmacol Ther. 2024 [cited 2025 May 18];80–8. Available from: http://www.ncbi.nlm.nih.gov/pubmed/39299227. S. Karger AG.
94. Lee PK, Jarosek SL, Virnig BA, Evasovich M, Tuttle TM. Trends in the incidence and treatment of parathyroid cancer in the United States. Cancer [Internet]. 2007 May 1 [cited 2025 May 26];109(9):1736–41. Available from: https://pubmed.ncbi.nlm.nih.gov/17372919/.
95. Leonard-Murali S, Ivanics T, Kwon DS, Han X, Steffes CP, Shah R. Local resection versus radical surgery for parathyroid carcinoma: a National Cancer Database analysis. Eur J Surg Oncol. 2021:2768–73. WB Saunders Ltd.
96. Li M, Lu H, Gao Y. FDG-anorectic parathyroid carcinoma with FDG-avid bone metastasis on PET/CT images. Clin Nucl Med. 2013;38(11):916–8.
97. Liberini V, Morand GB, Rupp NJ, Orita E, Deandreis D, Broglie Däppen M, et al. Histopathological features of parathyroid adenoma and 18F-Choline uptake in PET/MR of primary hyperparathyroidism. Clin Nucl Med [Internet]. 2022 Feb 1 [cited 2022 Jun 2];47(2):101–7. Available from: https://pubmed.ncbi.nlm.nih.gov/35006103/.
98. Limberg J, Stefanova D, Ullmann TM, Thiesmeyer JW, Bains S, Beninato T, et al. The use and benefit of adjuvant radiotherapy in parathyroid carcinoma: a National Cancer Database Analysis. Ann Surg Oncol [Internet]. 2021 Jan 1 [cited 2025 May 31];28(1):502–511. Available from: https://pubmed.ncbi.nlm.nih.gov/32661850/. Springer Science and Business Media Deutschland GmbH.
99. Liu J, Zhan WW, Zhou JQ, Zhou W. Role of ultrasound in the differentiation of parathyroid carcinoma and benign parathyroid lesions. Clin Radiol. 2020;75(3):179–84. W.B. Saunders Ltd.
100. Liu R, Gao L, Xia Y, Shi X, Lv K, Xia W, Qiu L, Hu Y, Jiang Y. Locoregional recurrence of parathyroid carcinoma: how to identify this rare but fatal condition using ultrasonography. Endocr J. 2021 Oct 28;68(10):1179-1186. https://doi.org/10.1507/endocrj.EJ21-0124. Epub 2021 May 8. PMID: 33967164.
101. Liu X, Yang W, Zhao T, Wang Q, Wang J, Feng D, et al. Development of a prediction model for recurrent parathyroid carcinoma lesions based on 3D-EnCT and ultrasound imaging features. Clin Transl Oncol [Internet]. 2024 Jun [cited 2025 May 18];27(6):2658–66. Available from: http://www.ncbi.nlm.nih.gov/pubmed/39565549. Springer Science and Business Media Deutschland GmbH.
102. Lo WM, Good ML, Nilubol N, Perrier ND, Patel DT. Tumor size and presence of metastatic disease at diagnosis are associated with disease-specific survival in parathyroid carcinoma. Ann Surg Oncol. 2018;25(9):2535–40. Springer New York LLC.

103. Long KL, Sippel RS. Current and future treatments for parathyroid carcinoma. Int J Endocr Oncol. 2018;5(1). Informa UK Limited.
104. Longo F, Sarubbi A, Palladino C, Palermo A, Naciu AM, Crescenzi A, et al. Two-step surgical strategy for parathyroid carcinoma: a single-center experience. Med [Internet]. 2024 Dec 13 [cited 2025 May 18];60(12). Available from: http://www.ncbi.nlm.nih.gov/pubmed/39768933. Multidisciplinary Digital Publishing Institute (MDPI).
105. Ma T, Zhao X, Zhang J, Zhao X. Differential diagnosis of Brown tumors and bone metastases in parathyroid carcinoma using 18F-FDG PET/CT and 99mTc-MIBI SPECT/CT: a case report [Internet]. Asian J Surg. 2024 [cited 2025 Jun 8]. Available from: http://www.ncbi.nlm.nih.gov/pubmed/39271342. Elsevier (Singapore) Pte Ltd.
106. Marini F, Giusti F, Palmini G, Aurilia C, Donati S, Brandi ML. Parathyroid carcinoma: molecular therapeutic targets [Internet]. Endocrine; 2023 [cited 2025 May 18];409–18. Available from: https://pubmed.ncbi.nlm.nih.gov/37160841/. Springer.
107. Marini F, Giusti F, Palmini G, Perigli G, Santoro R, Brandi ML. Genetics and epigenetics of parathyroid carcinoma [Internet]. Front Endocrinol (Lausanne). 2022 [cited 2025 May 18];834362. Available from: http://www.ncbi.nlm.nih.gov/pubmed/35282432. Frontiers Media SA.
108. Marx SJ. New concepts about familial isolated hyperparathyroidism [Internet]. J Clin Endocrinol Metab. 2019 [cited 2025 May 28];4058–66. Available from: https://pmc.ncbi.nlm.nih.gov/articles/PMC6684304/. Endocrine Society.
109. Matsui M, Jikuzono T, Kure S, Ishibashi O, Akasu H, Sugitani I. Usefulness of ultrasonographic detective flow imaging for detecting parathyroid tumors: a report of two cases. J Nippon Med Sch. 2023;90(6):460–4. Medical Association of Nippon Medical School.
110. Melloul M, Paz A, Koren R, Cytron S, Feinmesser R, Gal R. 99mTc-MIBI scintigraphy of parathyroid adenomas and its relation to tumour size and oxyphil cell abundance. Eur J Nucl Med [Internet]. 2001 [cited 2020 Mar 21];28(2):209–13. Available from: https://pubmed.ncbi.nlm.nih.gov/11303892/.
111. Merchavy S, Luckman J, Guindy M, Segev Y, Khafif A. 4D MRI for the localization of parathyroid adenoma. Otolaryngol - Head Neck Surg (United States). 2016;154:446–8. SAGE Publications Inc.
112. Moline J, Eng C. Multiple endocrine neoplasia type 2: an overview [Internet]. Genet Med. 2011 [cited 2025 May 28];755–64. Available from: https://www.nature.com/articles/gim2011127. Nature Publishing Group.
113. Morand GB, Helmchen BM, Steinert HC, Schmid C, Broglie MA. 18F-Choline-PET in parathyroid carcinoma [Internet]. Oral Oncol; 2018b [cited 2022 Jun 2];314–5. Available from: https://pubmed.ncbi.nlm.nih.gov/30274770/.
114. Morand GB, Rupp NJ, Huellner MW, Gerber PA, Soyka MB, Broglie MA, et al. Transnasal-transpterygoid endoscopic removal of an 18F-Choline-avid parathyroid carcinoma metastasis in the skull base [Internet]. JAMA Otolaryngol - Head Neck Surg. 2019 [cited 2025 Jun 8];978–80. Available from: https://jamanetwork.com/journals/jamaotolaryngology/fullarticle/2748899. American Medical Association.
115. Morris MA, Saboury B, Ahlman M, Malayeri AA, Jones EC, Chen CC, et al. Parathyroid imaging: past, present, and future. Front Endocrinol (Lausanne) [Internet]. 2022 Feb 25 [cited 2025 May 18];12:760419. Available from: https://www.frontiersin.org. Frontiers Media S.A.
116. Munson ND, Foote RL, Northcutt RC, Tiegs RD, Fitzpatrick LA, Grant CS, et al. Parathyroid carcinoma: is there a role for adjuvant radiation therapy? Cancer. 2003;98:2378–84.
117. Nael K, Hur J, Bauer A, Khan R, Sepahdari A, Inampudi R, et al. Dynamic 4D MRI for characterization of parathyroid adenomas: multiparametric analysis. AJNR Am J Neuroradiol [Internet]; 2015 Nov 1 [cited 2025 Jun 5];36(11):2147–52. Available from: https://www.ajnr.org/content/36/11/2147.
118. Nam M, Jeong HS, Shin JH. Differentiation of parathyroid carcinoma and adenoma by preoperative ultrasonography. Acta Radiol. 2017;58(6):670–5. SAGE Publications Inc.
119. Norman J, Politz D, Browarsky I. Diagnostic aspiration of parathyroid adenomas causes severe fibrosis complicating surgery and final histologic diagnosis. Thyroid. 2007;17(12):1251–5.
120. O'Neill CJ, Chan C, Symons J, Learoyd DL, Sidhu SB, Delbridge LW, et al. Parathyroid carcinoma encountered after minimally invasive focused parathyroidectomy may not require further radical surgery. World J Surg [Internet]. 2011 Jan [cited 2025 May 31];35(1):147–53. Available from: https://pubmed.ncbi.nlm.nih.gov/20981544/.
121. Ozturk M, Polat AV, Celenk C, Elmali M, Kir S, Polat C. The diagnostic value of 4D MRI at 3T for the localization of parathyroid adenomas. Eur J Radiol [Internet]. 2019 Mar 1 [cited 2025 Jun 5];112:207–13. Available from: https://www.ejradiology.com/action/showFullText?pii=S0720048X19300312. Elsevier Ireland Ltd.
122. Palestro CJ, Tomas MB, Tronco GG. Radionuclide imaging of the parathyroid glands. Semin Nucl Med [Internet]; 2005 [cited 2025 Jul 13];35(4):266–76. Available from: https://pubmed.ncbi.nlm.nih.gov/16150247/. WB Saunders.
123. Park D, Airi R, Sherman M. Microsatellite instability driven metastatic parathyroid carcinoma managed with the anti-PD1 immunotherapy, pembrolizumab. BMJ Case Rep [Internet]. 2020 Sep 23 [cited 2025 Jun 1];13(9). Available from: https://pubmed.ncbi.nlm.nih.gov/32967944/. BMJ Publishing Group.
124. Perrier N, Lang BH, Farias LCB, Poch LL, Sywak M, Almquist M, et al. Surgical aspects of pri-

mary hyperparathyroidism. J Bone Miner Res. 2022;37(11):2373–90. John Wiley and Sons Inc.
125. Petranović Ovčariček P, Campennì A, Giovanella L, Huellner MW. Parathyroid carcinoma: a comprehensive analysis with focus on molecular imaging [Internet]. Eur J Nucl Med Mol Imaging. 2025a [cited 2025 Jun 5];1–5. Available from: https://link.springer.com/article/10.1007/s00259-025-07162-w. Springer.
126. Petranović Ovčariček P, Giovanella L, Carrió Gasset I, Hindié E, Huellner MW, Luster M, et al. The EANM practice guidelines for parathyroid imaging. Eur J Nucl Med Mol Imaging. 2021a;48(9):2801–22. Springer Science and Business Media Deutschland GmbH.
127. Petranović Ovčariček P, Giovanella L, Carrió Gasset I, Hindié E, Huellner MW, Luster M, et al. The EANM practice guidelines for parathyroid imaging. Eur J Nucl Med Mol Imaging [Internet]; 2021b Aug 1 [cited 2022 Jun 2];48(9):2801–22. Available from: https://pubmed.ncbi.nlm.nih.gov/33839893/.
128. Petranović Ovčariček P, Schaab J, Beintner-Skawran S, Maurer A, Rupp NJ, Ikenberg K, et al. [18F] Fluorocholine PET/MRI and [18F]Fluorocholine PET/CT as first- and second-line imaging in primary hyperparathyroidism—who takes the lead? Eur J Nucl Med Mol Imaging [Internet]. 2025b [cited 2025 Jun 5]. Available from: https://pubmed.ncbi.nlm.nih.gov/40445316/. Springer.
129. Rager O, Radojewski P, Dumont RA, Treglia G, Giovanella L, Walter MA. Radioisotope imaging for discriminating benign from malignant cytologically indeterminate thyroid nodules. Gland Surg. 2019;8:S118–25. AME Publishing Company.
130. Roser P, Leca BM, Coelho C, Schulte KM, Gilbert J, Drakou EE, et al. Diagnosis and management of parathyroid carcinoma: a state-of-the-art review. Endocr Relat Cancer. 2023;30(4):e220287. BioScientifica Ltd.
131. Russell MD, Orloff LA. Ultrasonography of the thyroid, parathyroids, and beyond [Internet]. HNO. 2022 [cited 2025 Jun 2];70:333–44. Available from: https://pmc.ncbi.nlm.nih.gov/articles/PMC8974803/. Springer Medizin.
132. Sacconi B, Argirò R, Diacinti D, Iannarelli A, Bezzi M, Cipriani C, et al. MR appearance of parathyroid adenomas at 3 T in patients with primary hyperparathyroidism: what radiologists need to know for preoperative localization. Eur Radiol [Internet]. 2016 Mar 1 [cited 2025 Jun 5];26(3):664–73. Available from: https://pubmed.ncbi.nlm.nih.gov/26024849/. Springer Verlag.
133. Schulte KM, Gill AJ, Barczynski M, Karakas E, Miyauchi A, Knoefel WT, et al. Classification of parathyroid cancer. Ann Surg Oncol [Internet]; 2012 Aug 21 [cited 2025 May 28];19(8):2620–8. Available from: https://link.springer.com/article/10.1245/s10434-012-2306-6. Springer.
134. Schulte KM, Talat N, Miell J, Moniz C, Sinha P, Diaz-Cano S. Lymph node involvement and surgical approach in parathyroid cancer. World J Surg [Internet]. 2010 [cited 2025 May 26];34(11):2611–20. Available from: https://pubmed.ncbi.nlm.nih.gov/20640422/. Springer New York LLC.
135. Seki K, Hashimoto K, Hisada T, Maeda M, Satoh T, Uehara Y, et al. A patient with classic severe primary hyperparathyroidism in whom both Tc-99m MIBI scintigraphy and FDG-PET failed to detect the parathyroid tumor. Intern Med [Internet]; 2004 Sep [cited 2025 May 18];43(9):816–23. Available from: https://pubmed.ncbi.nlm.nih.gov/15497517/.
136. Selvan B, Paul MJ, Seshadri MS, Thomas N, Paul T, Abraham D, et al. High index of clinical suspicion with optimal surgical techniques and adjuvant radiotherapy is critical to reduce locoregional disease progression in parathyroid carcinoma. Am J Clin Oncol Cancer Clin Trials [Internet]; 2013 Feb [cited 2025 May 31];36(1):64–9. Available from: https://pubmed.ncbi.nlm.nih.gov/22270105/.
137. Sethi N, England JA. Parathyroid surgery: from inception to the modern day [Internet]. Br J Hosp Med; 2017 [cited 2025 May 31];333–7. Available from: https://pubmed.ncbi.nlm.nih.gov/28614027/. MA Healthcare Ltd.
138. Shane E. Clinical review 122: parathyroid carcinoma [Internet]. J Clin Endocrinol Metab 2001 [cited 2025 May 27];485–93. Available from: https://www.scopus.com/record/display.uri?eid=2-s2.0-0035097021&origin=inward.
139. Shim HK, Kim BS. 18F-FDG PET findings of a parathyroid cancer with cortical skeletal demineralization. Clin Nucl Med. 2012;37(3):293–5.
140. Sidhu PS, Talat N, Patel P, Mulholland NJ, Schulte KM. Ultrasound features of malignancy in the preoperative diagnosis of parathyroid cancer: a retrospective analysis of parathyroid tumours larger than 15 mm. Eur Radiol. 2011;21:1865–73.
141. Silva-Figueroa AM, Hess KR, Williams MD, Clarke CN, Christakis I, Graham PH, et al. Prognostic scoring system to risk stratify parathyroid carcinoma. J Am Coll Surg. 2017;224(5):980–7. Elsevier Inc.
142. Smit MA, Van Kinschot CMJ, Van Der Linden J, Van Noord C, Kos S. Clinical guidelines and PTH measurement: does assay generation matter? [Internet]. Endocr Rev. 2019 [cited 2025 May 29];1468–80. Available from: https://pubmed.ncbi.nlm.nih.gov/31081903/. Oxford University Press.
143. Song A, Yang Y, Liu S, Nie M, Jiang Y, Li M, et al. Prevalence of parathyroid carcinoma and atypical parathyroid neoplasms in 153 patients with multiple endocrine neoplasia type 1: case series and literature review. Front Endocrinol (Lausanne) [Internet]. 2020 Sep 30 [cited 2025 May 18];11:557050. Available from: http://www.ncbi.nlm.nih.gov/pubmed/33101196. Frontiers Media S.A.
144. Storvall S, Leijon H, Ryhänen E, Louhimo J, Haglund C, Schalin-Jäntti C, et al. Somatostatin receptor expression in parathyroid neoplasms. Endocr Connect [Internet]. 2019 Aug 1 [cited 2025 Jun

8];8(8):1213–23. Available from: https://pubmed.ncbi.nlm.nih.gov/31336364/. BioScientifica Ltd.
145. Su C, Zhang J, Yang H, Xu Y, Lu X. Diagnosis and treatment of liver metastases of parathyroid carcinoma. Front Endocrinol (Lausanne) [Internet]. 2022 Oct 11 [cited 2025 Jun 8];13:982972. Available from: https://pmc.ncbi.nlm.nih.gov/articles/PMC9592764/. Frontiers Media S.A.
146. Sun L, Yao J, Hao P, Yang Y, Liu Z, Peng R. Diagnostic role of four-dimensional computed tomography for preoperative parathyroid localization in patients with primary hyperparathyroidism: a systematic review and meta-analysis. Diagnostics [Internet]. 2021 Apr 1 [cited 2025 Jun 3];11(4):664. Available from: https://pubmed.ncbi.nlm.nih.gov/33917261/. Multidisciplinary Digital Publishing Institute (MDPI).
147. Takeuchi Y, Takahashi S, Miura D, Katagiri M, Nakashima N, Ohishi H, et al. Cinacalcet hydrochloride relieves hypercalcemia in Japanese patients with parathyroid cancer and intractable primary hyperparathyroidism. J Bone Miner Metab [Internet]. 2017 Nov 1 [cited 2025 May 31];35(6):616–22. Available from: https://pubmed.ncbi.nlm.nih.gov/27873072/. Springer Tokyo.
148. Talat N, Schulte KM. Clinical presentation, staging and long-term evolution of parathyroid cancer. Ann Surg Oncol [Internet]; 2010 Aug [cited 2025 May 28];17(8):2156–74. Available from: https://pubmed.ncbi.nlm.nih.gov/20221704/.
149. Thanseer NTK, Parihar AS, Sood A, Bhadada SK, Dahiya D, Singh P, et al. Evaluation of recurrent parathyroid carcinoma: a new imaging tool in uncommon entity. World J Nucl Med. 2019;18(02):198–200. Georg Thieme Verlag KG.
150. Torresan F, Iacobone M. Clinical features, treatment, and surveillance of hyperparathyroidism-jaw tumor syndrome: an up-to-date and review of the literature [Internet]. Int J Endocrinol; 2019 [cited 2025 May 28];1761030. Available from: https://doi.org/10.1155/2019/1761030. John Wiley & Sons, Ltd.
151. Treglia G, Piccardo A, Imperiale A, Strobel K, Kaufmann PA, Prior JO, et al. Diagnostic performance of choline PET for detection of hyperfunctioning parathyroid glands in hyperparathyroidism: a systematic review and meta-analysis. Eur J Nucl Med Mol Imaging. 2019;46(3):751–65. Springer Berlin Heidelberg.
152. Treglia G, Sadeghi R, Schalin-Jäntti C, Caldarella C, Ceriani L, Giovanella L. Detection rate of 99mTc-MIBI single photon emission computed tomography (SPECT)/CT in preoperative planning for patients with primary hyperparathyroidism: a meta-analysis. Head Neck. 2016;E2159–72. Wiley.
153. Truran PP, Johnson SJ, Bliss RD, Lennard TWJ, Aspinall SR. Parafibromin, galectin-3, PGP9.5, Ki67, and cyclin D1: using an immunohistochemical panel to aid in the diagnosis of parathyroid cancer. World J Surg. 2014;38(11):2845–54.
154. Tsai WH, Zeng YH, Lee CC, Tsai MC. Mortality factors in recurrent parathyroid cancer: a pooled analysis. J Bone Miner Metab. 2022;40(3):508–17. Springer Japan.
155. Tsukamoto S, Kawabata K, Kawamura H, Takata K, Hosono M. Differentiating brown tumor from bone metastasis in parathyroid cancer using 18F-FDG PET and 99mTc-MIBI SPECT. Clin Nucl Med. 2024;49(5):444–6. Lippincott Williams and Wilkins.
156. Ullah A, Khan J, Waheed A, Sharma N, Pryor EK, Stumpe TR, et al. Parathyroid carcinoma: incidence, survival analysis, and management: a study from the SEER database and insights into future therapeutic perspectives. Cancers (Basel). 2022;14(6). MDPI.
157. Ünlütürk U, Erdoğan MF, Demir Ö, Çulha C, Güllü S, Başkal N. The role of ultrasound elastography in preoperative localization of parathyroid lesions: a new assisting method to preoperative parathyroid ultrasonography. Clin Endocrinol (Oxf) [Internet]. 2012 Apr 1 [cited 2025 Jun 2];76(4):492–8. Available from: https://doi.org/10.1111/j.1365--2265.2011.04241.x. John Wiley & Sons, Ltd.
158. Do Vale RHB, Queiroz MA, Coutinho AMN, Buchpiguel CA, De Menezes MR. 18F-FDG PET/CT osteometabolic activity in metastatic parathyroid carcinoma. Clin Nucl Med. 2016;41(9):724–5. Lippincott Williams and Wilkins.
159. Vijayasarathi A, Karnezis S, Azizyan A, Salamon N, Sepahdari A. 4D CT parathyroid for the general radiologist: a pictorial essay of illustrative cases [Internet]. Curr Probl Diagn Radiol; 2022 [cited 2025 May 18];659–65. Available from: https://pubmed.ncbi.nlm.nih.gov/32216980/. Elsevier Inc.
160. Viswanath A, Drakou EE, Lajeunesse-Trempe F, Grossman AB, Dimitriadis GK. Parathyroid carcinoma: new insights [Internet]. Best Pract Res Clin Endocrinol Metab. 2025 [cited 2025 May 18];101966. Available from: https://www.sciencedirect.com/science/article/pii/S1521690X24001428. Elsevier B.V.
161. Walker MD, Silverberg SJ. Primary hyperparathyroidism [Internet]. Nat Rev Endocrinol. 2018 [cited 2025 May 26];115–25. Available from: https://pubmed.ncbi.nlm.nih.gov/28885621/. Nature Publishing Group.
162. Walton AR, Formby MR, Kumar ASR. Multimodality imaging in parathyroid carcinoma: a tale of two nodules. Radiol Case Reports. 2015;10(1):914. Elsevier Inc.
163. Wang L, Han D, Chen W, Zhang S, Wang Z, Li K, et al. Non-functional parathyroid carcinoma: a case report and review of the literature. Cancer Biol Ther. 2015;16(11):1569–76. Taylor and Francis Inc.
164. Wei B, Zhao T, Shen H, Jin M, Zhou Q, Liu X, et al. Extended en bloc reoperation for recurrent or persistent parathyroid carcinoma: analysis of 31 cases in a single institute experience. Ann Surg Oncol [Internet]. 2022 Feb 1 [cited 2025 Jun 2];29(2):1208–15. Available from: https://pubmed.

ncbi.nlm.nih.gov/34694522/. Springer Science and Business Media Deutschland GmbH.

165. Wei CH, Harari A. Parathyroid carcinoma: update and guidelines for management. Curr Treat Options in Oncol. 2012;13(1):11–23.
166. Wilkins BJ, Lewis JS. Non-functional parathyroid carcinoma: a review of the literature and report of a case requiring extensive surgery. Head Neck Pathol [Internet]. 2009 Jul [cited 2025 May 29];3(2):140–9. Available from: https://pubmed.ncbi.nlm.nih.gov/19644546/.
167. Wojtczak B, Syrycka J, Kaliszewski K, Rudnicki J, Bolanowski M, Barczynski M. Surgical implications of recent modalities for parathyroid imaging [Internet]. Gland Surg. 2020 [cited 2025 Jun 4];S86–94. Available from: https://pmc.ncbi.nlm.nih.gov/articles/PMC7044083/. AME Publishing Company.
168. Xue S, Chen H, Lv C, Shen X, Ding J, Liu J, et al. Preoperative diagnosis and prognosis in 40 parathyroid carcinoma patients. Clin Endocrinol (Oxf). 2016;85(1):29–36. Blackwell Publishing Ltd.
169. Yabanoglu H, Arer IM, Ozarslan F. Parathyroid cancer: review of uncommon disease [Internet]. Acta Endocrinol (Copenh). 2024 [cited 2025 May 14];212–21. Available from: https://pubmed.ncbi.nlm.nih.gov/39845763/. Acta Endocrinologica Foundation.
170. Yao XA, Jiang T, Wei BB, Chang H. Analysis of preoperative predictive factors and clinical characteristics in patients with parathyroid carcinoma. Zhonghua Zhong Liu Za Zhi. 2018;40(6):428–32.
171. Zhang A, Gao T, Wu S, You Z, Zhen J, Wan F. Feasibility of using colloidal gold immunochromatography for point-of-care identification of parathyroid glands during thyroidectomy. Biochem Biophys Res Commun [Internet]. 2018 Dec 9 [cited 2025 May 31];507(1–4):110–3. Available from: https://pubmed.ncbi.nlm.nih.gov/30420286/. Elsevier BV.
172. Zhang M, Sun L, Rui W, Guo R, He H, Miao Y, et al. Semi-quantitative analysis of 99mTc-sestamibi retention level for preoperative differential diagnosis of parathyroid carcinoma. Quant Imaging Med Surg [Internet]. 2019 [cited 2025 Jun 8];9(8):1394–401. Available from: https://pubmed.ncbi.nlm.nih.gov/31559168/. AME Publishing Company.
173. Zhou P, Xu J, Guo Y, Chen L, Liu Y, Guo H, et al. The role of anatomical and functional orientation in identification of parathyroid glands for patients with parathyroidectomy. Front Endocrinol (Lausanne). 2024:15. Frontiers Media SA.
174. Zhu Y, Wang L, You J, Deng S, Shi Y, Liu Z, et al. Diagnostic value of Tc-99m-MIBI SPECT/CT in parathyroid carcinoma with lung metastasis: a case report and literature review. Front Oncol [Internet]; 2024 [cited 2025 Jun 8];14:1501447. Available from: https://pmc.ncbi.nlm.nih.gov/articles/PMC11703706/. Frontiers Media SA.
175. Pathology Outlines [Internet]. [cited 2025 May 28]. Available from: https://www.pathologyoutlines.com/topic/parathyroidstaging.html.

Parathyroid Gland Surgery

12

Grégoire B. Morand and Michael. P. Hier

Definitions

Tetany—Involuntary muscle contractions and spasms due to low calcium levels, often seen after accidental removal or damage to parathyroid glands during thyroid surgery.

Von Recklinghausen's brown tumors—Bone lesions caused by excessive osteoclastic activity in hyperparathyroidism (osteitis fibrosa cystica), appearing as brownish cyst-like masses.

Primary hyperparathyroidism (pHPT)—Excess PTH secretion, usually due to a single adenoma, leading to hypercalcemia and symptoms like kidney stones, osteoporosis, and neurocognitive changes.

Tertiary hyperparathyroidism—Persistent PTH overproduction after long-standing secondary hyperparathyroidism, usually in patients with chronic kidney disease, requiring surgery.

Parathyroid hyperplasia—Enlargement of all parathyroid glands, sometimes linked to genetic syndromes like MEN (multiple endocrine neoplasia).

Focused parathyroidectomy—Minimally invasive surgical removal of a single enlarged gland, guided by preoperative imaging and intraoperative monitoring.

Intraoperative PTH monitoring—Real-time measurement of parathyroid hormone during surgery; a $\geq$ 50% drop in PTH within 10–15 minutes after gland removal indicates successful excision.

Frozen section analysis—Rapid intraoperative histology to confirm excised tissue is parathyroid, though it cannot reliably distinguish adenoma, hyperplasia, or carcinoma.

Recurrent laryngeal nerve (RLN) palsy—Injury to the nerve during surgery leading to hoarseness with vocal cord palsy.

Hungry bone syndrome—Postoperative hypocalcemia due to rapid bone remineralization after removal of hyperfunctioning parathyroid tissue.

Selective venous sampling—Interventional radiology technique where venous blood samples are taken from neck and mediastinal veins to localize hyperfunctioning parathyroid tissue when imaging is inconclusive.

Autofluorescence imaging—Intraoperative technique using near-infrared light to identify parathyroid glands based on their characteristic fluorescence, helping preserve them during surgery.

G. B. Morand (✉)
Department of Otorhinolaryngology - Head & Neck Surgery, University Hospital Zurich, University of Zurich, Zurich, Switzerland
e-mail: gregoire.morand@usz.ch

M. P. Hier
Department of Otolaryngology - Head and Neck Surgery, Jewish General Hospital, McGill University, Montreal, QC, Canada
e-mail: michael.hier@mcgill.ca

© The Author(s), under exclusive license to Springer Nature Switzerland AG 2026
P. Petranović Ovčariček et al. (eds.), *Parathyroid Imaging*,
https://doi.org/10.1007/978-3-032-14178-1_12

Learning Objectives

1. Understand the surgical anatomy and main indications for parathyroid surgery
2. Understand the surgical approaches to parathyroid disorders
   (a) Minimally invasive parathyroidectomy
   (b) Bilateral neck exploration
   (c) Approach to failed exploration/recurrent hyperparathyroidism
3. Understand the value and limitations of intraoperative tools such as
   (a) Intraoperative PTH assay
   (b) Frozen section analysis
   (c) Intraoperative imaging techniques (gamma probe, autofluorescence)

12.1 Introduction

12.1.1 Historical Perspective

The earliest known description of the parathyroid glands is believed to have followed the dissection of a deceased great Indian rhinoceros in London. In 1859, a report presented to the Zoological Society of London described "a small compact yellow glandular body attached to the thyroid at the point where the vein emerged" [1]. The term *glandulae parathyroideae* was later proposed by Ivar Sandström, a medical student from Uppsala, Sweden, who identified parathyroid glands in various animals and in human cadavers [2, 3].

William Halsted played a pivotal role in elucidating the function of the parathyroid glands. Having observed pioneering surgeons Billroth and Kocher performing thyroid surgery, he noted that Kocher's patients experienced a lower incidence of postoperative tetany. Kocher's slower yet more meticulous technique, which incorporated subcapsular dissection [4], likely preserved parathyroid tissue. Halsted is considered the first to recognize the connection between thyroid surgery, inadvertent removal of the parathyroid glands, and the development of postoperative tetany [5].

Von Recklinghausen, whose name remains associated with the syndrome known as neurofibromatosis type 1, published in 1891 on the condition later referred to as "von Recklinghausen brown tumors of the bone," or osteitis fibrosa cystica, observed in hyperparathyroidism. His case series appeared in a commemorative volume honoring the 72nd birthday of the German pathologist Rudolf Virchow [6].

The first successful parathyroidectomy is attributed to the Austrian surgeon Felix Mandl in 1925 [7]. His patient, Albert Gahne, a 34-year-old tram conductor, presented with bone pain and had a medical history notable for surviving World War I, tuberculosis, and syphilis. Radiographs led to a diagnosis of osteitis fibrosa cystica. Mandl removed a 2.5 cm tumor from the left lower pole of the thyroid, resulting in temporary left recurrent laryngeal palsy. Postoperatively, Gahne recovered well and was eventually able to walk without crutches again [7].

Gahne experienced a recurrence approximately 6 years after the initial surgery. Mandle reexplored the neck and upper mediastinum, removing the thyroid gland in the belief that intrathyroidal parathyroid tissue might be present. Histopathology confirmed the presence of two additional parathyroid glands—one located within the thyroid itself. Despite the surgery, Gahne's condition did not improve, and he died a few years later. Postmortem examination revealed no evidence of recurrent parathyroid adenoma in the neck or upper mediastinum. Given that he died from complications of hypercalcemia, some authors postulated that the underlying cause might have been distant, occult metastases from parathyroid carcinoma [7].

12.1.2 Surgical Anatomy

The embryology and general anatomy of the parathyroid glands are described in Chap. 1 in detail. It shall be noted that, in most cases (approximately 85%), patients have four parathyroid glands. About 13% of individuals have more than four parathyroid glands, while the remaining 2% have fewer than four.

From a surgical perspective, it is important to recognize that, owing to their embryology and development, the parathyroid glands maintain a close anatomical relationship with both the recurrent laryngeal nerve and the inferior thyroid artery.

The superior parathyroid glands originate from the fourth pharyngeal pouch, whereas the inferior parathyroid glands arise from the third pharyngeal pouch. Because of their longer embryological migration, anatomical variations are more common in the inferior parathyroid glands. Occasionally, parathyroid gland (usually inferior parathyroid) can be located within the thyroid gland itself [8]. In their typical, non-ectopic position, the inferior parathyroid glands are usually found in close association with the inferior pole of the thyroid, often on the posterolateral aspect of the thyroid capsule at the inferior pole or within 1–2 cm of it. They are frequently related to the thickened adipose tissue of the thyrothymic horn or thyrothymic ligament.

This relationship is also rooted in embryology, as the inferior parathyroid glands migrate together with the thymus during development. In some cases, the inferior parathyroids and thymus fail to separate completely, resulting in a parathyroid gland being located within the thymus.

Other potential sites for ectopic inferior parathyroid glands include any point along the thymic migration pathway, occasionally as far down as the mediastinum [9].

In contrast, the superior parathyroid glands, which originate from the fourth pharyngeal pouch, typically remain close to the thyroid gland because of their shorter migratory path [10].

Both the superior and inferior parathyroid glands receive their arterial blood supply and venous drainage primarily from the inferior thyroid artery and vein. Consequently, during central neck exploration, ligation of branches of the inferior thyroid pedicle can cause a drop in intraoperative PTH levels—changes that may not necessarily indicate the removal of an adenoma. Likewise, studies have shown that the incidence of postoperative hypoparathyroidism is higher following total thyroidectomy when the inferior thyroid artery has been ligated [11].

In terms of anatomical relationships, the inferior parathyroid gland is typically positioned more superficially than the recurrent laryngeal nerve in the coronal plane, whereas the superior parathyroid gland lies deeper than the nerve. This characteristic diagonal course of the nerve between the inferior and superior parathyroid glands has been likened to a "percent (%)" sign (Fig. 12.1, Panel A and B).

12.1.3 Indications for Parathyroid Surgery

Historically, the classical indication for parathyroid surgery was the treatment of symptomatic advanced hyperparathyroidism, typically manifesting as the triad of "stones, bones, and abdominal groans." The widespread adoption of routine laboratory testing has, however, shifted the focus toward detecting and managing earlier, often asymptomatic disease. Today, the primary indications for parathyroid surgery are primary and tertiary hyperparathyroidism. In cases of secondary hyperparathyroidism, the first-line approach is always to address the underlying condition, with the aim of achieving resolution of the hyperparathyroidism.

In primary hyperparathyroidism, the most frequent underlying cause is a single parathyroid adenoma. Multiple adenomas account for approximately 15% of cases [12]. Parathyroid carcinoma is exceptionally rare, representing less than 1% of all causes, and is almost invariably endocrinologically active [13–15].

Another manifestation of primary hyperparathyroidism is parathyroid hyperplasia, in which all glands are slightly enlarged, though often in an asymmetric and sometimes asynchronous fashion. Parathyroid hyperplasia is frequently associated with syndromes such as multiple endocrine neoplasia (MEN) type I and II, and familial hyperparathyroidism. Approximately

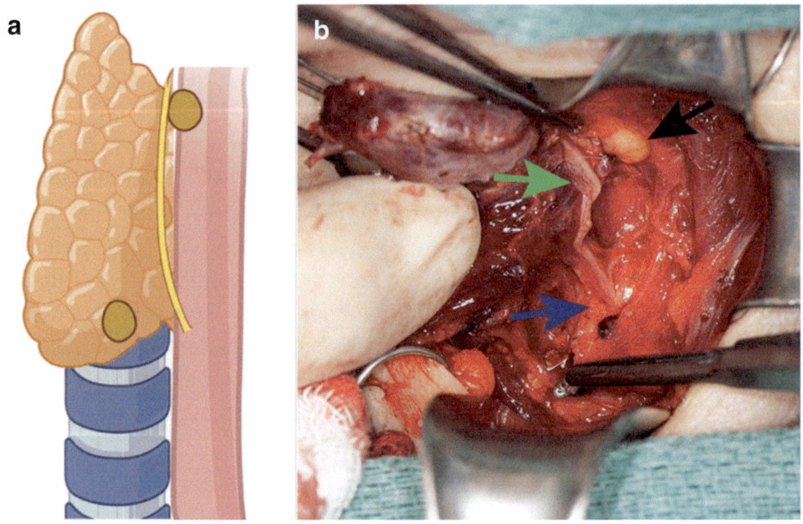

Fig. 12.1 Panel **A**: The "percent (%) sign." Schematic diagram of the left central neck compartment. The recurrent laryngeal nerve (yellow) is shown passing deep to the inferior parathyroid gland and superficial to the superior parathyroid gland. Panel **B**: Intraoperative photograph demonstrating the characteristic "percent (%) sign" configuration during left hemithyroidectomy. The recurrent laryngeal nerve is indicated by the green arrow, the left upper parathyroid gland by the black arrow, and the partially visible left inferior parathyroid gland by the blue arrow. The left thyroid lobe is retracted medially using Allis clamps and the surgeon's finger to expose the surgical field

25% of hyperplasia cases occur as part of a genetic syndrome, while the remaining 75% are sporadic [16]. Histologically, two main forms are recognized: chief cell hyperplasia and primary water-clear cell hyperplasia, the latter not being associated with congenital syndromes [17]. The surgical management of parathyroid hyperplasia generally parallels that tertiary hyperparathyroidism, as discussed below.

Some authors suggest that the patients labeled as "recurrent parathyroid adenoma" may in fact represent asynchronous or asymmetric hyperplasia, with true multiple parathyroid adenomas being exceedingly rare [17]. Their argument is supported by the fact that histologically, adenoma and hyperplasia are virtually the same.

According to the American guidelines for the management of primary hyperparathyroidism (pHPT) [12], indications for parathyroidectomy include symptomatic disease, such as nephrolithiasis, fragility fracture, or vertebral compression fractures identified on imaging, as well as neurocognitive and/or neuropsychiatric symptoms attributable to pHPT. Surgery is also indicated in patients with osteoporosis, defined as a bone mineral density T-score below −2.5 at any site, to prevent further skeletal deterioration. For asymptomatic patients, additional surgical indications include objective evidence of renal involvement, such as silent nephrolithiasis on imaging, nephrocalcinosis, hypercalciuria (24-hour urine calcium level >400 mg/dL) with an increased stone risk, or impaired renal function (glomerular filtration rate <60 mL/min), as well as age under 50 years, and/or a serum calcium level exceeding the upper limit of normal by more than 1 mg/dL [12].

For tertiary hyperparathyroidism, the decision for surgical intervention should always be made in close consultation with the treating nephrologist. As a general rule, surgery is considered in patients with end stage kidney disease who exhibit persistent hyperparathyroidism despite optimal medical management, including vitamin D supplementation and phosphate binders, when PTH levels exceed 1000 pg/dL in the absence of calcimimetic therapy, or remain above 500 pg/dl despite treatment with calcimimetics [18].

Historically, a four-gland parathyroidectomy was performed, followed by reimplantation of half a parathyroid gland into the forearm or strap muscles. However, this technique resulted in permanent hypoparathyroidism in approximately 20% of cases, as the free graft occasionally failed to survive. Consequently, this method has largely been abandoned [19]. The current standard approach to tertiary hyperparathyroidism and/or parathyroid hyperplasia is bilateral neck exploration with excision of three or three and a half glands. After inspecting all four glands, the decision to three or three-and-a-half glands depends on whether the smallest gland is enlarged. The objective is to preserve one normal-sized gland with an intact blood supply, thereby minimizing the risk of recurrence while avoiding permanent hypoparathyroidism. Many surgeons prefer to mark the remaining half or whole parathyroid gland with surgical clips or permanent sutures to facilitate identification in case reexploration is required. Similarly, when a parathyroid gland is implanted in the strap muscles or forearm, it is routinely tagged for the same reason.

12.1.4 From Routine Bilateral Neck Exploration to Focused Parathyroidectomy

In the early days of parathyroid surgery, once surgeons and endocrinologists could reliably identify patients requiring surgery, preoperative localization of the enlarged parathyroid(s) remained challenging. This was largely due to the technical limitations of available imaging modalities at the time, including ultrasonography, early generation CT scanners, and MRI. For ultrasonography, the main reason was comparably low spatial and contrast resolution at the time, while CT and MR suffered, and still suffer today, from a lack of functional capabilities necessary to identify hyperfunctioning parathyroid. As a result, the traditional approach to pHPT was bilateral neck exploration, since intraoperative evaluation of all four glands provided greater diagnostic accuracy than the available imaging modalities.

The technological advancements in preoperative imaging modalities (discussed in other chapters of this book), combined with the increased complexity and potential morbidity of routine bilateral neck exploration, have led to the widespread use of minimally invasive focused parathyroidectomy.

Given the diagnostic uncertainty associated with the "traditional" imaging methods (CT, MRI, scintigraphy, and/or ultrasonography), a common rule of thumb was to require two concordant imaging modalities—ideally an anatomic study such as CT or ultrasonography paired with a functional study such as [99mTc]sestamibi scintigraphy, to confidently proceed with focused parathyroidectomy [20].

With the introduction of highly very sensitive and specific techniques, such as hybrid [18F] fluorocholine-PET, some surgeons now rely on this single imaging modality before proceeding with focused parathyroidectomy [21]. Others, however, still prefer to complement [18F] fluorocholine-PET with dual energy CT or so-called 4D CT to aid in surgical planning and execution [22, 23].

12.2 Surgical Approach

Regardless of the intraoperative strategy, parathyroidectomy is usually performed through a 2–3 cm horizontal midline incision just below the cricoid cartilage. The incision length is primarily determined by the patient's cervical anatomy. After incising the skin, subcutaneous tissue, and fascia (note: in the midline, the platysma is often absent, though a clear fascial plane is usually visible), small inferior and superior subplastysmal-subfascial flaps are raised. The strap muscles are then separated in the midline, providing access to the anterior surface of the thyroid gland. Then the surgeon can follow the plane between the thyroid and the sternothyroid muscle, which forms the deep layer of the strap muscles.

For a lower parathyroid adenoma, the dissection proceeds toward the lower pole of the thyroid gland. In many cases, the adenoma is relatively superficial and encountered before the

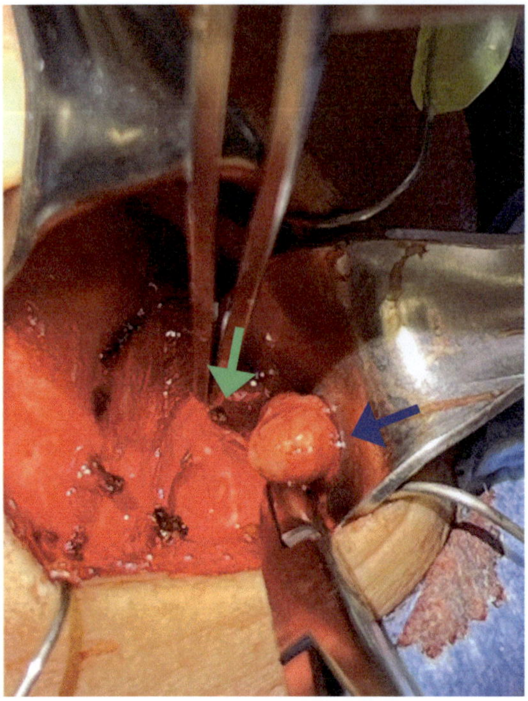

Fig. 12.2 Intraoperative photograph demonstrating a left inferior parathyroid adenoma (blue arrow). Deep to the adenoma, the recurrent laryngeal nerve is partially visible (green arrow)

recurrent laryngeal nerve is identified (Fig. 12.2), though this is not always the case. In contrast, excision of a superior parathyroid adenoma often requires ligation of the middle thyroid vein (Kocher's vein). The lateral thyroid surface is fully dissected, the recurrent laryngeal nerve identified and preserved, and the adenoma is usually encountered deep to the nerve.

During dissection, special care must be taken to avoid damaging the thin adenoma capsule. Capsular injury may cause diffuse, sometimes brisk bleeding that is difficult to control until the adenoma is fully removed. Furthermore, spillage of adenoma cells carries a risk of multifocal recurrence. Gentle, meticulous dissection along the adenoma capsule typically reveals a clear surgical plane. The safest technique relies on blunt dissection, often using a peanut (dental roll) mounted on a hemostat, and grasping tissues adjacent to the adenoma with forceps rather than the capsule itself.

The feeding vessel, usually a branch of the inferior thyroid artery, must always be ligated. In some cases, a rim of normal parathyroid tissue can be identified adjacent to the adenoma, appearing like a "cap" on it. Once hemostasis is secured, the strap muscles are re-approximated, and a double layered skin closure is performed. In most cases, drains are not required.

Several minimally invasive or minimal access techniques have been described for focused parathyroidectomy.

Minimally invasive video-assisted parathyroidectomy (MIVAP), introduced by Miccoli [24], employs a 1.5 cm midline incision. Standard zero-degree endoscopes (commonly used in endoscopic sinus surgery) are utilized to assist dissection through the small access point. The operative steps mirror those of the conventional open approach, with the main difference being endoscopic visualization through the limited incision.

An alternative approach is the *video-assisted parathyroidectomy via the lateral approach (VAPLA)*, described by Henry [25]. Here the incision is made along the anterior border of the sternocleidomastoid muscle. Carbon dioxide insufflation is used to enhance visualization, and two additional trocars are placed, employing technology similar to that used in laparoscopic surgery [25].

Robotic-assisted parathyroidectomy, using either transaxillary or retroauricular approaches, has also been reported. However, its application in parathyroid surgery remains rare, with only sporadic case reports published [26, 27], and it is not widely adopted in clinical practice.

More, recently the *transoral (transvestibular) robotic approach* has been introduced [28]. While large series of over 100 cases have been reported in thyroid surgery, its application in parathyroidectomy remains limited to institutional case reports [29]. The theoretical advantage of avoiding even a small scar (1.5–2 cm) in the midline of the neck must be carefully weighed against the increased cost, complexity, and potential risks of the robotic approach.

12.2.1 Frozen Section Analysis

Frozen section analysis is a commonly used adjunct in parathyroid surgery. Some authors recommend its use in all cases, even when preoperative imaging is concordant and the surgeon is confident in identifying a parathyroid adenoma intraoperatively. Frozen section typically takes 15–20 minutes to complete after excision of the suspected adenoma. In practice, both authors routinely send the specimen for frozen section, closing the strap muscles and skin incision while pathology is processing the tissue. This approach adds only about 5–10 minutes to the total operative time. Importantly, frozen section analysis cannot reliably distinguish hyperplasia, adenoma, or carcinoma. The pathologist can essentially only confirm the presence of "hypercellular parathyroid tissue." While limited, this information provides assurance that the surgery has achieved excision of parathyroid tissue rather than unrelated structures. Misidentification is possible; there are reported cases of lymph nodes, thymic tissue, thyroid nodules, or adipose tissue being excised under the mistaken assumption that they represented parathyroid adenoma [30]. Thus, although frozen section does not eliminate the possibility of recurrence due to asynchronous/asymmetric hyperplasia or the development of multiple adenomas, it provides critical confirmation that the abnormal parathyroid gland targeted at surgery has indeed been resected.

12.2.2 Intraoperative PTH Analysis

Intraoperative parathyroid hormone PTH testing takes advantage of the short half-life of biologically active forms of PTH in serum (approximately 2–5 minutes). The standard approach is to measure PTH levels about 10–15 minutes after removal of the suspected adenoma. A ≥50% drop from the preoperative baseline value is generally considered evidence of successful removal of hyperfunctioning parathyroid tissue (Miami criteria) [31]. Some authors recommend obtaining two intraoperative blood samples: one at the beginning of surgery (baseline) and one after removal of the diseased gland(s), providing real-time comparison. Alternatively, the most recent preoperative PTH value (e.g., from the clinic) can be used as reference, but given the natural fluctuations in PTH levels in individual patients, same-day intraoperative comparisons are preferable.

The use of intraoperative PTH is especially reasonable in cases of equivocal imaging or when multiglandular disease is suspected, where studies have shown higher cure rates with its application [32]. Its principal advantage lies in confirming achievement of the surgical goal—biochemical cure.

A potential pitfall, however, is the occurrence of false-positive results. A temporary drop in PTH may occur if surgical dissection devascularizes the true adenoma, while non-parathyroid tissue or a non-culprit parathyroid gland is excised. Once perfusion of the true adenoma is restored, PTH levels may rise again. To minimize this risk, unnecessary ligation of vessels near the adenoma should be avoided, especially when intraoperative PTH monitoring is relied upon to confirm cure.

Intraoperative PTH testing can also produce false negative results, where no intraoperative PTH drop is observed, yet postoperative levels decrease appropriately. This may occur when manipulation or excision of an adenoma causes spillage of stored hormone into the bloodstream, resulting in transiently elevated intraoperative PTH values. Measuring levels too soon (for example 10 minutes after extensive adenoma handling) may therefore lead to misleadingly high results. Additionally, some patients have physiologically prolonged PTH half-life—due to renal impairment, hepatic dysfunction, or genetic variability producing specific subsets of active PTH variants—which can delay the expected decline and mimic a false negative [33]. To minimize this risk, careful and atraumatic dissection is essential, with particular attention to avoiding compression of the adenoma.

A practical limitation of intraoperative PTH testing is the potential for intraoperative delays. If a false negative is suspected, repeat blood sampling is often required, further prolonging the procedure. In cases involving bilateral exploration, where both frozen section and intraoperative PTH assays are employed, surgical time can become significantly extended, creating logistical challenges in the context of tightly scheduled operating lists.

12.2.3 Intraoperative Gamma Probe

The *Intraoperative gamma probe* can assist surgeons in localizing hyperfunctioning parathyroid glands. Its effective use, however, requires that preoperative conventional scintigraphy demonstrates a clearly localized adenoma with distinct radiotracer uptake and minimal to no uptake in the thyroid gland.

Intraoperatively, the same radiotracer used during preoperative localization studies (see relevant chapters) is administered, and the gamma probe is employed to guide dissection. Of note, this technology is currently unavailable for PET radiotracers. The adoption of intraoperative gamma probe varies considerably worldwide—while some centers use it routinely, many do not incorporate it into standard practice. A commonly cited criterion for success, sometimes referred to as Norman's rule, is a decrease to $\leq 20\%$ of the initial baseline value following adenoma excision [34]. However, the validity and universal applicability of this threshold have been questioned in the literature [35].

An important technical consideration is that the probe used for parathyroidectomy must be highly collimated. This is because background activity in the central neck is significantly higher than in sentinel lymph node biopsies for early-stage oral squamous cell carcinoma [13]. Surgeons accustomed to the latter procedure should be aware of these differences when transitioning to the use of intraoperative gamma probes in parathyroid surgery.

12.2.4 Autofluorescence Imaging

Parathyroid autofluorescence can be used to preserve parathyroid glands during thyroid surgery and to facilitate intraoperative localization of parathyroid adenomas. Parathyroid tissue demonstrates characteristic autofluorescence at a wavelength of approximately 800 nm, which is physiologically than that of the thyroid, adipose tissue, or lymph nodes. An example of a commercially available near-infrared (NIR) system is the Fluobeam®, FDA-approved in 2018 [36]. In a large study including 137 patients undergoing bilateral exploration, 468 parathyroid glands were identified by surgeon recognition and/or pathologic confirmation. NIR correctly identified 451 (96.4%). In the subgroup with at least one positive preoperative localizing study (n = 115), NIR detected 17% (n = 39) of normal glands and 10% (n = 16) of abnormal glands before they were visually recognized by the surgeon. In patients with negative localizing studies (n = 22), NIR identified 12% (n = 4 of 33) of normal glands and 21% (7/34) of abnormal glands prior to visual recognition and subsequent dissection [36].

These findings suggest that autofluorescence may provide added value in parathyroid surgery, particularly when preoperative imaging is negative or equivocal. However, its utility remains debated. Experienced surgeon working in a clear, bloodless field may find that NIR adds little beyond their own recognition skills [37]. Furthermore, practical drawbacks exist: The need to darken the operating room, adjust equipment, and repeatedly alternate between NIR and standard lighting can introduce significant delays. Critics argue that this time might be better spent in careful surgical exploration.

12.2.5 Approach to Recurrent Hyperparathyroidism

In cases of revision surgery, careful planning based on preoperative imaging, prior history, and detailed operative reports is essential. For a successful outcome, a comprehensive personal and surgical history must be obtained, including full review of earlier operative notes. In addition, localization studies should be performed to their fullest extent. These include high-resolution cross-sectional imaging, [18F]fluorocholine PET imaging, and selective venous sampling where appropriate.

When addressing recurrent hyperparathyroidism, it is important to differentiate between true recurrence and failed initial exploration. In true recurrence, patients typically experience a longer interval of normocalcemia, as it may take time for a second adenoma to develop.

In contrast, failed exploration usually presents with a shorter interval before hypercalcemia reappears. The underlying causes of recurrence are diverse. Multiglandular disease is a common explanation, particularly when the initial operation was thought to address a solitary adenoma. In these cases, preoperative workup often reveals a new disease focus in a different anatomical location. By contrast, in failed explorations, the repeated workup is more likely to demonstrate residual or missed disease in close proximity to the original operative field. In situations requiring reexploration on the same side of the neck, some authors recommend obtaining consent for hemithyroidectomy should intraoperative PTH fail to drop, thereby enabling removal of potential intrathyroidal parathyroid tissue. Similarly, if preoperative findings suggest that disease persists in the central compartment, a formal central neck dissection should be considered.

When planning to reexplore a previously operated side, it is essential that the surgeon verify the integrity of the contralateral recurrent laryngeal nerve. This precaution helps avoid exposing the patient to the potentially devastating complications of bilateral vocal cord palsy. If reexploration must be performed in the setting of a contralateral nerve palsy, the risks of bilateral paralysis must be weighed carefully against the expected benefit of surgery.

Intraoperative PTH monitoring is particularly valuable during such complex reexplorations. Measuring PTH at critical steps of the procedure can prevent the surgeon from undertaking further, potentially morbid dissections if biochemical cure has already been achieved. In situations where nerve function is uncertain, many recommend aborting the procedure—even in the absence of a significant intraoperative PTH drop—and instead undertaking a thorough reevaluation. This includes reassessment of histopathology of the previous surgery or surgeries, or repeat high-quality imaging, and renewed surgical planning, rather than putting the contralateral nerve at risk.

A useful adjunct in revision cases is selective venous sampling, particularly if the source of the increased PTH could not be localized by preoperative imaging (Fig. 12.3). This technique takes advantage of the very short half-life of PTH: venous blood drawn from a vein draining a hyperfunctioning parathyroid gland will show elevated PTH compared with more remote sites. The procedure, performed by an interventional radiologist, begins with a baseline peripheral PTH measurement. Sequential samples are then drawn from the upper and lower internal jugular vein (bilaterally); subclavian veins (bilaterally); brachiocephalic (innominate) vein (bilaterally); superior vena cava; and azygos vein (Fig. 12.3). Comparing these values allows inference of the likely location of a hyperfunctioning gland, thereby narrowing the surgical field to a focused reexploration of one side of the neck or even the upper mediastinum.

While selective venous sampling remains a valuable salvage technique in challenging cases, its role may decline further in the future, as highly sensitive imaging methods such as [18F] fluorocholine PET become more widely available. Figure 12.3 illustrates a representative case in which, despite two previous operations including bilateral exploration, conventional imaging remained equivocal. Selective venous sampling clearly localized the adenoma to the upper mediastinum, enabling successful targeted resection.

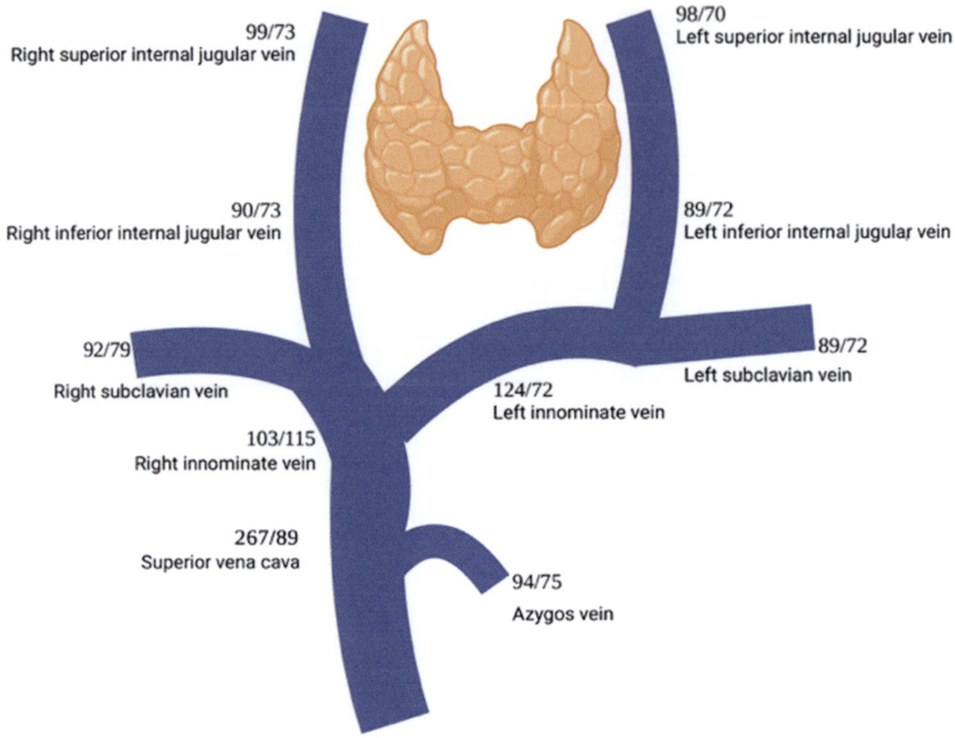

Fig. 12.3 Selective venous sampling in a 23-year-old female with primary hyperparathyroidism. Then patient had a 5-year history of primary hyperparathyroidism with urolithiasis and osteoporosis. She had previously undergone parathyroidectomy at another institution (without intraoperative PTH drop), followed by bilateral neck exploration with removal of three parathyroid glands (again, without PTH decrease). Subsequent diagnostic workup after failed exploration showed mild [99mTc]sestamibi uptake on SPECT imaging at the aortopulmonary location, which could not be confirmed on dual-energy CT. Selective venous sampling, however, localized a hyperfunctioning adenoma to the superior vena cava region. Based on these findings, mini-sternotomy was performed, and a 1.5 cm adenoma was identified and excised from the aortopulmonal window. Postoperatively, PTH dropped to 16 pg/ml, confirming biochemical cure
(All PTH values shown are in pg/ml. The numerator represents the PTH value at the sampled location; the denominator represents the simultaneous control value obtained from a peripheral vein.)

12.2.6 Complications

Besides the general complications of surgery (such as hematoma or surgical site infection) and the sequelae of any surgical intervention (including visible scarring and deep tissue fibrosis), there are several complications specific to parathyroidectomy.

The most significant is injury to the recurrent laryngeal nerve. As noted above, adenomas of the inferior parathyroid gland are less likely to endanger the nerve due to their more superficial location in relation to the nerve. In contrast, surgery of the superior parathyroid adenomas more often requires careful management of the RLN, as the superior glands are typically situated in a coronal plane deep to the nerve (Fig. 12.1). However, caution is warranted since superior adenomas can enlarge and displace the nerve anteriorly, bringing it into the field early during dissection of the anterolateral adenoma surface. Over time, superior adenomas may also descend along the tracheoesophageal groove and mimic inferior parathyroid adenomas on imaging in the axial plane. In such cases, dissection may require exposure not only of the RLN but also of the esophagus and, occasionally, even the prevertebral fascia.

In the event of RLN injury, it is crucial to distinguish between neurotmesis and neurapraxia. True transection (neurotmesis) should remain exceedingly rare in elective parathyroid surgery. If it occurs, a primary anastomosis of the transected ends is advisable, even though normal vocal cord mobility will not be restored. Nonetheless, reinnervation prevents atrophy of the vocalis muscle and improves voice quality, thereby facilitating rehabilitation. In cases of neurapraxia, spontaneous recovery of vocal function can be expected within 1–4 months. There is clear evidence showing that intraoperative neuromonitoring with RLN electrostimulation reduces the incidence of nerve injury in thyroid and parathyroid surgery [38, 39]. Furthermore, recent evidence data suggest improved surgical outcomes with the use of magnification (surgical loupes) in thyroid surgery [40]. While extrapolation of this evidence to parathyroid surgery remains unproven, it is reasonable to assume similar benefits.

Hematoma formation should also be exceedingly rare in parathyroid surgery. The branches of the inferior thyroid artery must be meticulously ligated, which not only reduces bleeding risk but also facilitates mobilization of the adenoma. The use of drains is rarely indicated, as they do not prevent hematoma formation [41].

Postoperatively, serum calcium and PTH levels must be monitored closely to detect and manage hypocalcemia, particularly due to hungry bone syndrome [42]. This complication most often arises in patients with markedly elevated preoperative PTH levels (≥200 pg/ml up). This occurs because PTH-driven osteoblastic activity persists for several hours to days (in some rare cases even weeks! [43]) following parathyroid adenoma or carcinoma removal, while the hypercalcemic effects of PTH cease immediately after removal of the hyperfunctioning gland [44].

References

1. Professor Owen FRS F, c. III. On the anatomy of the Indian Rhinoceros (Rh. unicornis, L.). Trans Zool Soc Lond. 1852;4(2):31–58.
2. On a new gland in man and several mammals (Glandulæ Parathyreoideæ). JAMA J Am Med Assoc. 1938;111(2):197. https://doi.org/10.1001/jama.1938.02790280087037.
3. Ivar Sandström (1852–1889) Witness to the parathyroids. JAMA. 1966;196(8):733. https://doi.org/10.1001/jama.1966.03100210103034.
4. The operative story of Goitre. The author's operation. JAMA J Am Med Assoc. 1920;74(10):693–4. https://doi.org/10.1001/jama.1920.02620100053037.
5. MacCallum WG, Voegtlin C. On the relation of tetany to the parathyroid glands and to calcium metabolism. J Exp Med. 1909;11(1):118–51.
6. von Recklinghausen F. Die fibrose oder deformierende Ostitis, die Osteomalacic und die osteoplastische Carcinose, in ihren gegenseitigen Beziehungen. Rudolf Virchow Festschriften. 1891:1–89.
7. Mandl F. Clinical and experimental questions about localised and generalised osteitis fibrosa [in German]. Arch Klin Chir. 1926;143:245.
8. Gowrishankar SV, Bidaye R, Das T, Majcher V, Fish B, Casey R, et al. Intrathyroidal parathyroid adenomas: scoping review on clinical presentation, preoperative localization, and surgical treatment. Head Neck. 2023;45(3):706–20. https://doi.org/10.1002/hed.27287.
9. Marzouki HZ, Chavannes M, Tamilia M, Hier MP, Black MJ, Levental M, et al. Location of parathyroid adenomas: 7-year experience. J Otolaryngol--Head & Neck Surg. 2010;39(5)
10. Mansberger AR, Wei JP. Surgical embryology and anatomy of the thyroid and parathyroid glands. Surg Clin N Am. 1993;73(4):727–46. https://doi.org/10.1016/S0039-6109(16)46082-2.
11. Thomusch O, Machens A, Sekulla C, Ukkat J, Brauckhoff M, Dralle H. The impact of surgical technique on postoperative hypoparathyroidism in bilateral thyroid surgery: a multivariate analysis of 5846 consecutive patients. Surgery. 2003;133(2):180–5.
12. Wilhelm SM, Wang TS, Ruan DT, Lee JA, Asa SL, Duh Q-Y, et al. The American Association of Endocrine Surgeons Guidelines for definitive management of primary hyperparathyroidism. JAMA Surg. 2016;151(10):959–68. https://doi.org/10.1001/jamasurg.2016.2310.
13. Rubello D, Kapse N, Grassetto G, Massaro A, Al-Nahhas A. Minimally invasive radio-guided surgery for primary hyperparathyroidism: from preoperative to intraoperative localization imaging. Ann Endocrinol. 2010;71(6):511–8. https://doi.org/10.1016/j.ando.2010.08.001.
14. Morand GB, Helmchen BM, Steinert HC, Schmid C, Broglie MA. 18F-Choline-PET in parathyroid carcinoma. Oral Oncol. 2018;86:314–5. https://doi.org/10.1016/j.oraloncology.2018.09.009.
15. Morand GB, Rupp NJ, Huellner MW, Gerber PA, Soyka MB, Broglie MA, et al. Transnasal-transpterygoid endoscopic removal of an 18F-choline-avid parathyroid carcinoma metastasis in the skull base. JAMA Otolaryngol Head

Neck Surg. 2019;145(10):978–80. https://doi.org/10.1001/jamaoto.2019.2352.
16. Marx SJ, Simonds WF, Agarwal SK, Burns AL, Weinstein LS, Cochran C, et al. Hyperparathyroidism in hereditary syndromes: special expressions and special managements. J Bone Miner Res. 2002;17:N37–43.
17. DeLellis RA. Parathyroid tumors and related disorders. Mod Pathol. 2011;24(2):S78–93. https://doi.org/10.1038/modpathol.2010.132.
18. Delos Santos R, Rossi A, Coyne D, Maw TT. Management of post-transplant hyperparathyroidism and bone disease. Drugs. 2019;79(5):501–13. https://doi.org/10.1007/s40265-019-01074-4.
19. Gagné ER, Ureña P, Leite-Silva S, Zingraff J, Chevalier A, Sarfati E, et al. Short- and long-term efficacy of total parathyroidectomy with immediate autografting compared with subtotal parathyroidectomy in hemodialysis patients. J Am Soc Nephrol. 1992;3(4):1008–17. https://doi.org/10.1681/asn.V341008.
20. Munk RS, Payne RJ, Luria BJ, Hier MP, Black MJ. Preoperative localization in primary hyperparathyroidism. J Otolaryngol Head Neck Surg. 2008;37(3):347–54.
21. Ferrari SB, Morand GB, Rupp NJ, Krutzfeldt J, Vetter D, Hullner MW, et al. Clinical predictors of negative/equivocal SPECT imaging outcomes in primary hyperparathyroidism: factors calling for (18)F-choline-PET. Am J Otolaryngol. 2024;45(4):104315. https://doi.org/10.1016/j.amjoto.2024.104315.
22. Roskies M, Liu X, Hier MP, Payne RJ, Mlynarek A, Forest V, et al. 3-phase dual-energy CT scan as a feasible salvage imaging modality for the identification of non-localizing parathyroid adenomas: a prospective study. J Otolaryngol-Head & Neck Surg. 2015;44(1):44.
23. Forghani R, Roskies M, Liu X, Tan X, Mlynarek A, Payne RJ, et al. Dual-energy CT characteristics of parathyroid adenomas on 25-and 55-second 4D-CT acquisitions: preliminary experience. J Comput Assist Tomogr. 2016;40(5):806–14.
24. Miccoli P, Berti P, Materazzi G, Donatini G. Minimally invasive video assisted parathyroidectomy (MIVAP). Eur J Surg Oncol. 2003;29(2):188–90. https://doi.org/10.1053/ejso.2002.1313.
25. Henry JF, Iacobone M, Mirallie E, Deveze A, Pili S. Indications and results of video-assisted parathyroidectomy by a lateral approach in patients with primary hyperparathyroidism. Surgery. 2001;130(6):999–1004. https://doi.org/10.1067/msy.2001.119112.
26. Lee JM, Byeon HK, Choi EC, Koh YW. Robotic excision of a huge parathyroid adenoma via a retroauricular approach. J Craniofac Surg. 2015;26(1):e55–8. https://doi.org/10.1097/scs.0000000000001308.
27. Paspala A, Spartalis E, Nastos C, Tsourouflis G, Dimitroulis D, Pikoulis E, et al. Robotic-assisted parathyroidectomy and short-term outcomes: a systematic review of the literature. J Robot Surg. 2020;14(6):821–7. https://doi.org/10.1007/s11701-020-01119-x.
28. Ozdenkaya Y, Ersavas C, Arslan NC. Robotic transoral vestibular parathyroidectomy: two case reports and review of literature. World J Clin Cases. 2018;6(12):542.
29. Tae K, Ji YB, Song CM, Park JS, Park JH, Kim DS. Safety and efficacy of transoral robotic and endoscopic thyroidectomy: the first 100 cases. Head Neck. 2020;42(2):321–9.
30. Johnson SJ, Sheffield EA, McNicol AM. Best practice no 183. Examination of parathyroid gland specimens. J Clin Pathol. 2005;58(4):338–42. https://doi.org/10.1136/jcp.2002.002550.
31. Barczynski M, Konturek A, Hubalewska-Dydejczyk A, Cichon S, Nowak W. Evaluation of Halle, Miami, Rome, and Vienna intraoperative iPTH assay criteria in guiding minimally invasive parathyroidectomy. Langenbeck's Arch Surg. 2009;394(5):843–9. https://doi.org/10.1007/s00423-009-0510-z.
32. Bilezikian JP, Khan AA, Silverberg SJ, Fuleihan GE, Marcocci C, Minisola S, et al. Evaluation and management of primary hyperparathyroidism: summary statement and guidelines from the fifth international workshop. J Bone Miner Res. 2022;37(11):2293–314. https://doi.org/10.1002/jbmr.4677.
33. Graves CE, Campbell MJ. Variation in PTH levels and kinetics after parathyroidectomy. Am J Surg. 2025;239:116010. https://doi.org/10.1016/j.amjsurg.2024.116010.
34. Murphy C, Norman J. The 20% rule: a simple, instantaneous radioactivity measurement defines cure and allows elimination of frozen sections and hormone assays during parathyroidectomy. Surgery. 1999;126(6):1023–8; discussion 8-9. https://doi.org/10.1067/msy.2099.101578.
35. Friedman M, Gurpinar B, Schalch P, Joseph NJ. Guidelines for radioguided parathyroid surgery. Arch Otolaryngol Head Neck Surg. 2007;133(12):1235–9. https://doi.org/10.1001/archotol.133.12.1235.
36. Kose E, Rudin AV, Kahramangil B, Moore E, Aydin H, Donmez M, et al. Autofluorescence imaging of parathyroid glands: an assessment of potential indications. Surgery. 2020;167(1):173–9. https://doi.org/10.1016/j.surg.2019.04.072.
37. Lerchenberger M, Al Arabi N, Gallwas JKS, Stepp H, Hallfeldt KKJ, Ladurner R. Intraoperative near-infrared autofluorescence and indocyanine green imaging to identify parathyroid glands: a comparison. Int J Endocrinol. 2019;2019(1):4687951. https://doi.org/10.1155/2019/4687951.
38. Kim J, Graves CE, Jin C, Duh QY, Gosnell JE, Shen WT, et al. Intraoperative nerve monitoring is associated with a lower risk of recurrent laryngeal nerve injury: a national analysis of 17,610 patients. Am J Surg. 2021;221(2):472–7. https://doi.org/10.1016/j.amjsurg.2020.10.013.

39. Scharpf J, Liu JC, Sinclair C, Singer M, Liddy W, Orloff L, et al. Critical review and consensus statement for neural monitoring in otolaryngologic head, neck, and endocrine surgery. Otolaryngol Head Neck Surg. 2022;166(2):233–48.
40. Rao KN, Zafereo M, Rao AN, Nixon I, Robbins KT, Sreeram MP, et al. Implication of surgical loupes on complications following thyroidectomy: a meta-analysis. Eur Arch Otorrinolaringol. 2025;282(3):1159–69. https://doi.org/10.1007/s00405-024-09003-2.
41. Corsten M, Johnson S, Alherabi A. Is suction drainage an effective means of preventing hematoma in thyroid surgery? A meta-analysis. J Otolaryngol. 2005;34(6):415.
42. Graf C, Huellner M, Tschopp O, Bode-Lesniewska B, Schmid C. (18)F-NaF-PET/CT in patients with primary hyperparathyroidism and brown tumors. J Bone Miner Metab. 2020;38(3):299–309. https://doi.org/10.1007/s00774-019-01059-z.
43. Juárez-León ÓA, Gómez-Sámano MÁ, Cuevas-Ramos D, Almeda-Valdés P, López-Flores A, La Torre MA, Reza-Albarrán AA, et al. Atypical parathyroid adenoma complicated with protracted hungry bone syndrome after surgery: a case report and literature review. Case Rep Endocrinol. 2015;2015(1):757951. https://doi.org/10.1155/2015/757951.
44. Jain N, Reilly RF. Hungry bone syndrome. Curr Opin Nephrol Hypertens. 2017;26(4):250–5.

Brown Tumors

13

Sonya Joy, Martin W. Huellner, and Bert-Ram Sah

Definitions

- Brown tumor: A reactive, osteolytic bone lesion driven by excess PTH with osteoclast activation; composed of fibrovascular stroma with hemorrhage and hemosiderin.
- Prevalence (brown tumors): <5% in primary, <2% in secondary hyperparathyroidism.
- Giant cell-rich lesion (histology): Proliferation of osteoclast-type multinucleated giant cells within a hemorrhagic fibrous stroma containing hemosiderin-laden macrophages.
- Skeletal predilection of brown tumors: Any bone may be affected, but facial bones (including mandible), ribs, clavicles, pelvis, and femur are common locations.
- Radiographic appearance of brown tumors: Well-defined, lytic, expansile lesions, typically solitary or few; often occur with generalized osteopenia and other signs of hyperparathyroidism.
- Differential diagnosis for brown tumors: Includes giant cell tumor, central giant cell granuloma, aneurysmal bone cyst, lytic metastasis. Accurate identification relies on a comprehensive imaging strategy integrating morphological and functional modalities; correlation with laboratory values is necessary.
- Post-parathyroidectomy regression: Brown tumors typically regress after correction of hyperparathyroidism.
- Hungry bone syndrome (HBS): Rapid, profound, and prolonged hypocalcemia with hypophosphatemia and hypomagnesemia after parathyroidectomy in patients with high preoperative bone turnover, necessitating intensive calcium and active vitamin D replacement.

S. Joy
Department of Diagnostic, Interventional, and Pediatric Radiology, Inselspital, and University of Bern, Bern, Switzerland

M. W. Huellner
Department of Nuclear Medicine, University Hospital Zurich / University of Zurich, Zurich, Switzerland
e-mail: martin.huellner@usz.ch

B.-R. Sah (✉)
Department of Diagnostic, Interventional, and Pediatric Radiology, Inselspital, and University of Bern, Bern, Switzerland

Department of Nuclear Medicine, University Hospital Zurich, and University of Zurich, Zurich, Switzerland

Learning Objectives

After completing this chapter, readers will be able to:

- Explain the pathophysiologic mechanisms by which elevated PTH leads to the development of brown tumors.
- Describe the radiologic characteristics that distinguish brown tumors from primary bone neoplasms and other osteolytic bone lesions.

© The Author(s), under exclusive license to Springer Nature Switzerland AG 2026
P. Petranović Ovčariček et al. (eds.), *Parathyroid Imaging*,
https://doi.org/10.1007/978-3-032-14178-1_13

- Correlate laboratory parameters (including serum calcium, phosphate, and PTH levels) with imaging findings to support diagnostic accuracy.
- Outline therapeutic strategies for hyperparathyroidism and discuss their impact on the regression of brown tumors.
- Identify key considerations in the differential diagnosis of osteolytic bone lesions in endocrine disorders.

13.1 Introduction

Brown tumors are rare, reactive, and non-neoplastic bone lesions that can develop in the context of hyperparathyroidism [1–3]. Elevated parathyroid hormone levels stimulate osteoclastic bone resorption, leading to loss of both cortical and trabecular bone, and consequently, hypercalcemia in primary or tertiary hyperparathyroidism [4–6]. In secondary hyperparathyroidism serum calcium may be normal or low. In response, fibroblastic proliferation and woven bone formation occur as part of a reparative process [1, 3, 6]. Collectively, these changes represent focal areas of severe osteitis fibrosa cystica within a high-turnover remodeling state [3]. Since brown tumors do not contain parathyroid cells, they do not synthesize PTH and therefore do not contribute to elevated PTH levels in patients with hyperparathyroidism.

Brown tumors may develop in primary, secondary, and tertiary hyperparathyroidism [1, 2]. In adults, primary hyperparathyroidism is most commonly caused by a solitary parathyroid adenoma, less frequently by multiglandular disease, and only rarely by parathyroid carcinoma [6, 7]. These conditions can also be part of hereditary syndromes. Secondary hyperparathyroidism typically arises as part of chronic kidney disease-mineral and bone disorder (CKD-MBD). Over time, persistent stimulation can lead to autonomous parathyroid activity, resulting in tertiary hyperparathyroidism [8, 9].

Management depends on the underlying cause. Treatment of secondary hyperparathyroidism focuses on correcting abnormalities in calcium, phosphorus, and vitamin D [3]. Parathyroidectomy remains the definitive therapy for primary hyperparathyroidism, while surgical intervention may also be indicated for refractory secondary or tertiary disease.

Epidemiology

In modern clinical series, the prevalence of brown tumors in primary hyperparathyroidism is reported to be less than 5%, while in secondary hyperparathyroidism it is below 2% [2, 9]. The prevalence in tertiary hyperparathyroidism remains uncertain due to limited data [8]. The classical skeletal manifestations of primary hyperparathyroidism have become increasingly uncommon due to earlier biochemical detection and timely surgical intervention [9, 10]. Despite overall declines, regional variations persist. Advanced skeletal disease continues to occur in resource-limited settings, where routine screening and access to early treatment is limited [11]. Brown tumors can affect both sexes but demonstrate a female predominance, consistent with the higher prevalence of primary hyperparathyroidism among women. Most reported cases involve adult patients in contemporary institutional cohorts, though pediatric and adolescent presentations may also occur.

Pathophysiology and Histology

Persistent parathyroid hormone (PTH) excess stimulates osteoclastogenesis and shifts bone remodeling toward resorption rather than formation, resulting in diffuse osteopenia. Focally, this overactivity produces bone marrow expansion and lytic change, with cortical thinning and replacement of normal marrow by fibrovascular tissue, but notably without malignant infiltration (also in the presence of a parathyroid carcinoma being responsible for the hyperparathyroidism) [5, 6, 10, 12]. These processes underlie the development of subperiosteal bone erosions and cystic excavations [3]. In more detail, osteoclasts resorb the trabecular bone in areas of excessive remodeling, and this cycle of disproportionate resorption and reparative stromal proliferation may extend beyond the bone's normal contours, leading to expansile remodeling of the affected region.

Histologically, brown tumors consist of a fibroblastic stroma interspersed with numerous osteoclast-type multinucleated giant cells [8]. Areas of hemorrhage and hemosiderin deposition impart the distinctive brown coloration of the lesion [1, 3]. The coexistence of active osteoclastic resorption and surrounding osteoblastic repair reflects the high-turnover state of osteitis fibrosa cystica. Importantly, the absence of cytologic atypia distinguishes this (tumor-like) reactive process from a true neoplasm.

13.2 Clinical Implications

Brown tumors can arise in virtually any skeletal site, though certain patterns of distribution are recognized across clinical cohorts. Extra-craniofacial lesions most frequently involve the ribs, clavicles, pelvis, femur, tibia, and proximal humerus [1, 2, 4]. Within the oral and maxillofacial region, the mandible is most commonly affected, followed by the maxilla [9]. Brown tumors may occur as solitary or multifocal lesions.

Patients may present with localized bone pain, swelling, or pathologic fractures at the time of diagnosis [13]. Some individuals experience symptoms of hypercalcemia or neurologic deficits secondary to compressive lesion growth. In many cases, brown tumors are discovered incidentally during imaging performed for unrelated complaints [1, 2]. Because their radiologic appearance can closely mimic malignancy, there is a significant risk of misclassification and even inappropriate oncologic intervention [9]. Accurate diagnosis therefore relies on multidisciplinary evaluation, integrating biochemical, radiologic, and clinical data to prevent diagnostic delays and ensure appropriate management.

The clinical symptoms depend on the specific bones that are affected. Pelvic and sacral lesions may compromise acetabular support or manifest in the sacral region, where neurologic complications might arise from local mass effect [2]. Femoral involvement increases the risk of pathologic fracture due to focal expansile osteolysis [1]. Rib and clavicular lesions can cause chest wall pain or present as palpable masses [2]. Although spinal epidural extension of vertebral lesions is rare, it necessitates vigilance for signs of progressive neurologic deficit. In the absence of appropriate treatment, continued catabolic activity leads to bone fragility, deformity, and recurrent fractures [5, 14]. Consequently, diagnostic delay can result in preventable morbidity and increase procedural risk.

Radiologists and nuclear medicine physicians play a central role in preventing these outcomes. Comprehensive anatomic mapping and whole-skeleton functional imaging help delineate lesion extent, assess cortical stability, and evaluate overall disease burden, while also aiding in the exclusion of malignant mimics. Prompt biochemical assessment, including serum calcium and PTH levels, is essential to avoid misclassification. Timely interpretation and referral facilitate endocrine correction and substantially reduce cumulative skeletal morbidity.

Post-therapeutic Clinical Implications/ Hungry Bone Syndrome

Most brown tumors regress following correction of hyperparathyroidism, although complete resolution may take several months, and some destructive structural defects can persist despite normalization of biochemical markers [12]. Historical reports indicate that extensive bone involvement and older age are associated with a slower or incomplete rate of brown tumor regression after parathyroidectomy [12].

Rapid skeletal remineralization following parathyroidectomy can trigger Hungry Bone Syndrome (HBS), a potentially severe hypocalcemic condition commonly seen in patients with hyperparathyroidism (HPT), particularly those with brown tumors, especially after secondary hyperparathyroidism [7, 15]. The abrupt postoperative decline in PTH shifts bone remodeling toward osteoblastic dominance, while osteoclast activity remains normal or reduced [16]. As remineralization consumes calcium, clinically significant hypocalcemia can develop, potentially leading to tetany or even acute cardiac symptoms [7, 15]. HBS is typically accompanied by normal or high PTH levels, distinguishing it from hypocalcemia caused by hypoparathyroidism [7]. Hypocalcemia generally begins between postoperative days 3 and 5, and is usually temporary, but may persist if all parathyroid glands are removed or devascularized [7]. In severe cases, continuous i.v. replacement of calcium can be necessary. Multidisciplinary monitoring is critical to minimize morbidity and support optimal recovery.

Preoperative risk stratification for HBS incorporates biochemical and skeletal markers. Elevated PTH and alkaline phosphatase (ALP), together with low 25-hydroxyvitamin D, indicate a higher risk [7]. The presence of preoperative parathyroid-related bone lesions is also significantly associated with the development of postoperative HBS [15]. HBS occurs more frequently after parathyroidectomy for renal hyperparathyroidism, where the clinical manifestation of HBS is more severe [15].

13.3 Imaging

Baseline Imaging

Whole-body cross-sectional and molecular imaging allows mapping of brown tumor distribution, quantification of skeletal activity, guidance of treatment, and monitoring of therapeutic response. However, morphological features across imaging modalities are not fully specific, and tracer uptake primarily reflects non-specific bone remodeling, limiting standalone diagnostic certainty. Therefore, imaging interpretation must be correlated with biochemical parameters, especially serum calcium and parathyroid hormone, and considered in the clinical context. Multimodal integration enhances specificity and reduces the risk of misclassification. When imaging and laboratory findings remain inconclusive, image-guided biopsy can confirm the diagnosis and inform management [17].

Post-therapeutic Imaging

After parathyroidectomy, radiologists and nuclear medicine physicians must distinguish healing changes from residual or recurrent brown tumors to guide management and avoid unnecessary interventions. Following endocrine correction, radiotracer uptake (particularly FDG) typically declines, indicating metabolic resolution, and also distinguishing these bone lesions from metastases due to parathyroid carcinoma, which would not respond to normalization of serum calcium levels [1]. Nevertheless, brown tumors can maintain elevated bone turnover for extended periods, and lesions may appear "active" during early postoperative remodeling, particularly with bone-seeking radiotracers, making single time-point assessment unreliable [18]. Structural changes evolve in parallel, with increased mineralization and partial lesion shrinkage [12]. Lack of size regression should not be overinterpreted as persistent disease without biochemical confirmation [1]. Conversely, uptake that plateaus or rises against expected trends may indicate incomplete biochemical control or different pathology. Consequently, imaging integrated with biochemical context and assessment of morphologic remodeling provides the most reliable differentiation between post-therapeutic healing, residual/recurrent disease, and coincident malignancy. A summary of the different modalities can be found in Table 13.1.

13.3.1 Conventional Radiography

On radiographs, decreased bone density appears as increased lucency, cortical thinning, and trabecular rarefaction. An early hallmark of hyperparathyroidism is subperiosteal erosion, presenting as localized, irregular cortical resorption, most apparent at the phalanges. In the skull, the characteristic salt-and-pepper appearance may be found [9].

Brown tumors are often expansile, and may show cortical thinning or extension beyond normal bone contours [2].

Table 13.1 Comparative utility of different radionuclide imaging studies in detecting brown tumors and related findings

	Sensitivity for BT	Specificity for BT	Changes after therapy	Diagnostic clues
^{99m}Tc-MIBI Scintigraphy / SPECT/CT	*Low*—variable or absent osseous uptake on whole-body MIBI despite parathyroid localization properties	*Low*—lack of MIBI in bone lesions is nonspecific; many metastases also lack uptake	Parathyroid adenoma MIBI uptake disappears Brown tumor foci, if faint on MIBI, resolve Post-surgery bone healing is better monitored on CT or FDG-PET than on MIBI	Known parathyroid pathology: FDG-positive/ MIBI-negative bone lesions favor brown tumors
^{99m}Tc-MDP Bone Scintigraphy / SPECT/CT	*High*—reflects increased osteoblastic activity	*Low*—overlaps with fractures, metabolic bone disease, and other benign and malignant processes Superscan with diffuse, symmetric skeletal uptake may indicate brown tumors	Transient rise of bone-scan activity with healing or decline as lesions re-ossify, reflecting variable post-treatment kinetics. Persistent generalized uptake for months in patients with hungry bone syndrome	In biochemically proven HPT, diffuse metabolic uptake with superimposed focal MDP hot spots indicate brown tumors rather than metastases
^{18}F-FDG PET/ CT	*High*—multiple hypermetabolic bone lesions, including small ones Intense FDG uptake, comparable to malignant lesions	*Low*—increased skeletal tracer uptake may mimic metastatic disease Clinical correlation required	FDG uptake in brown tumors usually decreases or resolves, and lesions become sclerotic on CT	FDG-avid lytic lesions in a hypercalcemic, high-PTH patient should trigger a work-up for brown tumors and prompt targeted parathyroid imaging to prevent misclassification as metastatic disease
^{18}F-NaF PET/ CT	*High*—avid uptake on NaF PET/CT, may mimic metastases	*Low*—increased skeletal tracer uptake may mimic metastatic disease Clinical correlation required	NaF uptake usually resolves NaF metrics correlate with PTH and ALP	NaF PET/CT may quantify skeletal disease burden and guide risk assessment in severe HPT, interpreting skeletal foci as brown tumors if CT morphology and laboratory parameters support the diagnosis
^{18}F-FCH PET/ CT	*High*—superior to ^{99m}Tc-MIBI Superior performance for localizing hyperfunctioning parathyroid tissue	*Low*—increased skeletal tracer uptake may mimic metastatic disease Clinical correlation required	FCH uptake in brown tumors resolves, but FCH-specific longitudinal response evidence is limited	May identify parathyroid adenoma and simultaneous skeletal lesions in a single examination, indicating brown tumors rather than metastases

Radiographs serve as a first-line modality, offering accessible and cost-effective information. Multiple lytic lesions in the absence of known malignancy should prompt biochemical evaluation for hyperparathyroidism. Radiographs also document lesion size and location and facilitate fracture-risk assessment [19]. Following parathyroidectomy, lesions gradually calcify and re-densify over months [1, 4]. Limitations of radiographs include low sensitivity in early disease and limited specificity, as radiographic features may mimic other pathologies [5].

Nonetheless, conventional radiography remains central to initial evaluation, skeletal mapping, treatment planning, and monitoring post-parathyroidectomy response.

13.3.2 Computed Tomography (CT)

CT provides detailed evaluation of bone morphology and architecture, enhancing diagnostic accuracy and supporting treatment planning. Diffuse osteopenia appears as generalized reduced attenuation, cortical thinning, and trabecular rarefaction. Early disease manifests as subperiosteal erosions with irregular cortical resorption and discontinuity, most apparent along the radial aspects of the phalanges [1]. Brown tumors present as osteolytic lesions that may show "ground glass opacification", marginal sclerosis and internal septa [1, 12]. Cortical involvement ranges from thinning to rare cortical breakthrough [2]. Lesion size varies from millimeters to several centimeters, occasionally producing expansile mass effect [1].

CT is particularly valuable for incidental identification of multiple well-defined lytic lesions, prompting timely biochemical testing. It also serves as an anatomic roadmap for surgical planning, stabilization decisions, and biopsy guidance. Compared with radiography, CT has higher sensitivity for subtle cortical erosions and quantitative assessment of cortical thickness, improving diagnostic confidence.

After parathyroidectomy, CT often demonstrates progressive sclerosis and partial shrinkage of brown tumors. However, morphologic evaluation alone cannot reliably distinguish brown tumors from bone metastases [4]. Correlation with laboratory parameters remains essential, and sometimes only histology can establish a definitive diagnosis [17].

Hybrid imaging strategies, such as bone scintigraphy with SPECT/CT or PET/CT, integrate functional and anatomic data, further improving lesion attribution and diagnostic confidence [20, 21].

In practice, CT remains indispensable in the multidisciplinary workup of brown tumors, offering high-resolution morphologic assessment, guidance for treatment planning, and monitoring of post-parathyroidectomy remodeling, especially when combined with advanced hybrid imaging.

13.3.3 Magnetic Resonance Imaging (MRI)

As already outlined above in more detail, brown tumors arise from excessive focal osteoclastic activity, resulting in lesions composed of vascular fibrous tissue, cystic change, and hemorrhagic components [9]. On MRI, signal patterns yield three main lesion types: (1) solid fibrous lesions (iso- to hypointense), (2) mixed solid-cystic, and (3) purely cystic lesions (T2 hyperintense) [6]. The solid portions are iso- to hypointense on T1- and T2-weighted images, and well enhanced [6]. Cystic regions are T2 hyperintense, with possible T2 shortening due to hemosiderin and fluid-fluid levels from recurrent intralesional hemorrhage [6], and contrast enhancement from the periphery and septa. In mixed lesions, enhancement involves both the solid fibrous tissue and the internal septa within cystic areas [6].

MRI is particularly valuable in complex locations or when neurological compromise is suspected [17]. It allows precise delineation of spinal cord or nerve root compression, soft-tissue extension, and relationships with adjacent structures. Additionally, MRI may identify incidental lesions during evaluation of pain or unrelated indications, highlighting the need for biochemical correlation.

In practice, MRI is central to the multidisciplinary workup of brown tumors, providing detailed anatomical and neurological evaluation and is especially helpul in surgically challenging lesions.

13.3.4 ^{99m}Tc-Sestamibi (MIBI) Parathyroid Scintigraphy

MIBI is a lipophilic cationic tracer distributed according to tissue perfusion and accumulates in mitochondria-rich cells. In brown tumors, uptake is heterogeneous, reflecting variable histology from metabolically active multinucleated giant cells to low-mitochondrial fibrous tissue. Clinically, MIBI uptake in brown tumors is inconsistent. Some lesions demonstrate moderate-to-high uptake, whereas others, particularly established osteolytic lesions, may show absent uptake [1]. In patients with parathyroid disease, MIBI-negative bone lesions with FDG uptake may favor a diagnosis of brown tumors [22]. Incidentally, MIBI may also display brown tumors, although skeletal uptake should not be relied upon for diagnosis. Because MIBI uptake does not reliably reflect the metabolic activity of brown tumors, bone healing is better monitored using CT or FDG-PET/CT than MIBI.

Despite these limitations, MIBI still serves as the first-line functional imaging for primary hyperparathyroidism in the absence of ^{18}F-Fluorocholine PET because it localizes the abnormal PTH source, guiding curative parathyroidectomy.

13.3.5 ^{99m}Tc-methylene diphosphonates (MDP) Bone Scintigraphy and Bone-SPECT/CT

^{99m}Tc-MDP adsorbs to hydroxyapatite surfaces, proportional to local vascularity and osteoblastic activity [20]. Localization occurs via chemisorption, as phosphate groups form coordination bonds with calcium on exposed hydroxyapatite surfaces. This process highlights immature mineralization with increased osteoblastic activity, particularly at brown tumor margins, resulting in intense peripheral tracer accumulation.

On planar ^{99m}Tc-MDP bone scintigraphy, brown tumors appear as areas of increased skeletal uptake, often mimicking metastatic lesions [5]. Three-phase bone scintigraphy increases sensitivity for brown tumor detection [5]. Biochemical correlation is essential to establish the correct diagnosis. In very advanced disease, a metabolic superscan may be observed, showing diffuse, symmetric skeletal uptake with diminished renal and soft-tissue retention, while focal bone lesions may still be evident. Hybrid single photon emission computed tomography/computed tomography (SPECT/CT) improves lesion conspicuity and anatomic localization in complex skeletal regions [20, 21]. After parathyroidectomy, avid lesions generally decrease in uptake and demonstrate progressive sclerosis, consistent with healing [5]. However, a transient rise of bone-scan activity with healing or persistent generalized uptake for months in patients with hungry bone syndrome may also occur.

Despite limited specificity, ^{99m}Tc-MDP scintigraphy and SPECT/CT remain valuable tools for quantifying skeleton burden andmonitoring treatment response in patients with hyperparathyroidism.

13.3.6 ^{18}F-Fluorodeoxyglucose (FDG) PET

FDG is a radiolabeled glucose analog that images cellular glucose metabolism. FDG enters cells via GLUT transporters and is phosphorylated by hexokinase to FDG-6-phosphate, which becomes trapped intracellularly [23]. Brown tumors are rich in multinucleated giant cells and macrophages, which display high hexokinase activity, leading to avid FDG uptake.

On FDG-PET, uptake patterns include generalized skeletal hyperactivity from hyperparathyroid bone turnover, with superimposed focal hot spots at brown tumor sites [24]. FDG-PET allows whole-body imaging, increases overall sensitivity and is able to detect smaller lesions than bone scintigraphy or ^{99m}Tc-MIBI imaging. It may also identify a hypermetabolic parathyroid adenoma, although other tracers may be preferable for precise parathyroid localization.

Although benign, brown tumors can demonstrate FDG avidity comparable to malignant lesions, sometimes with multiple coalescent FDG-avid sites and aggressive CT features, which may mimic metastases (Fig. 13.1a). Biochemical testing is important to avoid misclassification. After parathyroidectomy, lesions become sclerotic, and FDG uptake diminishes or resolves, with normalization often occurring earlier on ^{18}F-FCH PET than on FDG-PET (Fig. 13.1c) [22].

In practice, FDG-PET is valuable in delineating disease extent and monitoring treatment response, though differentiation between benign and malignant bone lesions may be challenging in patients with known malignancy [24].

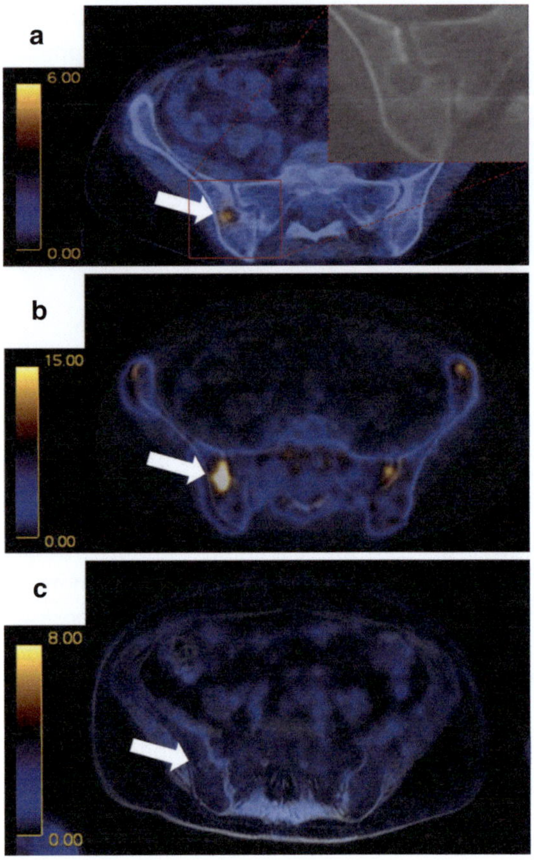

Fig. 13.1 Patient with breast cancer and brown tumors. (**a**) First surveillance ^{18}F-FDG PET/CT, 6 months after right-sided breast-conserving surgery (T2N1M0). A newly appearing FDG-avid bone lesion (arrow) with lytic correlate on CT is seen. (**b**) On ^{18}F-sodium fluoride PET/CT, the lesion (arrow) shows intense uptake. The patient also had several other brown tumors, e.g., in the left iliac crest; nonspecific bone uptake with no corresponding findings on CT is seen in the left sacroiliac joint. Laboratory results revealed elevated parathyroid hormone serum levels as well as hypercalcemia. (**c**) On follow-up ^{18}F-FDG-PET/MR a few weeks after parathyroid adenoma resection, the lesion demonstrates complete metabolic resolution, being consistent with a brown tumor

13.3.7 ^{18}F-Sodium Fluoride (NaF) PET

^{18}F-NaF targets the bone mineralization phase by substituting hydroxyl ion (OH^-) with fluoride ions (F^-) in newly forming hydroxyapatite crystals, producing fluoroapatite [18]. Owing to fluoride's high electronegativity, small ionic radius, and strong charge density, it competitively replaces hydroxyl groups at actively remodeling bone surfaces. Brown tumors, characterized by extraordinarily high bone turnover, demonstrate intense peripheral osteoblastic activity, making them highly conspicuous on NaF imaging.

On NaF PET, brown tumors appear as highly avid foci corresponding to osteolytic skeletal lesions. Reported maximum standardized uptake values average 17 to 18, reflecting vigorous osteoblastic bone formation at lesion margins [18] (Fig. 13.1b).

Because NaF uptake reflects osteoblastic activity, it is highly sensitive for detecting skeletal disease but nonspecific without biochemical and clinical correlation. The imaging appearance can vary depending on the osteolytic-to-osteoblastic ratio within each lesion, from absent uptake in purely lytic areas to peripheral rim activity or markedly increased tracer accumulation [21]. Extensive skeletal involvement may produce a metabolic superscan pattern, with diffuse, homogeneous skeletal uptake throughout the axial and appendicular skeleton and absent renal visualization [25]. This appearance must be distinguished from metastatic superscans, which typically demonstrate heterogeneous axial and proximal appendicular-predominant uptake [25]. After parathyroidectomy, NaF uptake of brown tumors usually declines as bone metabolism normalizes, though persistent activity may remain for several months, particularly in large destructive lesions [18].

In clinical practice, ^{18}F-NaF PET provides a high-sensitivity quantitative assessment of skeletal involvement in brown tumors [18]. Whole-skeleton metrics, such as total metabolically active bone volume, correlate with parathyroid hormone and alkaline phosphatase levels, supporting their use in Hungry Bone Syndrome risk assessment [18]. Combination with other tracers, especially FDG, can enhance diagnostic accuracy and disease characterization.

13.3.8 ^{18}F-Fluorocholine (FCH) PET

^{18}F-FCH is a synthetic choline analog taken up by cells with high cellular membrane turnover [26]. After transport into the cytoplasm, choline is phosphorylated by choline kinase and incorporated into phosphatidylcholine, a major phospholipid component of cell membranes [26]. Consequently, tissues undergoing active proliferation or repair exhibit increased FCH uptake on PET (Fig. 13.2). In brown tumors, the fibroblastic reparative tissue and osteoblastic activity drive enhanced tracer accumulation.

On FCH-PET, multiple choline-avid foci correspond to lytic skeletal lesions [27], typically requiring biochemical confirmation of hyperparathyroidism. Beyond skeletal mapping, FCH-PET simultaneously localizes parathyroid adenomas or hyperplasia, linking etiology and skeletal sequelae within a single examination [27]. For example, a patient presenting with a painful tibial mass, later confirmed as a brown tumor, was found on FCH-PET to harbor a hyperfunctioning parathyroid adenoma and multiple additional brown tumors [27]. After parathyroidectomy, FCH uptake of brown tumors typically declines more rapidly than FDG-PET uptake, but FCH-specific longitudinal response evidence is limited [1].

In clinical practice, FCH-PET currently shows great promise for comprehensive evaluation of brown tumors. It offers simultaneous localization of hyperfunctioning parathyroid tissue and skeletal lesions, supporting integrated diagnostic and therapeutic planning in both primary and non-primary hyperparathyroidism.

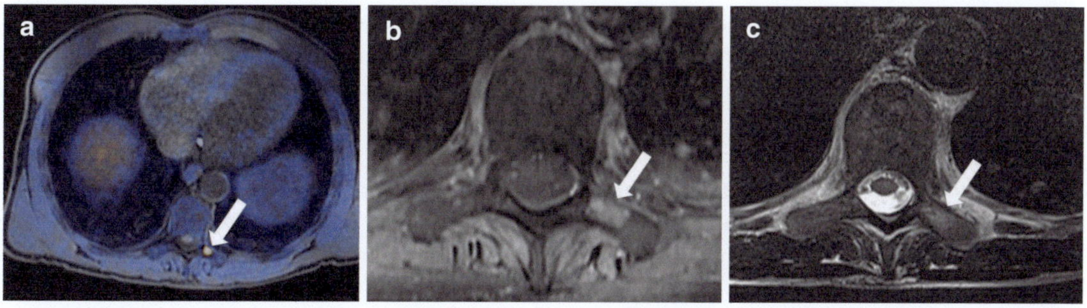

Fig. 13.2 ^{18}F-fluorocholine PET/MRI carried out for localization diagnostics in a patient hyperparathyroidism. (**a**) A brown tumor (arrow) is seen in the 12th thoracic vertebra, with intense tracer uptake. The brown tumor (arrow) is well seen on the T1w fs post-contrast image (**b**) as a well-defined hyperintense lesion, and on the T2w image as an intermediate intense to hyperintense alteration of bone marrow (**c**)

13.3.9 Comparison of Different Tracers Used for Brown Tumor Assessment

13.4 Differential Diagnosis

Brown tumors are focal osteolytic lesions occuring in patients with hyperparathyroidism, and they can closely mimic a wide range of lytic skeletal pathologies across multiple imaging modalities [6, 12]. This overlap may complicate the differential diagnosis, delay appropriate endocrine therapy, and even misdirect oncologic management [9]. Accurate differentiation requires systematic correlation of imaging findings with biochemical markers and parathyroid-focused molecular imaging (Table 13.2). Such correlation is essential to avoid unnecessary biopsy, inappropiriate oncologic work-up, or unwarranted surgery [2, 13].

13.4.1 Osteolytic Metastases

Osteolytic metastases are malignant deposits within bone, most commonly originating from lung cancer, breast cancer, thyroid carcinoma, or renal cell carcinoma, preferentially involving the axial skeleton. These lesions induce osteoclastic activation and trabecular destruction, producing imaging appearances that can closely resemble brown tumors, particularly in oncology patients where hyperparathyroidism is often not initially suspected based on imaging results [25]. A key distinguishing feature lies in biochemical findings: Brown tumors occur in the setting of elevated PTH, whereas osteolytic metastases do not elevate PTH and often present with suppressed levels in malignancy-related hypercalcemia.

In many malignancies, FDG-PET/CT is used for staging or surveillance imaging, but FDG avidity alone lacks specificity. Discordance of FDG-PET results with parathyroid-directed imaging and/or laboratory verification of hyperparathyroidism should guide diagnosis. However, a definitive characterization of specific lesions often requires biopsy [4]. Potential diagnostic imaging clues on FDG-PET/CT are:

Diagnostic clue:

In patients with "metastatic-appearing" osteolytic lesions, especially without a known primary malignancy, it is critical to measure serum calcium and PTH and perform parathyroid-targeted imaging before labeling lesions as metastases.

13.4.2 Multiple Myeloma

Multiple myeloma is a plasma-cell neoplasm characterized by overproduction of monoclonal immunuoglobulins or free light chains, bone marrow infiltration, and multifocal osteolytic destruction [28]. Its imaging appearance can mimic brown tumors, particularly when both present as multiple lytic lesions [12].

However, several distinguishing clinical and biochemical features are key: Brown tumors occur in hyperparathyroid patients with elevated PTH and calcium levels, whereas multiple myeloma is associated with monoclonal protein (M-protein) on serum or urine electrophoresis and bone marrow plasmacytosis. Multiple myeloma typically affects older adults, while brown tumors may occur at any age depending on the endocrine etiology [28].

Whole-body MRI and FDG-PET are preferred for staging and response assessment in patients with multiple myeloma but cannot reliably distinguish between brown tumors and multiple myeloma lesions without further clinical context [28]. Diagnostic imaging features on whole-body MRI and FDG-PET are:

Diagnostic clues:

Unlike the T2-hyperintense appearance of myeloma, brown tumors are typically iso- to hypointense [28]. In patients with multiple osteolytic lesions, the presence of monoclonal gammopathy supports a diagnosis of multiple myeloma, whereas elevated PTH and calcium indicate brown tumors [28].

Clinical pitfall:

Misdiagnosing brown tumors as myeloma may expose patients to unnecessary cytotoxic

Table 13.2 Overview of differential diagnosis of brown tumors

	Brown tumor	Fibrous dysplasia	Giant cell tumor / Central giant cell Granuloma	Aneurysmal bone cyst	Lytic metastasis	Multiple myeloma	Osteomyelitis
Features upon presentation	Often solitary or few; predilection for mandible, ribs, clavicle, pelvis; Thinned or preserved cortical bone	Usually solitary; ribs, femur, craniofacial bones, in children and young adults	Typically solitary; GCC: Epiphyseal region of long bones, especially around the knee; CGCG: Predominantly anterior mandible; often crosses midline, in children and young adults	Usually solitary	Typically multifocal; preferentially involves axial skeleton	Typically multiple, diffuse "punched-out" foci; predilection for pelvis and vertebral column. Typically not expansile	Fever, elevated WBC and ESR, often localized tenderness and soft-tissue inflammation
X-ray	Well defined lytic lesions, radiolucent; thin or broken cortex; expansile with cortical thinning; generally no periosteal reaction	Focal lytic, mixed or sclerotic lesion	Solid or mixed well defined solid-cystic lesion; bone expansion; cortical thinning; non-sclerotic margins	Focal, multi lobulated pseudocyst; lytic lesions; thin sclerotic margins	Focal, lytic lesions: bone destruction; narrow zones of transition; periosteal reaction	Lytic expansive lesions; prominent cortical thinning; well defined, non-sclerotic margins	Osteopenia, periosteal reaction; peripheral sclerosis possible
CT	Irregular, multi-loculated lytic lesions; ground glass opacification and interruption of the cortex; contrast enhancement	Ground-glass matrix; mixed pattern of ground glass, lytic or sclerotic appearance	Solid or mixed solid/cystic lesion; bone expansion; hyperdense solid components with contrast enhancement	Focal, multi-lobulated pseudocyst; lytic lesions with fluid-fluid levels; cortical thinning; no contrast enhancement	Lytic lesions; poorly defined margins; bone destruction	Punched-out expansive lytic lesions	Osteopenia, periosteal reaction, cortical erosion, sequestra; contrast enhanced CT may show abscess formation

(continued)

Table 13.2 (continued)

	Brown tumor	Fibrous dysplasia	Giant cell tumor / Central giant cell Granuloma	Aneurysmal bone cyst	Lytic metastasis	Multiple myeloma	Osteomyelitis
MRI	Iso- to hypointense signal on T1w and T2w; contrast enhancement of the solid portions and septa of cystic lesions; T2w hyperintense in cystic lesion and contrast enhancement from the periphery and septa	Low signal intensity on T1w and T2w images in ossified or fibrous portions; heterogeneous enhancement and signal intensity in the active phase	Hypoisointense signal on T1w; hypointensity on T2w; heterogeneous contrast enhancement	Variable T1w and T2w intensity signal of intracavitary fluid-fluid levels; surrounding rim of low T1w and T2w signal; possible septa enhancement	Soft hypointense tissue on T1w replacing bone marrow; heterogeneous contrast enhancement	Hypointense to isointense signal on T1w; hyperintense signal on T2w fat suppression sequences; early contrast enhancement; diffuse bone marrow infiltration ("pepper-pot skull")	Low T1w and high STIR signal; often with adjacent soft-tissue cellulitis or diffuse marrow edema in acute infection; abscess formation possible
Bone scintigraphy: DPD	Increased focal uptake	Increased focal uptake	Increased peripheral uptake with central photopenia (donut sign)	Homogeneous increased of mild uptake	Increased or diffuse uptake	Increased uptake	Increased uptake (in blood pool and delayed views)
PET: FDG	Moderate to high	Low to moderate	High	Mild to moderate	High	Absent to moderate seldom high	High
PET: Choline	Moderate to high	Low	Intermediate	Low	High	High	Variable
PET: Fluoride	Moderate to high	Moderate	Mild to moderate	Low to mild	Moderate to high	Variable	Variable to high
Total calcium	High	Normal	Normal	Normal	High	High/Normal	Normal
PTH	High	High/Normal	Normal	Normal	Low	Low/Normal	Normal
Alkaline phosphatase	High	High/Normal	Normal	Normal	High	Normal	Normal

Adapted from Diacinti et al. [12]: https://doi.org/10.1016/j.bonr.2020.100745, Bone Reports, © *2021 The Authors. Published by Elsevier Inc.*, OA article under the CC BY-NC-ND license (http://creativecommons.org/licenses/by-nc-nd/4.0/) with Permission therapy. Integration of patient history as well as biochemical parameters (PTH, calcium, phosphate) with imaging patterns remains the most effective safeguard against such diagnostic errors.

13.4.3 Giant Cell Lesions

13.4.3.1 Giant Cell Tumor (GCT)

GCT of bone is a typically solitary, benign but locally aggressive neoplasm that arises after skeletal maturity, most commonly in the epiphyseal region of long bones, particularly around the knee (distal femur, proximal tibia) [29]. Histologically, GCT is characterized by osteoclast-type multinucleated giant cells interspersed among mononuclear stromal cells [29].

Brown tumors may closely mimic GCT both histologically and radiographically. In some cases, fluid-fluid levels can appear due to secondary aneurysmal bone cyst formation, further blurring the distinction between the two [29]. Unlike brown tumors, GCTs occur in patients with normal serum calcium and PTH levels [12]. Failure to recognize underlying hyperparathyroidism may result in unnecessary medical or surgical treatment for presumed neoplasia. Potential diagnostic features are:

Diagnostic clue:

All giant-cell–rich osteolytic lesions should prompt serum calcium and PTH testing before definitive diagnosis or therapy.

13.4.3.2 Central Giant Cell Granuloma (CGCG)

CGCG is a usually solitary, benign but sometimes locally aggressive intraosseous lesion of the jaw, most frequently occurring in the anterior mandible and often crossing the midline [30]. Histology reveals areas of hemorrhage, aggregates of multinucleated giant cells, and irregular trabeculae of woven bone [30].

Brown tumors may closely resemble CGCG in both histologic pattern and radiographic appearance, particularly when the jaw is involved. The two entities share overlapping morphology, but their clinical contexts differ: CGCG predominantly affects adults up to their forties [30]. Brown tumors typically occur in adults with biochemical evidence of hyperparathyroidism. Mistaking a brown tumor for CGCG can lead to unnecessary surgical curettage or resection, whereas biochemical correction of hyperparathyroidism alone typically induces regression of brown tumors.

Diagnostic clue:

Any giant-cell–rich lytic jaw lesion should trigger serum calcium and PTH assessment before invasive management.

13.4.3.3 Aneurysmal Bone Cyst (ABC)

ABC is a typically solitary, benign, locally destructive, expansile bone neoplasm characterized by multiloculated, blood-filled cystic spaces, separated by fibrous septa containing fibroblast-like stromal cells, osteoclast-like giant cells and reactive woven bone [31]. ABCs may arise de novo (primary ABC) or secondary to an underlying bone tumor such as giant cell tumor or chondroblastoma.

They most frequently occur in the metadiaphysis of the long bones and the posterior elements of vertebrae, with a predilection for children and adolescents [31].

Brown tumors may mimic ABC, particularly in long bones, due to their cystic morphology and presence of hemorrhagic components, including occasional fluid-fluid levels. As MRI is the modality of choice for evaluating ABCs, these overlapping features can complicate interpretation. However, ABCs typically occur in younger patients, whereas brown tumors are most commonly found in adults with biochemical HPT, making clinical and biochemical correlation essential. Misdiagnosing a brown tumor as ABC can lead to unnecessary surgical intervention rather than appropriate endocrine management. Potential diagnostic imaging features on MRI:

Diagnostic clue:

In adults, a giant-cell–rich lesion resembling ABC should prompt serum calcium and PTH measurement before confirming the diagnosis.

13.4.4 Fibrous Dysplasia

Fibrous dysplasia is a benign intramedullary fibro-osseous lesion caused by postzygotic activating mutation of the GNAS gene, leading to abnormal bone remodeling and replacement of normal bone marrow with fibro-osseous tissue. Histologically, fibrous dysplasia consists of a fibroblastic stroma containing irregularly shaped woven bone trabeculae that lack osteoblastic rimming.

Fibrous dysplasia can present as monostotic or polyostotic disease and typically affects children and young adults. Commonly involved sites include the ribs, femur, and craniofacial bones.

Brown tumors can simulate fibrous dysplasia both clinically and radiographically, especially when multiple skeletal sites are involved [32].

Incorrectly diagnosing fibrous dysplasia in a patient with HPT may delay appropriate endocrine treatment and lead to unnecessary surgical management.

CT is the preferred imaging modality for fibrous dysplasia, as it delineates the characteristic ground-glass matrix within the bone, cortical thinning, and endosteal scalloping.

13.4.5 Osteomyelitis

Osteomyelitis is an infection-induced inflammation of the bone and bone marrow, most often caused by hematogenous bacterial seeding or contiguous spread from adjacent soft tissues [33]. The inflammatory process leads to marrow edema, trabecular and cortical destruction and, in chronic stages, reactive sclerosis and new bone formation [33].

Brown tumors may closely mimic osteomyelitis, presenting as painful, expansile osteolytic lesions with possible surrounding soft-tissue reaction.

However, unlike infectious osteolysis, brown tumors lack systemic inflammatory signs such as fever, elevated white blood cell count, or raised erythrocyte sedimentation rate (ESR). MRI is the imaging modality of choice for suspected osteomyelitis, owing to its sensitivity for detecting bone marrow edema, cortical changes, abscesses, and sinus tracts. Integrating MRI findings with clinical and biochemical parameters is essential to prevent unnecessary surgical debridement in patients with underlying hyperparathyroidism.

Diagnostic clue:

> When osteomyelitis is suspected but imaging and clinical infection markers are inconclusive, biochemical screening for hyperparathyroidism (serum calcium and PTH) is recommended before initiating surgical debridement.

13.5 Conclusion

Brown tumors remain a clinically significant manifestation within the spectrum of hyperparathyroidism. Although their incidence has declined with earlier biochemical screening and improved endocrine management, they continue to present diagnostic challenges due to their ability to mimic malignant and other benign osteolytic lesions.

Accurate identification relies on a comprehensive imaging strategy integrating morphological and functional modalities. Advanced nuclear medicine techniques, particularly FCH-PET/CT and NaF-PET/CT, provide valuable insight into disease extent, metabolic activity, and treatment response. Equally important is an understanding of the temporal evolution of imaging findings following parathyroidectomy, to differentiate physiologic healing from residual or recurrent disease and to prevent premature or unnecessary interventions.

Ultimately, successful management depends on maintaining a high index of suspicion for brown tumors in patients presenting with osteolytic bone lesions, particularly when multifocal or located in characteristic skeletal regions. Integration of clinical, biochemical, and multimodal imaging data, combined with a multidisciplinary approach involving endocrinology, nuclear medicine, and orthopedic surgery, ensures timely diagnosis, targeted therapy, and optimal patient outcomes while avoiding invasive or inappropriate procedures.

References

1. Jacquet-Francillon N, Prevot N. Brown tumors in nuclear medicine: a systematic review. Ann Nucl Med. 2023;37(5):255–70. https://doi.org/10.1007/s12149-023-01832-1.
2. Xie C, Tsakok M, Taylor N, Partington K. Imaging of brown tumours: a pictorial review. Insights Imaging. 2019;10(1):75. https://doi.org/10.1186/s13244-019-0757-z.
3. Santoso D, Thaha M, Empitu MA, Kadariswantiningsih IN, Suryantoro SD, Haryati MR, et al. Brown tumour in chronic kidney disease: revisiting an old disease with a new perspective. Cancers (Basel). 2023;15(16):4107. https://doi.org/10.3390/cancers15164107.
4. Dinoi E, Prete A, Sardella C, Pierotti L, Della Valentina S, Dal Lago A, et al. The challenge of the differential diagnosis between brown tumors and metastases in parathyroid carcinoma: a case report. Front Endocrinol (Lausanne). 2024;15:1414896. https://doi.org/10.3389/fendo.2024.1414896.
5. van der Bruggen W, Bulten BF. Use of bone-SPECT/CT and Na[(18)F]F-PET/CT in hyperparathyroidism. Front Nucl Med. 2025;5:1565906. https://doi.org/10.3389/fnume.2025.1565906.
6. Hong WS, Sung MS, Chun KA, Kim JY, Park SW, Lee KH, et al. Emphasis on the MR imaging findings of brown tumor: a report of five cases. Skeletal Radiol. 2011;40(2):205–13. https://doi.org/10.1007/s00256-010-0979-0.
7. Bollerslev J, Rejnmark L, Zahn A, Heck A, Appelman-Dijkstra NM, Cardoso L, et al. European expert consensus on practical management of specific aspects of parathyroid disorders in adults and in pregnancy: recommendations of the ESE Educational Program of Parathyroid Disorders. Eur J Endocrinol. 2022;186(2):R33–63. https://doi.org/10.1530/EJE-21-1044.
8. Bransky N, Iyer NR, Cannon SM, Tyan AH, Mylavarapu P, Orosco R, et al. Three rare concurrent complications of tertiary hyperparathyroidism: maxillary brown tumor, uremic leontiasis ossea, and hungry bone syndrome. J Bone Metab. 2020;27(3):217–26. https://doi.org/10.11005/jbm.2020.27.3.217.
9. Karaca MO, Ozyildiran M, Savran MD, Basarir K, Yildiz HY. Brown tumors: retrospective analysis of 26 cases. Arch Orthop Trauma Surg. 2024;144(7):2927–34. https://doi.org/10.1007/s00402-024-05372-9.
10. Misiorowski W, Czajka-Oraniec I, Kochman M, Zgliczynski W, Bilezikian JP. Osteitis fibrosa cystica-a forgotten radiological feature of primary hyperparathyroidism. Endocrine. 2017;58(2):380–5. https://doi.org/10.1007/s12020-017-1414-2.
11. Govind K, Paruk IM, Motala AA. Characteristics, management and outcomes of primary hyperparathyroidism from 2009 to 2021: a single centre report from South Africa. BMC Endocr Disord. 2024;24(1):53. https://doi.org/10.1186/s12902-024-01583-8.
12. Diacinti D, Cipriani C, Biamonte F, Pepe J, Colangelo L, Kripa E, et al. Imaging technologies in the differential diagnosis and follow-up of brown tumor in primary hyperparathyroidism: case report and review of the literature. Bone Rep. 2021;14:100745. https://doi.org/10.1016/j.bonr.2020.100745.
13. Hamidi S, Mottard S, Berthiaume MJ, Doyon J, Begin MJ, Bondaz L. Brown tumor of the iliac crest initially misdiagnosed as a giant cell tumor of the bone. Endocrinol Diabetes Metab Case Rep. 2020:2020. https://doi.org/10.1530/EDM-20-0029.
14. Bilezikian JP, Khan AA, Silverberg SJ, Fuleihan GE, Marcocci C, Minisola S, et al. Evaluation and management of primary hyperparathyroidism: summary statement and guidelines from the fifth international workshop. J Bone Miner Res. 2022;37(11):2293–314. https://doi.org/10.1002/jbmr.4677.
15. Radu CP, Daniealopol V, Santini A, Darie R, Sala DT. Fatal hypocalcaemia due to hungry bone syndrome with secondary refractory hyperparathyroidism after parathyroidectomy: a case report. J Crit Care Med (Targu Mures). 2019;5(4):140–4. https://doi.org/10.2478/jccm-2019-0021.
16. Carsote M, Nistor C. Forestalling hungry bone syndrome after parathyroidectomy in patients with primary and renal hyperparathyroidism. Diagnostics (Basel). 2023;13(11):1953. https://doi.org/10.3390/diagnostics13111953.
17. Hu J, He S, Yang J, Ye C, Yang X, Xiao J. Management of brown tumor of spine with primary hyperparathyroidism: a case report and literature review. Medicine (Baltimore). 2019;98(14):e15007. https://doi.org/10.1097/MD.0000000000015007.
18. Graf C, Huellner M, Tschopp O, Bode-Lesniewska B, Schmid C. (18)F-NaF-PET/CT in patients with primary hyperparathyroidism and brown tumors. J Bone Miner Metab. 2020;38(3):299–309. https://doi.org/10.1007/s00774-019-01059-z.
19. Expert Panel on Musculoskeletal I, Ahlawat S, Lenchik L, Baker JC, Allen H, Banks J, et al. ACR Appropriateness Criteria(R) suspected primary bone tumors: 2024 update. J Am Coll Radiol. 2025;22(5S):S440–S54. https://doi.org/10.1016/j.jacr.2025.02.020.
20. Bartel TB, Kuruva M, Gnanasegaran G, Beheshti M, Cohen EJ, Weissman AF, Yarbrough TL. SNMMI procedure standard for bone scintigraphy 4.0. J Nucl Med Technol. 2018;46(4):398–404.
21. Beheshti M, Mottaghy FM, Paycha F, Behrendt FFF, Van den Wyngaert T, Fogelman I, et al. (18)F-NaF PET/CT: EANM procedure guidelines for bone imaging. Eur J Nucl Med Mol Imaging. 2015;42(11):1767–77. https://doi.org/10.1007/s00259-015-3138-y.
22. Tsukamoto S, Kawabata K, Kawamura H, Takata K, Hosono M. Differentiating brown tumor from bone metastasis in parathyroid cancer using 18 F-FDG PET and 99m Tc-MIBI SPECT. Clin Nucl Med. 2024;49(5):444–6. https://doi.org/10.1097/RLU.0000000000005115.
23. Abikhzer G, Treglia G, Pelletier-Galarneau M, Buscombe J, Chiti A, Dibble EH, et al. EANM/

SNMMI guideline/procedure standard for [(18)F] FDG hybrid PET use in infection and inflammation in adults v2.0. Eur J Nucl Med Mol Imaging. 2025;52(2):510–38. https://doi.org/10.1007/s00259-024-06915-3.
24. Geysen A, Van Laere K, Verscuren R. Detection of unexpected brown tumors due to hyperparathyroidism diagnosed by 18F-FDG PET/CT. Clin Nucl Med. 2021;46(1):e16–e7. https://doi.org/10.1097/RLU.0000000000003380.
25. Edamadaka Y, Parghane RV, Basu S. Complimentary role of [18F]FDG and [18F]NaF-PET/CT in evaluating synchronous thyroid carcinoma and parathyroid adenoma with brown tumors. World J Nucl Med. 2024;23(3):220–4. https://doi.org/10.1055/s-0044-1787732.
26. Leung K. [(18)F]Fluorocholine. Bethesda (MD): Molecular Imaging and Contrast Agent Database (MICAD); 2004.
27. Werner J, Grunig H, Loher H, Fischli S, Strobel K, Wicke C. Localization of brown tumors with 18 F-fluorocholine PET/CT imaging in severe primary hyperparathyroidism. Clin Nucl Med. 2023;48(8):e387–e9. https://doi.org/10.1097/RLU.0000000000004718.
28. Healy CF, Murray JG, Eustace SJ, Madewell J, O'Gorman PJ, O'Sullivan P. Multiple myeloma: a review of imaging features and radiological techniques. Bone Marrow Res. 2011;2011:583439. https://doi.org/10.1155/2011/583439.
29. Chakarun CJ, Forrester DM, Gottsegen CJ, Patel DB, White EA, Matcuk GR Jr. Giant cell tumor of bone: review, mimics, and new developments in treatment. Radiographics. 2013;33(1):197–211. https://doi.org/10.1148/rg.331125089.
30. Aliu F, Shabani DB, Aliu I, Qeli ED, Kacani G, Fiorillo L, Meto A. Evaluating treatment modalities for reducing recurrence in central giant cell granuloma: a narrative review. Dent J (Basel). 2024;12(9):295. https://doi.org/10.3390/dj12090295.
31. Nasri E, Reith JD. Aneurysmal bone cyst: a review. J Pathol Transl Med. 2023;57(2):81–7. https://doi.org/10.4132/jptm.2023.02.23.
32. Shah ZK, Peh WC, Koh WL, Shek TW. Magnetic resonance imaging appearances of fibrous dysplasia. Br J Radiol. 2005;78(936):1104–15. https://doi.org/10.1259/bjr/73852511.
33. Lee YJ, Sadigh S, Mankad K, Kapse N, Rajeswaran G. The imaging of osteomyelitis. Quant Imaging Med Surg. 2016;6(2):184–98. https://doi.org/10.21037/qims.2016.04.01.

14 Unmet Needs and Future Perspectives in Parathyroid Imaging

Petra Petranović Ovčariček, Frederik Anton Verburg, Luca Giovanella, and Martin W. Huellner

Definitions *Primary hyperparathyroidism:* An endocrine disorder characterized by the overproduction of parathyroid hormone from one or more hyperfunctioning parathyroid glands and associated hypercalcemia. In some cases, parathyroid hormone levels may be in a higher reference range, while in other instances, calcium levels may be normal (normocalcemic hyperparathyroidism).

Multiglandular disease: Hyperparathyroidism caused by hyperfunction of more than one parathyroid gland.

Ectopic parathyroid gland: A parathyroid gland located outside the typical anatomical position adjacent to the thyroid, found along the embryologic migration path from the angle of the mandible to the mediastinum.

[^{99m}Tc]Tc-MIBI: A radiopharmaceutical that accumulates in mitochondria-rich cells, used for functional imaging of hyperfunctioning parathyroid glands.

SPECT/CT: Single-photon emission computed tomography combined with computed tomography, providing both functional and anatomical imaging information.

4D-CT: Four-dimensional computed tomography, a multiphase contrast-enhanced CT technique that provides anatomical and functional information about parathyroid glands.

Discordant imaging: Conflicting results between different imaging modalities (typically [^{99m}Tc]Tc-MIBI SPECT/CT and cervical ultrasonography) regarding the presence or location of hyperfunctioning parathyroid glands.

Minimally invasive parathyroidectomy: A focused surgical approach to remove hyperfunctioning parathyroid gland based on preoperative

P. Petranović Ovčariček (✉)
Department of Oncology and Nuclear Medicine, University Hospital Center Sestre Milosrdnice, Zagreb, Croatia

School of Medicine, University of Zagreb, Zagreb, Croatia
e-mail: p.petranovic@gmail.com

F. A. Verburg
Department of Radiology and Nuclear Medicine, Erasmus Medical Centre Rotterdam, Rotterdam, The Netherlands
e-mail: f.verburg@erasmusmc.nl

L. Giovanella
Department of Nuclear Medicine, University Hospital of Zurich, University of Zurich, Zurich, Switzerland

Department of Nuclear Medicine, Gruppo Ospedaliero Moncucco SA, Clinica Moncucco, Lugano, Switzerland

Department of Clinical Chemistry and Endocrinology, Medysin, Luzern, Switzerland
e-mail: luca.giovanella@moncucco.ch

M. W. Huellner
Department of Nuclear Medicine, University Hospital of Zurich / University of Zurich, Zurich, Switzerland
e-mail: martin.huellner@usz.ch

© The Author(s), under exclusive license to Springer Nature Switzerland AG 2026

P. Petranović Ovčariček et al. (eds.), *Parathyroid Imaging*,
https://doi.org/10.1007/978-3-032-14177-8-1_14

localization, offering advantages over traditional bilateral neck exploration.

Parathyroid carcinoma: A rare malignant tumor of the parathyroid gland, accounting for less than 1% of primary hyperparathyroidism cases.

^{18}F-fluorocholine PET/CT: Positron emission tomography combined with computed tomography using ^{18}F-labeled choline analogs, an advanced imaging technique for detecting hyperfunctioning parathyroid glands.

^{18}F-fluorocholine PET/MR: Positron emission tomography combined with magnetic resonance imaging using ^{18}F-labeled choline analogs, an advanced imaging technique with low radiation exposure for detecting hyperfunctioning parathyroid glands.

Learning Objectives

1. Identify the major limitations of historical first-line parathyroid imaging modalities, including [^{99m}Tc]Tc-MIBI SPECT/CT and cUS.
2. Identify limitations remaining with ^{18}F-fluorocholine PET/CT and PET/MR imaging.
3. Understand the specific challenges in detecting multiglandular disease and explain why current imaging techniques show reduced sensitivity.
4. Recognize the clinical importance of accurate ectopic parathyroid gland localization and describe the limitations of various imaging modalities in detecting ectopic glands.
5. Analyze the clinical implications of discordant imaging results and evaluate strategies for managing inconclusive findings between different imaging modalities.
6. Distinguish the imaging characteristics that may suggest parathyroid carcinoma and understand the limitations of current techniques in differentiating malignant from benign lesions.
7. Compare the advantages and limitations of different imaging modalities in parathyroid imaging.
8. Discuss the clinical consequences of unmet needs in parathyroid imaging and their impact on patient care and surgical outcomes.
9. Integrate understanding of current imaging challenges to critically evaluate diagnostic results and recognize scenarios requiring additional or alternative imaging approaches.

14.1 Introduction

Primary hyperparathyroidism is the third most common endocrine disorder, affecting 16–90 per 100,000 people annually [3]. While solitary parathyroid adenomas account for the majority of cases, the clinical spectrum includes multiglandular disease, parathyroid hyperplasia, and, rarely, parathyroid carcinoma [64, 88, 92]. The improvement in parathyroid imaging over the past several decades has changed the surgical approach from routine bilateral neck exploration to targeted, focused, even minimally invasive parathyroidectomy. However, despite technological advances, significant challenges persist in achieving optimal detection and characterization of hyperfunctioning parathyroid glands [63].

The success of parathyroid surgery depends on accurate preoperative localization. Focused approaches offer substantial advantages over traditional bilateral exploration, including reduced operative time, fewer complications, improved cosmetic outcomes, and lower overall healthcare costs [22, 38, 43, 72, 77, 85, 90]. These benefits have probably driven the development of various imaging modalities. However, substantial limitations still impact clinical decision-making and surgical outcomes [63].

This chapter examines the persistent challenges and unmet needs in parathyroid imaging, exploring current limitations within clinical practice.

14.2 SPECT Tracers

[^{99m}Tc]Tc-MIBI has been the most widely used radiopharmaceutical for parathyroid scintigraphy since its introduction in 1989 [18]. The tracer accumulates in mitochondria-rich cells, with hyperfunctioning parathyroid glands typically demonstrating higher uptake and slower washout than thyroid tissue. The integration of SPECT/CT has further improved diagnostic accuracy by enabling precise anatomical localization and reducing false-positive findings from adjacent structures [63, 66].

Despite its widespread adoption and proven clinical utility, [^{99m}Tc]Tc-MIBI SPECT/CT has notable limitations. Its sensitivity is markedly reduced in multiglandular disease, with detection rates falling from approximately 88% for single-gland disease to as low as 26.7–61% for multiple adenomas [48, 54]. However, detection rates are consistently higher in dual-tracer protocols compared with dual-phase studies [27–30, 79]. Small parathyroid lesions, particularly those under 500 mg, frequently fall below the resolution limits of conventional SPECT systems. Factors such as rapid tracer washout, high expression of P-glycoprotein and multidrug resistance proteins, and variable thyroid uptake patterns further contribute to false-negative results [65]. False-positive findings also pose a significant challenge, particularly in patients with concomitant thyroid disease. Both benign and malignant thyroid nodules may demonstrate [^{99m}Tc]Tc-MIBI uptake in dual-phase imaging, mimicking parathyroid adenomas. These pitfalls can be mitigated by using dual-tracer parathyroid scintigraphy [28, 30, 80] and by performing fine-needle aspiration cytology with measurement of the parathyroid hormone (PTH) levels in the aspirate [11, 84]. Additionally, inflammatory lymph nodes, particularly in the setting of thyroiditis, can cause misleading uptake patterns.

Furthermore, patient movement between sequential acquisitions can create subtraction artifacts when using ^{99m}Tc-pertechnetate instead of ^{123}I in the dual tracer method, while the limited availability of ^{123}I in some centers constrains its full implementation. These technical limitations, along with reduced sensitivity for small parathyroid glands under 300 mg, are effectively addressed by [^{18}F]fluorocholine PET/CT or PET/MR, which eliminates the need for subtraction imaging and demonstrates superior detection of small lesions through its higher spatial resolution and presumably more pronounced metabolic targeting.

These limitations underline the necessity of complementary imaging techniques and underscore the importance of expert interpretation.

[^{99m}Tc]Tc-tetrofosmin, although demonstrating comparable overall performance to [^{99m}Tc]Tc-MIBI, has not achieved widespread use in parathyroid imaging [7, 25, 31, 36, 86]. Its primary limitation is the lack of differential washout between thyroid and parathyroid tissue, which necessitates dual-tracer subtraction imaging with either [^{99m}Tc]pertechnetate or ^{123}I. This requirement restricts its utility, particularly in patients undergoing thyroid hormone replacement therapy or with recent iodine exposure, thereby limiting its broader clinical applicability.

14.3 Cervical Ultrasonography

Cervical ultrasonography serves as a valuable mandatory first-line imaging modality for patients with hyperparathyroidism. It is widely accessible, involves no radiation exposure, offers real-time visualization of neck anatomy, and allows simultaneous assessment of thyroid pathology [50, 78]. Modern high-frequency linear transducers (10–14 MHz) provide excellent spatial resolution, while advanced Doppler techniques enable identification of characteristic polar feeding vessels that help distinguish parathyroid glands from adjacent structures such as lymph nodes [52]. However, cUS also has notable limitations. Its performance is highly operator-dependent, leading to significant variability in diagnostic sensitivity, which has been reported to range from 55% to 87% [49, 61].

Anatomical limitations are especially pronounced with ectopic parathyroid glands, which constitute approximately 20% of cases in treatment-naive patients and up to 66% in reoperative cases [60]. Many ectopic glands, particularly those located in the mediastinum, remain inaccessible to sonographic evaluation.

Distinguishing parathyroid lesions from their mimics presents an additional challenge. Cervical lymph nodes, particularly those related to chronic lymphocytic thyroiditis, can closely resemble parathyroid adenomas. Although the presence of a central fatty hilum and hilar vascularity can theoretically help differentiate lymph nodes from parathyroid glands, which typically exhibit characteristic polar feeding vessels, these distinguishing features may be subtle or absent in many lymph nodes [63].

Limitations of cUS are especially evident in detecting multiglandular disease. Sensitivity significantly decreases from 78% for single adenomas to approximately 35% for multiglandular involvement, likely due to challenges in identifying smaller hyperplastic glands [76], particularly when situated in difficult anatomical locations. Additionally, hyperplastic glands often exhibit less prominent vascular patterns compared to large adenomas, complicating their differentiation from normal thyroid tissue or small lymph nodes.

Concurrent thyroid pathology, present in approximately 18% of patients with pHPT, poses additional diagnostic challenges [8]. Multinodular goiter can distort normal cervical anatomy, displacing parathyroid glands posteriorly into locations that are difficult to visualize with cUS. Hypoechoic thyroid nodules near the thyroid capsule may be indistinguishable from parathyroid adenomas, while intrathyroidal parathyroid adenomas might be misinterpreted as benign thyroid nodules [50, 63]. These factors can result in both false-positive and false-negative findings, potentially complicating surgical planning.

Advanced cUS techniques may help overcome some diagnostic challenges. Contrast-enhanced cUS uses the distinct vascular patterns of parathyroid tissue, i.e., adenomas show rapid arterial enhancement progressing from the periphery to the center, followed by characteristic washout patterns that differ from both thyroid nodules and lymph nodes. Early studies indicate improved sensitivity with this approach [62]. Similarly, cUS elastography quantifies tissue stiffness, with parathyroid adenomas exhibiting lower elastic modulus values than thyroid nodules, but higher values than normal thyroid parenchyma. Reported shear wave velocities of around 2.02 m/sec for adenomas versus 2.77 m/sec for thyroid nodules are promising for improved differential diagnosis [5]. However, these techniques are largely confined to specialized centers. Limited availability of contrast agents in many regions, the lack of training, and cost-effectiveness concerns have restricted widespread clinical adoption. Moreover, these methods cannot reliably detect very small parathyroid lesions.

These limitations can significantly impact further patient management. False-negative cUS results may lead to more invasive bilateral neck explorations instead of focused surgeries with fewer complications and other shortcomings. Conversely, false-positive interpretations may lead to unnecessary removal of normal thyroid tissue or lymph nodes, while hyperfunctioning parathyroid glands remain untreated. Additionally, the inability to accurately identify multiglandular disease may result in inappropriate use of focused surgical approaches in patients who would benefit from open-neck exploration.

Training and standardization can help overcome many of these challenges. Unlike thyroid nodule assessment, where structured reporting systems such as TI-RADS provide clear guidelines, parathyroid ultrasonography interpretation is largely subjective and heavily reliant on individual experience.

The integration of artificial intelligence and machine learning technologies presents promising solutions to some of these interpretive difficulties. Computer-aided detection systems could reduce operator dependence and improve consistency in lesion identification and characterization.

Novel transducers and contrast agents may improve lesion detection in cUS. However, cUS remains suboptimal for identifying deep and many ectopic parathyroid lesions, and its operator dependence is unlikely to be entirely eliminated.

Recognizing these limitations should not decrease the value of cUS in parathyroid imaging or the importance of concurrent thyroid gland evaluation. When performed by experienced operators within an appropriate clinical context, cUS provides invaluable anatomical information that aids surgical planning and improves patient outcomes. The key is to understand when cUS findings are reliable and when additional imaging modalities are needed to offer complementary diagnostic data.

14.4 PET Tracers

Choline PET/CT and PET/MR, using tracers such as [^{18}F]fluorocholine and [^{11}C]choline, represent the most significant advancement in parathyroid imaging since the introduction of [^{99m}Tc]Tc-MIBI scintigraphy decades ago. Parathyroid adenomas demonstrate increased choline kinase activity, attributed to the translocation of this enzyme from the cytosol to the cell membrane, a process stimulated by high PTH secretion [37]. This dual uptake mechanism, consisting of both mitochondrial accumulation and incorporation into phospholipid membrane synthesis, provides theoretical advantages over traditional scintigraphic techniques that primarily depend on mitochondrial localization. [^{18}F]fluorocholine is the predominant radiotracer in this category. It benefits from a physical half-life of approximately 110 minutes that facilitates regional distribution and practical clinical implementation. This longer half-life compared to carbon-11 labeled alternatives (half-life: 20 minutes) allows more flexible scheduling and broader accessibility. Imaging protocols typically balance diagnostic accuracy with operational efficiency, with standard acquisition performed 45–60 minutes postinjection. In selected cases, earlier dynamic imaging around 5 minutes postinjection can provide additional diagnostic information [74]. The superior diagnostic performance of [^{18}F]fluorocholine PET/CT (and PET/MR) has been consistently demonstrated in multiple studies and meta-analyses in both first-line and second-line imaging settings. Reported patient-based sensitivities exceed 95%, with positive predictive values approaching 97% [67, 70, 82]. This high diagnostic accuracy in the second-line setting has significantly impacted clinical management by reducing the need for bilateral neck exploration, previously required in patients with negative or inconclusive cUS and [^{99m}Tc]Tc-MIBI studies, by approximately 75% [70]. Furthermore, detection rates with [^{18}F]fluorocholine PET/CT or PET/MR exceed 90% even in challenging clinical scenarios involving multiglandular disease [9, 23, 33, 34, 81]. The modality demonstrates particular strength in detecting smaller lesions, reliably identifying adenomas under 10 mm in diameter that may be missed by other imaging approaches. In some series of confirmed multiglandular disease, sensitivity reaches 100%, markedly surpassing the performance of other available techniques [9]. In the context of secondary and tertiary hyperparathyroidism associated with chronic kidney disease, choline PET/CT shows significantly better detection in tertiary compared to secondary hyperparathyroidism [4]. This enhanced performance is especially important for patients requiring parathyroidectomy, as supernumerary and ectopic glands, which can be present in up to a quarter of cases, may be detected [73]. Despite its superior sensitivity, some hyperplastic glands remain unlocalized, especially in secondary hyperparathyroidism [13]. Accurate localization of all abnormal glands is critical in these patients to avoid incomplete parathyroidectomy, which can lead to persistent disease and necessitate reoperation.

The quantitative capabilities of PET imaging provide additional valuable information beyond simple lesion detection. Standardized uptake values correlate with disease severity, with higher SUVmax associated with elevated parathyroid hormone levels [1] and decreased bone mineral density [2]. This relationship suggests that tracer uptake intensity reflects the metabolic activity within abnormal parathyroid tissue, potentially offering prognostic information.

The clinical benefits of superior imaging extend beyond improved surgical outcomes to healthcare economics [83]. Several cost-effectiveness analyses have demonstrated that, despite higher initial costs, [^{18}F]fluorocholine PET/CT is a cost-effective strategy when considering the entire care pathway [47, 53, 91]. Improved diagnostic accuracy leads to reduced operative risks, shorter surgery times, decreased hospital stays, and, most importantly, a lower need for reoperations.

Operational advantages of choline PET/CT and PET/MR include substantial reductions in imaging time compared to conventional scintigraphy, with some studies reporting an 83% decrease in total imaging duration, an 89% reduction in radiopharmaceutical preparation time, and a 75% decrease in quality control requirements [75].

Despite these significant benefits, choline PET/CT and PET/MR also have some limitations. False-positive findings may result from uptake in inflammatory lymph nodes, thyroid nodules, or other pathological processes [63]. Therefore, careful correlation with corresponding CT or MR images is important to minimize misinterpretation.

Despite these facts, the initially higher cost of choline PET/CT and PET/MR compared to conventional imaging is still a barrier to widespread adoption. Additionally, availability and reimbursement issues further limit access in many healthcare systems. Choline PET requires dedicated PET/CT or PET/MR equipment and established radiopharmaceutical supply chains, which are not available in many medical centers.

The limitations of [^{11}C]choline underscore the advantages of the [^{18}F]fluorocholine. The short physical half-life of carbon-11 (20 minutes) necessitates on-site cyclotron facilities and specialized radiochemistry expertise, severely restricting accessibility for most patients [63]. From a physical standpoint, the higher average positron energy of carbon-11 compared to fluorine-18 increases positron range and consequently reduces spatial resolution, which can impair the detection of small parathyroid lesions, where precise localization is critical. Furthermore, the absence of standardized protocols for [^{11}C]choline has led to inconsistencies across centers, with studies reporting variable acquisition times [56, 63]. Such variability complicates direct comparison of diagnostic performance between different institutions. Moreover, most published research on [^{11}C]choline consists of single-center experiences involving relatively small patient cohorts, which limits the ability to determine true diagnostic accuracy in diverse clinical settings, although currently available data show comparable results to [^{18}F]fluorocholine [16, 57, 58, 71]. Local reimbursement restrictions and regulatory approval issues further obstruct its implementation.

Although false-negative findings are less frequent than with conventional imaging, they may still occur with choline PET/CT and PET/MR. Patients with mild biochemical abnormalities can have lower tracer uptake that falls below detection thresholds. Similarly, very small adenomas or cystic parathyroid lesions may demonstrate insufficient tracer accumulation for reliable detection, particularly when situated in anatomically challenging locations.

Another valuable application of choline PET/CT and PET/MR is the detection of brown tumors, the skeletal manifestations of severe hyperparathyroidism [89, 93]. These osteitis fibrosa cystica lesions, caused by chronic PTH-driven bone resorption, can be visualized throughout the skeleton via whole-body PET imaging.

Emerging technologies may address some current limitations. Artificial intelligence and deep learning have demonstrated promise in enhancing the visualization of small parathyroid glands and in standardizing image interpretation across different centers and reader expertise levels [10]. Deep learning-based tools could improve the detection of subtle lesions and reduce false-positive rates by providing quantitative assessments of uptake patterns and morphological features.

Hybrid imaging approaches combining choline PET with 4D-CT or MRI may offer further potential gains in diagnostic performance. Four-dimensional CT integrated with PET imaging can provide both metabolic and perfusion information in a single examination, potentially enhancing lesion characterization and surgical planning [24, 69]. PET/MRI, with its superior soft tissue contrast, may provide complementary anatomical and functional information [1, 44, 67].

PET/MR is preferred when imaging younger patients who would benefit from minimizing ionizing radiation, patients requiring follow-up imaging or repeat scans, and cases where the almost exclusively benign nature of parathyroid disease makes additional CT radiation unnecessary [1, 44, 67]. Superior soft-tissue contrast is needed, especially in reoperative necks with postoperative fibrosis and distorted anatomy, complex anatomical scenarios where precise tissue differentiation is crucial, and cases requiring detailed assessment of the relationship between lesions and surrounding structures like the thyroid capsule, major vessels, and the supposed course of the recurrent laryngeal nerve. Comprehensive neck evaluation is desired, such as when simultaneous assessment of incidental thyroid nodules, lymphadenopathy, or other structural abnormalities is valuable, and in cases where high-resolution MR sequences can provide additional diagnostic information.

PET/CT remains appropriate when PET/MR is not available due to limited institutional access to PET/MR scanners. It's also suitable in specific clinical scenarios where bone details are relevant, though this is uncommon in parathyroid imaging.

Diagnostic performance appears equivalent between PET/CT and PET/MR, with studies demonstrating no statistically significant differences in sensitivity, positive predictive value, or overall accuracy in both first-line and second-line imaging settings [67]. The choice, therefore, often depends on availability, institutional preference, and patient-specific considerations rather than inherent diagnostic superiority, with PET/MR, however, providing the added benefits of lower radiation exposure and enhanced soft-tissue contrast, which can be particularly valuable in complex anatomical settings.

Standardization of imaging protocols and interpretation criteria remains essential for the optimal use of choline PET/CT and PET/MR. Structured reporting systems similar to those established in other nuclear medicine domains could improve reproducibility.

Finally, dual-tracer approaches, such as combining choline with other metabolic tracers, may improve sensitivity and specificity, especially in suspected parathyroid carcinoma [68]. In parallel, the development of novel radiotracers targeting different metabolic pathways, including [^{18}F]-FAPI, [^{68}Ga]Ga-Trivehexin, and [^{18}F]flurpiridaz is promising for overcoming current limitations and providing complementary diagnostic insights [14, 21, 42].

[^{11}C]methionine PET/CT faces logistical challenges comparable to those of [^{11}C]choline, primarily due to the short physical half-life of ^{11}C, which necessitates on-site production. The radiochemical synthesis of [^{11}C]methionine is technically complex, requiring advanced radiochemistry infrastructure and highly skilled personnel. These demands contribute to elevated operational costs and limit its availability for routine clinical application.

Considerable variability in imaging protocols is evident across institutions, with reported acquisition times ranging from immediately postinjection to up to 40 minutes thereafter [17, 55, 59, 87]. This lack of standardization complicates the comparison between different studies.

14.5 Four-Dimensional Computed Tomography and Magnetic Resonance Imaging

The principle underlying 4D-CT lies in its ability to capture the dynamic enhancement characteristics of parathyroid tissue through multiple contrast-enhanced phases acquired at predetermined intervals following intravenous contrast administration. This technique typically encompasses non-contrast, arterial, venous, and delayed phases, though considerable institutional variability exists in protocol implementation [32]. The temporal dimension added by this multiphase approach allows radiologists to characterize tissue perfusion patterns that have been reported to distinguish parathyroid adenomas from potential mimics such as lymph nodes and exophytic thyroid nodules [12, 24, 40].

Diagnostic superiority over traditional imaging modalities was reported for 4D-CT. In direct comparative studies, 4D-CT demonstrated sensitivities of over 90% for parathyroid adenoma localization when used as a first-line study, substantially exceeding the performance of cUS and [^{99m}Tc]Tc-MIBI scintigraphy [41]. Even more importantly, when conventional imaging proves non-localizing or inconclusive, 4D-CT maintains reasonable diagnostic performance with sensitivities reaching 89%, potentially providing a valuable alternative imaging option [19].

However, 4D-CT carries significant radiation exposure compared to conventional imaging. Depending on the specific protocol implementation and number of phases acquired, patients may receive radiation doses ranging from 4 to 26 mSv, with optimized four-phase protocols typically delivering approximately 10.4 mSv [39]. The radiation dose to the thyroid is especially high, i.e., up to 57 times higher than that received during [^{99m}Tc]Tc-MIBI imaging [46]. Institutions are trying to balance diagnostic performance and radiation safety. Studies investigating two-phase and three-phase protocols have demonstrated that diagnostic performance remains robust even with less acquisition phases, with pooled sensitivities of 71% for two-phase studies, 76% for three-phase studies, and 80% for four-phase studies [39].

The interpretation of 4D-CT studies requires an understanding of parathyroid enhancement patterns. The idealized enhancement pattern of hypoattenuation on non-contrast imaging, followed by arterial hyperattenuation with rapid washout on venous and delayed phases, occurs in only approximately 20% of cases. Instead, at least three distinct enhancement patterns have been characterized, with the most common pattern showing no arterial hyperattenuation but demonstrating washout on delayed phases [6].

It should be acknowledged, however, that even standalone CT with late-arterial phase imaging has substantial potential for detecting diseased parathyroid glands. This capability is largely due to their often-pronounced arterial hyperenhancement compared with lymph nodes, as well as the occasional visualization of polar vessels, which can help differentiate adenomas from lymph nodes. By contrast, 4D-CT essentially requires prior knowledge of the adenoma's exact location in order to place a voxel and analyze the lesion's enhancement and washout pattern, which might not be as expected.

Protocol variability among institutions represents a persistent challenge in the clinical implementation of 4D-CT. The lack of standardized acquisition parameters, contrast timing, and interpretation criteria creates inconsistencies in diagnostic performance that may limit the generalizability of published results. 4D-CT may therefore be considered if appropriate nuclear medicine techniques, particularly choline-PET, are unavailable and both ultrasound and late-arterial phase CT yield inconclusive results.

Four-dimensional magnetic resonance imaging (4D-MRI) represents an alternative that theoretically addresses some of the limitations of 4D-CT, mainly radiation exposure, while introducing its own unique challenges. By enabling near-continuous acquisition of contrast perfusion information, 4D-MRI can generate high-resolution perfusion curves that provide more detailed characterization of tissue enhancement patterns than the snapshot-like timing of 4D-CT. The technique combines this temporal resolution with excellent soft tissue contrast and high spatial resolution.

The theoretical advantages of 4D-MRI compared to 4D-CT are particularly compelling considering there is no radiation exposure, which is especially important in younger patients or those requiring repeat imaging. However, the clinical implementation of 4D-MRI faces significant practical obstacles that have limited its widespread adoption [26]. It requires longer acquisition time than 4D-CT and has increased susceptibility to motion artifacts from breathing, swallowing, and vascular pulsation. These artifacts can degrade image quality, particularly in the lower neck and mediastinal regions where many ectopic parathyroid glands are located.

Patient selection is also an important factor in choosing the optimal imaging approach. While 4D-CT is unsuitable for patients with significant renal impairment or contrast allergies,

MRI is not suitable for patients with certain metallic implants, pacemakers, or severe claustrophobia [63].

14.6 Parathyroid Carcinoma Imaging

Parathyroid carcinoma is one of the most challenging entities in endocrine imaging. The primary difficulty lies in the substantial overlap between the imaging appearances of malignant and benign disease. On the other hand, fine needle aspiration cytology is strongly discouraged due to the risk of seeding, so the diagnosis relies on a combination of laboratory findings (prominent hypercalcemia and very high PTH levels), clinical signs, and imaging [63].

Although cUS is typically used as first-line imaging, the morphological features associated with malignancy (lesions >15–30 mm, irregular margins, heterogeneous echotexture, capsular disruption) lack the sensitivity and specificity required for confident preoperative diagnosis [68]. The conventional 30 mm size threshold has been called into question, as up to one-third of carcinomas present below this cutoff [45]. CT and MRI provide excellent anatomical detail but offer limited ability to differentiate carcinoma from benign adenoma. Similarly, four-dimensional CT demonstrates that enhancement patterns in carcinomas may closely resemble those of benign adenomas, with only subtle distinctions in washout kinetics [15].

Traditional [^{99m}Tc]Tc-MIBI imaging can reveal increased tracer retention in malignant lesions, yet small carcinomas often show considerable overlap with benign adenomas [68]. Choline PET/CT has demonstrated superior performance compared with conventional imaging, and even [^{18}F]FDG PET/CT, in detecting both primary tumors and metastatic disease [20, 35, 51, 68]. However, uptake intensity alone does not reliably distinguish malignancy from benign lesions.

These diagnostic limitations have a direct impact on surgical planning. Whereas parathyroid carcinoma requires en bloc resection with wide margins, a markedly different approach from the minimally invasive techniques used for benign lesions, the inability to distinguish between these entities preoperatively creates a dilemma. This can result in either unnecessarily aggressive surgery for benign disease or inadequate resection of malignant lesions. Optimal management, therefore, depends on a multimodal strategy integrating clinical assessment, biochemical markers, and imaging findings. No single imaging modality currently offers reliable discrimination between benign and malignant parathyroid lesions, except in the presence of metastatic spread, underscoring the importance of clinical correlation over imaging features alone.

14.7 Conclusions

Despite remarkable technological advances in recent decades, substantial unmet needs remain in parathyroid imaging, with potential implications for both clinical care and surgical outcomes. The evolution from routine bilateral neck exploration to targeted, minimally invasive approaches has created new opportunities but also introduced challenges that underscore the critical importance of accurate preoperative lesion localization.

Traditional first-line imaging modalities perform well for most patients with single-gland disease; however, their effectiveness diminishes considerably in more complex clinical scenarios. A persistent difficulty lies in the detection of multiglandular disease, where sensitivity drops markedly compared with single adenomas—a limitation that can significantly influence surgical strategy and patient outcomes. Equally important is the ongoing challenge of localizing ectopic parathyroid glands, particularly those situated in mediastinal or otherwise anatomically complex locations, where reliable detection remains difficult.

[^{18}F]fluorocholine PET/CT and PET/MR demonstrate superior performance precisely in those clinical scenarios where conventional imaging fails. Nonetheless, its broader clinical adoption is hindered by substantial barriers, including high initial costs, limited availability, and variable reimbursement policies.

Furthermore, clearer guidelines are needed regarding when surgical intervention, and consequently imaging, is truly indicated, particularly in cases of normocalcemic pHPT and mild biochemical abnormalities where surgery may not provide clinical benefit despite positive imaging findings. It is important to ensure that advanced imaging serves appropriate patient populations and improves surgical outcomes rather than simply detecting parathyroid lesions of uncertain clinical significance.

The diagnostic challenge of parathyroid carcinoma underscores the limitations of current imaging approaches: all available modalities show considerable overlap in the appearances of malignant and benign disease. This requires an integrated approach combining clinical, biochemical, and imaging data.

The standardization of imaging protocols and interpretation criteria is important for achieving consistent diagnostic performance across different institutions. In addition, the development of structured reporting systems could further improve reproducibility.

The integration of artificial intelligence and machine learning is promising for addressing interpretive challenges, reducing operator dependence, and improving diagnostic consistency.

Progress in parathyroid imaging will depend on close collaboration among endocrinologists, radiologists, nuclear medicine physicians, surgeons, and pathologists. The recognition that no single imaging modality offers a universal solution underscores the need for multimodal strategies, tailored to the patient's clinical profile and the resources of each institution.

References

1. Alharbi AA, Alshehri FM, Albatly AA, Sah B-R, Schmid C, Huber GF, Huellner MW. [18F] Fluorocholine uptake of parathyroid adenoma is correlated with parathyroid hormone level. Mol Imaging Biol. 2018;20:857–67. https://doi.org/10.1007/s11307-018-1179-x.
2. Araz M, Soydal Ç, Özkan E, Kır MK, İbiş E, Güllü S, Erdoğan MF, Emral R, Küçük ÖN. The efficacy of fluorine-18-choline PET/CT in comparison with 99mTc-MIBI SPECT/CT in the localization of a hyperfunctioning parathyroid gland in primary hyperparathyroidism. Nucl Med Commun. 2018;39:989–94. https://doi.org/10.1097/MNM.0000000000000899.
3. Arjunan D, Minisola S, Rao SD, Bhadada SK. Changing trends in clinical presentation of primary hyperparathyroidism across countries over time. Best Pract Res Clin Endocrinol Metab. 2025;39:101980. https://doi.org/10.1016/J.BEEM.2025.101980.
4. Aymard S, Leroy-Freschini B, Kaseb A, Marx D, Helali M, Averous G, Betz V, Riehm S, Vix M, Perrin P, et al. 18F-Fluorocholine PET/CT compared with current imaging procedures for preoperative localization of hyperfunctioning parathyroids in patients with chronic kidney disease. Diagnostics (Basel, Switzerland). 2023;13:1374. https://doi.org/10.3390/DIAGNOSTICS13081374.
5. Azizi G, Piper K, Keller JM, Mayo ML, Puett D, Earp KM, Malchoff CD. Shear wave elastography and parathyroid adenoma: a new tool for diagnosing parathyroid adenomas. Eur J Radiol. 2016;85:1586–93. https://doi.org/10.1016/j.ejrad.2016.06.009.
6. Bahl M, Sepahdari AR, Sosa JA, Hoang JK. Parathyroid adenomas and hyperplasia on four-dimensional CT scans: three patterns of enhancement relative to the thyroid gland justify a three-phase protocol. Radiology. 2015;277:454–62. https://doi.org/10.1148/radiol.2015142393.
7. Beheshti M, Hehenwarter L, Paymani Z, Rendl G, Imamovic L, Rettenbacher R, Tsybrovskyy O, Langsteger W, Pirich C. 18F-Fluorocholine PET/CT in the assessment of primary hyperparathyroidism compared with 99mTc-MIBI or 99mTc-tetrofosmin SPECT/CT: a prospective dual-centre study in 100 patients. Eur J Nucl Med Mol Imaging. 2018;45:1762–71. https://doi.org/10.1007/S00259-018-3980-9/FIGURES/3.
8. Bentrem DJ, Angelos P, Talamonti MS, Nayar R. Is preoperative investigation of the thyroid justified in patients undergoing parathyroidectomy for hyperparathyroidism? Thyroid. 2002;12:1109–12. https://doi.org/10.1089/105072502321085207.
9. Boucher A, Delabie J, Lussey-Lepoutre C, Haissaguerre M, Ouvrard E, Lavinia V, Le Bras M, Batisse-Lignier M, Cuny T, Jacquet-Francillon N, et al. Performance of [18F]fluorocholine PET/CT in MEN1-related primary hyperparathyroidism before initial surgery or for persistent/recurrent disease. Eur J Nucl Med Mol Imaging. 2024;51:1349–60. https://doi.org/10.1007/S00259-023-06537-1/TABLES/5.
10. Bradley KM, McGowan DR, Bartley L, Scott-Coombes D, Rees JI. Ectopic, intra-thyroid parathyroid adenoma better visualised by deep learning enhanced choline PET/CT. QJM: Mon J Assoc Physicians. 2025; https://doi.org/10.1093/QJMED/HCAF057.

11. Castellana M, Virili C, Palermo A, Giorgino F, Giovanella L, Trimboli P. Primary hyperparathyroidism with surgical indication and negative or equivocal scintigraphy: safety and reliability of PTH washout. A systematic review and meta-analysis. Eur J Endocrinol. 2019;181:245–53. https://doi.org/10.1530/EJE-19-0160.
12. Chazen JL, Gupta A, Dunning A, Phillips CD. Diagnostic accuracy of 4D-CT for parathyroid adenomas and hyperplasia. AJNR Am J Neuroradiol. 2012;33:429–33. https://doi.org/10.3174/ajnr.A2805.
13. Chen YH, Chen HT, Lee MC, Liu SH, Wang LY, Lue KH, Chan SC. Preoperative F-18 fluorocholine PET/CT for the detection of hyperfunctioning parathyroid glands in patients with secondary or tertiary hyperparathyroidism: comparison with Tc-99m sestamibi scan and neck ultrasound. Ann Nucl Med. 2020;34:527–37. https://doi.org/10.1007/S12149-020-01479-2.
14. Chen J, Zhao M, An Q, Wei L, Chen B. Detection of muscular metastasis in a case of parathyroid carcinoma using 18 F-FAPI-04 PET/CT. Clin Nucl Med. 2024;49:e501–2. https://doi.org/10.1097/RLU.0000000000005425.
15. Christakis I, Vu T, Chuang HH, Fellman B, Silva-Figueroa AM, Williams MD, Busaidy NL, Perrier ND. The diagnostic accuracy of neck ultrasound, 4D-Computed tomographyand sestamibi imaging in parathyroid carcinoma. Eur J Radiol. 2017;95:82–8. https://doi.org/10.1016/J.EJRAD.2017.07.026.
16. Christensen JW, Ismail A, Søndergaard SB, Bennedbæk FN, Nygaard B, Jensen LT, Trolle W, Holst-Hahn C, Zerahn B, Kristensen B, et al. Preoperative imaging in primary hyperparathyroidism: Are 11C-Choline PET/CT and 99mTc-MIBI/123Iodide subtraction SPECT/CT interchangeable or do they supplement each other? Clin Endocrinol. 2022;97:258–67. https://doi.org/10.1111/CEN.14688.
17. Chun IK, Cheon GJ, Paeng JC, Kang KW, Chung J-K, Lee DS. Detection and characterization of parathyroid adenoma/hyperplasia for preoperative localization: comparison between (11)C-Methionine PET/CT and (99m)Tc-sestamibi scintigraphy. Nucl Med Mol Imaging. 2013;47:166–72. https://doi.org/10.1007/s13139-013-0212-x.
18. Coakley AJ, Kettle AG, Wells CP, O'Doherty MJ, Collins RE. 99Tcm sestamibi--a new agent for parathyroid imaging. Nucl Med Commun. 1989;10:791–4. https://doi.org/10.1097/00006231-198911000-00003.
19. Day KM, Elsayed M, Beland MD, Monchik JM. The utility of 4-dimensional computed tomography for preoperative localization of primary hyperparathyroidism in patients not localized by sestamibi or ultrasonography. Surgery (United States). 2015;157:534–9. https://doi.org/10.1016/j.surg.2014.11.010.
20. Deandreis D, Terroir M, Al Ghuzlan A, Berdelou A, Lacroix L, Bidault F, Troalen F, Hartl D, Lumbroso J, Baudin E, et al. 18Fluorocholine PET/CT in parathyroid carcinoma: a new tool for disease staging? Eur J Nucl Med Mol Imaging. 2015;42:1941–2. https://doi.org/10.1007/s00259-015-3130-6.
21. Derlin T, Bengel FM, Kleine-Döpke D, Schmelzle M, Ringe BP. Value of [18F]flurpiridaz PET/CT for preoperative localization of atypical parathyroid tumors in primary hyperparathyroidism. Eur J Nucl Med Mol Imaging. 2025; https://doi.org/10.1007/S00259-025-07487-6.
22. Desiato V, Melis M, Amato B, Bianco T, Rocca A, Amato M, Quarto G, Benassai G. Minimally invasive radioguided parathyroid surgery: a literature review. Int J Surg. 2016;28:S84–93. https://doi.org/10.1016/J.IJSU.2015.12.037.
23. Ferrari SB, Morand GB, Rupp NJ, Krützfeldt J, Vetter D, Hüllner MW, Broglie MA. Clinical predictors of negative/equivocal SPECT imaging outcomes in primary hyperparathyroidism: factors calling for 18F-choline-PET. Am J Otolaryngol. 2024;45:104315. https://doi.org/10.1016/J.AMJOTO.2024.104315.
24. Fiz F, Bottoni G, Massollo M, Trimboli P, Catrambone U, Bacigalupo L, Righi S, Treglia G, Imperiale A, Piccardo A. [18F]F-Choline PET/CT and 4D-CT in the evaluation of primary hyperparathyroidism: rivals or allies? Q J Nucl Med Mol Imaging. 2023;67:130–7. https://doi.org/10.23736/S1824-4785.23.03514-8.
25. Fröberg AC, Valkema R, Bonjer JH, Krenning EP. 99mTc-tetrofosmin or 99mTc-sestamibi for double-phase parathyroid scintigraphy? Eur J Nucl Med Mol Imaging. 2003;30:193–6. https://doi.org/10.1007/s00259-002-1030-z.
26. Grayev AM, Gentry LR, Hartman MJ, Chen H, Perlman SB, Reeder SB. Presurgical localization of parathyroid adenomas with magnetic resonance imaging at 3.0 T: an adjunct method to supplement traditional imaging. Ann Surg Oncol. 2012;19:981–9. https://doi.org/10.1245/S10434-011-2046-Z.
27. Hindié E, Mellière D, Jeanguillaume C, Perlemuter L, Chéhadé F, Galle P. Parathyroid imaging using simultaneous double-window recording of technetium-99m-sestamibi and iodine-123. J Nucl Med. 1998;39:1100–5.
28. Hindié E, Zanotti-Fregonara P, Tabarin A, Rubello D, Morelec I, Wagner T, Henry J-F, Taïeb D. The role of radionuclide imaging in the surgical management of primary hyperparathyroidism. J Nucl Med. 2015;56:737–44. https://doi.org/10.2967/JNUMED.115.156018.
29. Hindié E, Ureña-Torres PA, Taïeb D. Parathyroid imaging in patients with renal hyperparathyroidism. In: Parathyroid glands in chronic kidney disease. Cham: Springer International Publishing; 2020. p. 35–49. https://doi.org/10.1007/978-3-030-43769-5_3.
30. Hindié E, Schwartz P, Avram AM, Imperiale A, Sebag F, Taïeb D. Primary hyperparathyroidism: defining the appropriate preoperative imaging algorithm. J Nucl Med. 2021;62:3S–12S. https://doi.org/10.2967/JNUMED.120.245993.
31. Hiromatsu Y, Ishibashi M, Nishida H, Okuda S, Miyake I. Technetium-99 m tetrofosmin parathy-

roid imaging in patients with primary hyperparathyroidism. Intern Med. 2000;39:101–6. https://doi.org/10.2169/internalmedicine.39.101.
32. Hoang JK, Williams K, Gaillard F, Dixon A, Sosa JA. Parathyroid 4D-CT: multi-institutional international survey of use and trends. Otolaryngol Head Neck Surg. 2016;155:956–60. https://doi.org/10.1177/0194599816655311.
33. Huber GF, Hüllner M, Schmid C, Brunner A, Sah B, Vetter D, Kaufmann PA, von Schulthess GK. Benefit of 18F-fluorocholine PET imaging in parathyroid surgery. Eur Radiol. 2018;28:2700–7. https://doi.org/10.1007/s00330-017-5190-4.
34. Huellner MW, Aberle S, Sah BR, Veit-Haibach P, Bonani M, Schmid C, Steinert H. Visualization of parathyroid hyperplasia using 18F-fluorocholine PET/MR in a patient with secondary hyperparathyroidism. Clin Nucl Med. 2016;41:e159–61. https://doi.org/10.1097/RLU.0000000000001053.
35. Iacovitti CM, Cuzzocrea M, Gianola L, Paone G, Treglia G. Dual-tracer positron emission tomography/computed tomography with [18F]FDG and [18F]fluorocholine in a patient with metastatic parathyroid carcinoma. Diagnostics (Basel, Switzerland). 2024;14:1548. https://doi.org/10.3390/DIAGNOSTICS14141548.
36. Ishibashi M, Nishida H, Hiromatsu Y, Kojima K, Tabuchi E, Hayabuchi N. Comparison of technetium-99m-MIBI, technetium-99m-tetrofosmin, ultrasound and MRI for localization of abnormal parathyroid glands. J Nucl Med. 1998;39:320–4.
37. Ishizuka T, Kajita K, Kamikubo K, Komaki T, Miura K, Nagao S, Nozawa Y. Phospholipid/Ca2+-dependent protein kinase activity in human parathyroid adenoma. Endocrinologia Japonica. 1987;34:965–8. https://doi.org/10.1507/ENDOCRJ1954.34.965.
38. Jinih M, O'Connell E, O'Leary DP, Liew A, Redmond HP. Focused versus bilateral parathyroid exploration for primary hyperparathyroidism: a systematic review and meta-analysis. Ann Surg Oncol. 2017;24:1924–34. https://doi.org/10.1245/S10434-016-5694-1.
39. Kluijfhout WP, Pasternak JD, Beninato T, Drake FT, Gosnell JE, Shen WT, Duh Q-Y, Allen IE, Vriens MR, de Keizer B, et al. Diagnostic performance of computed tomography for parathyroid adenoma localization; a systematic review and meta-analysis. Eur J Radiol. 2017;88:117–28. https://doi.org/10.1016/j.ejrad.2017.01.004.
40. Krakauer M, Wieslander B, Myschetzky PS, Lundstrøm A, Bacher T, Sørensen CH, Trolle W, Nygaard B, Bennedbæk FN. A prospective comparative study of parathyroid dual-phase scintigraphy, dual-Isotope subtraction scintigraphy, 4D-CT, and ultrasonography in primary hyperparathyroidism. Clin Nucl Med. 2016;41:93–100. https://doi.org/10.1097/RLU.0000000000000988.
41. Kukar M, Platz TA, Schaffner TJ, Elmarzouky R, Groman A, Kumar S, Abdelhalim A, Cance WG. The use of modified four-dimensional computed tomography in patients with primary hyperparathyroidism: an argument for the abandonment of routine sestamibi single-positron emission computed tomography (SPECT). Ann Surg Oncol. 2015;22:139–45. https://doi.org/10.1245/S10434-014-3940-Y.
42. Kuyumcu S, Denizmen D, Has-Simsek D, Poyanli A, Uzum AK, Buyukkaya F, Isik EG, Onder S, Aksakal N, Ozkan ZG, et al. 68Ga-Trivehexin PET/CT: a promising novel tracer for primary hyperparathyroidism. Eur J Nucl Med Mol Imaging. 2024:1–12. https://doi.org/10.1007/S00259-024-06846-Z/FIGURES/4.
43. Lebastchi AH, Donovan PI, Udelsman R. Paradigm shift in the surgical management of multigland parathyroid hyperplasia: An individualized approach. JAMA Surg. 2014;149:1133–7. https://doi.org/10.1001/jamasurg.2014.1296.
44. Liberini V, Morand GB, Rupp NJ, Orita E, Deandreis D, Broglie Däppen M, Hofbauer M, Maurer A, Husmann L, Mader CE, et al. Histopathological features of parathyroid adenoma and 18F-choline uptake in PET/MR of primary hyperparathyroidism. Clin Nucl Med. 2022;47:101–7. https://doi.org/10.1097/RLU.0000000000003987.
45. Lo WM, Good ML, Nilubol N, Perrier ND, Patel DT. Tumor size and presence of metastatic disease at diagnosis are associated with disease-specific survival in parathyroid carcinoma. Ann Surg Oncol. 2018;25:2535–40. https://doi.org/10.1245/S10434-018-6559-6.
46. Mahajan A, Starker LF, Ghita M, Udelsman R, Brink JA, Carling T. Parathyroid four-dimensional computed tomography: evaluation of radiation dose exposure during preoperative localization of parathyroid tumors in primary hyperparathyroidism. World J Surg. 2012;36:1335–9. https://doi.org/10.1007/s00268-011-1365-3.
47. Mamou A, Chkair S, Gilly O, Maimoun L, Mamou Y, Sheppard SC, Kotzki PO, Lallemant B, Boudousq V. Economic evaluation of [18F]fluorocholine PET/CT in pre operative assessment of hyperfunctional parathyroids in primary hyperparathyroidism: a cost effectiveness analysis. EJNMMI Rep. 2025;9:11. https://doi.org/10.1186/S41824-025-00244-W.
48. Medas F, Erdas E, Longheu A, Gordini L, Pisano G, Nicolosi A, Calò PG. Retrospective evaluation of the pre- and postoperative factors influencing the sensitivity of localization studies in primary hyperparathyroidism. Int J Surg. 2016;25:82–7. https://doi.org/10.1016/J.IJSU.2015.11.045.
49. Moghadam RN, Amlelshahbaz AP, Namiranian N, Sobhan-Ardekani M, Emami-Meybodi M, Dehghan A, Rahmanian M, Razavi-Ratki SK. Comparative diagnostic performance of ultrasonography and 99mTc-Sestamibi scintigraphy for parathyroid adenoma in primary hyperparathyroidism; Systematic review and meta-analysis. Asian Pac J Cancer Prev. 2017;18:3195–200. https://doi.org/10.22034/APJCP.2017.18.12.3195.
50. Mohammadi A, Moloudi F, Ghasemi-rad M. The role of colour Doppler ultrasonography in the preopera-

tive localization of parathyroid adenomas. Endocr J. 2012;59:375–82. https://doi.org/10.1507/endocrj.EJ11-0351.

51. Morand GB, Rupp NJ, Huellner MW, Gerber PA, Soyka MB, Broglie MA, Holzmann D. Transnasal-transpterygoid endoscopic removal of an ^{18} F–choline-avid parathyroid carcinoma metastasis in the skull base. JAMA Otolaryngol–Head Neck Surg. 2019;145:978. https://doi.org/10.1001/jamaoto.2019.2352.
52. Morris MA, Saboury B, Ahlman M, Malayeri AA, Jones EC, Chen CC, Millo C. Parathyroid imaging: past, present, and future. Front Endocrinol. 2022;12:760419. https://doi.org/10.3389/FENDO.2021.760419.
53. van Mossel S, Saing S, Appelman-Dijkstra N, Quak E, Schepers A, Smit F, de Geus-Oei LF, Vriens D. Cost-effectiveness of one-stop-shop [18F]Fluorocholine PET/CT to localise parathyroid adenomas in patients suffering from primary hyperparathyroidism. Eur J Nucl Med Mol Imaging. 2024;51:3585–95. https://doi.org/10.1007/S00259-024-06771-1/FIGURES/4.
54. Nichols KJ, Tomas MB, Tronco GG, Palestro CJ. Sestamibi parathyroid scintigraphy in multigland disease. Nucl Med Commun. 2012;33:43–50. https://doi.org/10.1097/MNM.0b013e32834bfeb1.
55. Noltes ME, Coester AM, van der Horst-Schrivers ANA, Dorgelo B, Jansen L, Noordzij W, Lemstra C, Brouwers AH, Kruijff S. Localization of parathyroid adenomas using 11C-methionine pet after prior inconclusive imaging. Langenbeck's Arch Surg. 2017;402:1109–17. https://doi.org/10.1007/s00423-017-1549-x.
56. Noltes ME, Kruijff S, Noordzij W, Telenga ED, Vállez García D, Trofimiuk-Müldner M, Opalińska M, Hubalewska-Dydejczyk A, Luurtsema G, Dierckx RAJO, et al. Optimization of parathyroid 11C-choline PET protocol for localization of parathyroid adenomas in patients with primary hyperparathyroidism. EJNMMI Res. 2019;9:73. https://doi.org/10.1186/s13550-019-0534-5.
57. Noltes ME, Kruijff S, Jansen L, Westerlaan HE, Zandee WT, Dierckx RAJO, Brouwers AH. A retrospective analysis of the diagnostic performance of 11C-choline PET/CT for detection of hyperfunctioning parathyroid glands after prior negative or discordant imaging in primary hyperparathyroidism. EJNMMI Res. 2021;11:1–9. https://doi.org/10.1186/S13550-021-00778-7.
58. Noltes ME, Kruijff S, Appelman APA, Jansen L, Zandee WT, Links TP, van Hemel BM, Schouw HM, Dierckx RAJO, Francken AB, et al. Head-to-head comparison of [11C]methionine PET, [11C]choline PET, and 4-dimensional CT as second-line scans for detection of parathyroid adenomas in primary hyperparathyroidism. Eur J Nucl Med Mol Imaging. 2024;51:1050–9. https://doi.org/10.1007/S00259-023-06488-7.
59. Otto D, Boerner AR, Hofmann M, Brunkhorst T, Meyer GJ, Petrich T, Scheumann GF, Knapp WH. Pre-operative localisation of hyperfunctional parathyroid tissue with 11C-methionine PET. Eur J Nucl Med Mol Imaging. 2004;31:1405–12. https://doi.org/10.1007/s00259-004-1610-1.
60. Parikh AM, Suliburk JW, Morón FE. Imaging localization and surgical approach in the management of ectopic parathyroid adenomas. Endocr Pract. 2018;24:589–98. https://doi.org/10.4158/EP-2018-0003.
61. Park HS, Hong N, Jeong JJ, Yun M, Rhee Y. Update on preoperative parathyroid localization in primary hyperparathyroidism. Endocrinol Metab. 2022;37:744. https://doi.org/10.3803/ENM.2022.1589.
62. Parra Ramírez P, Santiago Hernando A, Barquiel Alcalá B, Martín Rojas-Marcos P, Lisbona Catalán A, Álvarez Escolá C. Potential utility of contrast-enhanced ultrasound in the preoperative evaluation of primary hyperparathyroidism. J Ultrasound Med. 2019;38:2565–71. https://doi.org/10.1002/JUM.14949.
63. Petranović Ovčariček P, Giovanella L, Carrió Gasset I, Hindié E, Huellner MW, Luster M, Piccardo A, Weber T, Talbot JN, Verburg FA. The EANM practice guidelines for parathyroid imaging. Eur J Nucl Med Mol Imaging. 2021;48:2801–22. https://doi.org/10.1007/S00259-021-05334-Y/TABLES/1.
64. Petranović Ovčariček P, Giovanella L, Hindie E, Huellner MW, Talbot JN, Verburg FA. An essential practice summary of the new EANM guidelines for parathyroid imaging. Q J Nucl Med Mol Imaging. 2022;66:93–103. https://doi.org/10.23736/S1824-4785.22.03427-6.
65. Petranović Ovčariček P, Giovanella L, Vrachimis A. Parathyroid imaging. Q J Nucl Med Mol Imaging. 2023;67:93–5. https://doi.org/10.23736/S1824-4785.23.03511-2.
66. Petranović Ovčariček P, Calderoni L, Campenni A, Fanti S, Giovanella L. Molecular imaging of thyroid and parathyroid diseases. Expert Rev Endocrinol Metab. 2024;19:317–33. https://doi.org/10.1080/17446651.2024.2365776.
67. Petranović Ovčariček P, Schaab J, Beintner-Skawran S, Maurer A, Rupp NJ, Ikenberg K, Morand GB, Mueller SA, Vetter D, Liberini V, et al. [18F]Fluorocholine PET/MRI and [18F]Fluorocholine PET/CT as first- and second-line imaging in primary hyperparathyroidism – who takes the lead? Eur J Nucl Med Mol Imaging. 2025:1–10. https://doi.org/10.1007/S00259-025-07373-1/TABLES/5.
68. Petranović Ovčariček P, Campennì A, Giovanella L, Huellner MW. Parathyroid carcinoma: a comprehensive analysis with focus on molecular imaging. Eur J Nucl Med Mol Imaging. 2025:1–5. https://doi.org/10.1007/S00259-025-07162-W/FIGURES/2.
69. Piccardo A, Bottoni G, Boccalatte LA, Camponovo C, Musumeci M, Bacigalupo L, Collaud C, Ugolini M, Fiz F, Trimboli P. Head-to-head comparison among 18 F-choline PET/CT, 4D contrast-enhanced CT, and 18 F-choline PET/4D contrast-enhanced

CT in the detection of hyperfunctioning parathyroid glands: a systematic review and meta-analysis. Endocrine. 2021;74:404–12. https://doi.org/10.1007/S12020-021-02798-8.
70. Quak E, Blanchard D, Houdu B, Le Roux Y, Ciappuccini R, Lireux B, de Raucourt D, Grellard JM, Licaj I, Bardet S, et al. F18-choline PET/CT guided surgery in primary hyperparathyroidism when ultrasound and MIBI SPECT/CT are negative or inconclusive: the APACH1 study. Eur J Nucl Med Mol Imaging. 2018;45:658. https://doi.org/10.1007/S00259-017-3911-1.
71. Raitza M, Alshalali AAN, Glaudemans AWJM, Gans ROB, Slart RHJA. Use of [11C]choline PET/CT for visualization of four hyperactive parathyroid glands in a patient with renal hyperparathyroidism. Eur J Nucl Med Mol Imaging. 2022;49:4750–1. https://doi.org/10.1007/S00259-022-05885-8.
72. Ramonell KM, Fazendin J, Lindeman B, Chen H. My surgical practice: Radioguided parathyroid surgery, how and why we use it. Am J Surg. 2021; https://doi.org/10.1016/J.AMJSURG.2021.06.001.
73. Reitz RJ, Dreimiller A, Khil A, Horwitz E, McHenry CR. Ectopic and supernumerary parathyroid glands in patients with refractory renal hyperparathyroidism. Surgery. 2021;169:513–8. https://doi.org/10.1016/J.SURG.2020.08.007.
74. Rep S, Lezaic L, Kocjan T, Pfeifer M, Sever MJ, Simoncic U, Tomse P, Hocevar M. Optimal scan time for evaluation of parathyroid adenoma with [(18)F]-fluorocholine PET/CT. Radiol Oncol. 2015;49:327–33. https://doi.org/10.1515/raon-2015-0016.
75. Rep S, Sirca K, Lezaic EM, Zaletel K, Hocevar M, Lezaic L. fluorocholine PET vs. [99mTc]sestamibi scintigraphy for detection and localization of hyperfunctioning parathyroid glands in patients with primary hyperparathyroidism: outcomes and resource efficiency. Radiol Oncol. 2024;58:486–93. https://doi.org/10.2478/RAON-2024-0058.
76. Ruda JM, Hollenbeak CS, Stack BC. A systematic review of the diagnosis and treatment of primary hyperparathyroidism from 1995 to 2003. Otolaryngol Head Neck Surg. 2005;132:359–72. https://doi.org/10.1016/j.otohns.2004.10.005.
77. Singh Ospina NM, Rodriguez-Gutierrez R, Maraka S, Espinosa de Ycaza AE, Jasim S, Castaneda-Guarderas A, Gionfriddo MR, Al Nofal A, Brito JP, Erwin P, et al. Outcomes of parathyroidectomy in patients with primary hyperparathyroidism: a systematic review and meta-analysis. World J Surg. 2016;40:2359–77. https://doi.org/10.1007/s00268-016-3514-1.
78. Sukan A, Reyhan M, Aydin M, Yapar AF, Sert Y, Canpolat T, Aktas A. Preoperative evaluation of hyperparathyroidism: the role of dual-phase parathyroid scintigraphy and ultrasound imaging. Ann Nucl Med. 2008;22:123–31. https://doi.org/10.1007/s12149-007-0086-z.
79. Taïeb D, Hassad R, Sebag F, Colavolpe C, Guedj E, Hindié E, Henry J-F, Mundler O. Tomoscintigraphy improves the determination of the embryologic origin of parathyroid adenomas, especially in apparently inferior glands: imaging features and surgical implications. J Nucl Med Technol. 2007;35:135–9. https://doi.org/10.2967/JNMT.107.039743.
80. Taïeb D, Ureña-Torres P, Zanotti-Fregonara P, Rubello D, Ferretti A, Henter I, Henry J-F, Schiavi F, Opocher G, Blickman JG, et al. Parathyroid scintigraphy in renal hyperparathyroidism: the added diagnostic value of SPECT and SPECT/CT. Clin Nucl Med. 2013;38:630. https://doi.org/10.1097/RLU.0B013E31829AF5BF.
81. Talbot JN, Périé S, Tassart M, Delbot T, Aveline C, Zhang-Yin J, Kerrou K, Gaujoux S, Wagner I, Bennis M, et al. 18F-fluorocholine PET/CT detects parathyroid gland hyperplasia as well as adenoma: 401 PET/CTs in one center. Q J Nucl Med Mol Imaging. 2023;67:96–113. https://doi.org/10.23736/S1824-4785.23.03513-6.
82. Treglia G, Piccardo A, Imperiale A, Strobel K, Kaufmann PA, Prior JO, Giovanella L. Diagnostic performance of choline PET for detection of hyperfunctioning parathyroid glands in hyperparathyroidism: a systematic review and meta-analysis. Eur J Nucl Med Mol Imaging. 2019;46:751–65. https://doi.org/10.1007/S00259-018-4123-Z/FIGURES/4.
83. Treglia G, Piccardo A, Paone G, Trimboli P, Imperiale A. [18F]Fluorocholine PET/CT as First-Line vs. Second-Line Imaging Method to localize parathyroid adenomas in primary hyperparathyroidism: "Game, Set, and Match". Eur J Nucl Med Mol Imaging. 2024;51:3596–9. https://doi.org/10.1007/S00259-024-06772-0.
84. Trimboli P, D'Aurizio F, Tozzoli R, Giovanella L. Measurement of thyroglobulin, calcitonin, and PTH in FNA washout fluids. Clin Chem Lab Med. 2017;55:914–25. https://doi.org/10.1515/cclm-2016-0543.
85. Udelsman R, Lin Z, Donovan P. The superiority of minimally invasive parathyroidectomy based on 1650 consecutive patients with primary hyperparathyroidism. Ann Surg. 2011;253:585–91. https://doi.org/10.1097/SLA.0b013e318208fed9.
86. Wakamatsu H, Noguchi S, Yamashita H, Yamashita H, Tamura S, Jinnouchi S, Nagamachi S, Futami S. Technetium-99m tetrofosmin for parathyroid scintigraphy: a direct comparison with 99mTc-MIBI, 201Tl, MRI and US. Eur J Nucl Med. 2001;28:1817–27. https://doi.org/10.1007/s002590100627.
87. Weber T, Gottstein M, Schwenzer S, Beer A, Luster M. Is C-11 methionine PET/CT able to localise sestamibi-negative parathyroid adenomas? World J Surg. 2017;41:980–5. https://doi.org/10.1007/s00268-016-3795-4.
88. Weber T, Dotzenrath C, Dralle H, Niederle B, Riss P, Holzer K, Kußmann J, Trupka A, Negele T, Kaderli R, et al. Management of primary and renal hyperparathyroidism: guidelines from the German Association of Endocrine Surgeons (CAEK). Langenbeck's Arch

Surg. 2021;406:571–85. https://doi.org/10.1007/S00423-021-02173-1.

89. Werner J, Grünig H, Loher H, Fischli S, Strobel K, Wicke C. Localization of brown tumors with 18 F-fluorocholine PET/CT imaging in severe primary hyperparathyroidism. Clin Nucl Med. 2023;48:E387–9. https://doi.org/10.1097/RLU.0000000000004718.
90. Wilhelm SM, Wang TS, Ruan DT, Lee JA, Asa SL, Duh Q-Y, Doherty GM, Herrera MF, Pasieka JL, Perrier ND, et al. The American Association of Endocrine Surgeons guidelines for definitive management of primary hyperparathyroidism. JAMA Surg. 2016;151:959–68. https://doi.org/10.1001/jamasurg.2016.2310.
91. Yap A, Hope TA, Graves CE, Kluijfhout W, Shen WT, Gosnell JE, Sosa JA, Roman SA, Duh QY, Suh I. A cost-utility analysis of 18F-fluorocholine-positron emission tomography imaging for localizing primary hyperparathyroidism in the United States. Surgery. 2022;171:55–62. https://doi.org/10.1016/J.SURG.2021.03.075.
92. Yu N, Donnan PT, Murphy MJ, Leese GP. Epidemiology of primary hyperparathyroidism in Tayside, Scotland, UK. Clin Endocrinol. 2009;71:485–93. https://doi.org/10.1111/J.1365-2265.2008.03520.X.
93. Zhang-Yin J, Gaujoux S, Delbot T, Gauthé M, Talbot J-N. 18F-fluorocholine PET/CT imaging of brown tumors in a patient with severe primary hyperparathyroidism. Clin Nucl Med. 2019;44:971–4. https://doi.org/10.1097/RLU.0000000000002814.

Index

© The Editor(s) (if applicable) and The Author(s), under exclusive license to Springer Nature Switzerland AG 2026
P. Petranović Ovčariček et al. (eds.), *Parathyroid Imaging*,
https://doi.org/10.1007/978-3-032-14178-1

MIX
Papier aus verantwortungsvollen Quellen
Paper from responsible sources
FSC® C105338
FSC
www.fsc.org

If you have any concerns about our products,
you can contact us on
ProductSafety@springernature.com

In case Publisher is established outside the EU,
the EU authorized representative is:
Springer Nature Customer Service Center GmbH
Europaplatz 3, 69115 Heidelberg, Germany

Printed by Libri Plureos GmbH
in Hamburg, Germany